Frontiers in Cardiovascular Drug Discovery

(*Volume 6*)

Edited by

M. Iqbal Choudhary

H.E.J. Research Institute of Chemistry
International Center for Chemical and Biological Sciences
University of Karachi, Karachi
Pakistan

Frontiers in Cardiovascular Drug Discovery

Volume # 6

Editor: M. Iqbal Choudhary

ISSN (Online): 1879-6648

ISSN (Print): 2452-3267

ISBN (Online): 978-981-5036-90-9

ISBN (Print): 978-981-5036-91-6

ISBN (Paperback): 978-981-5036-92-3

First published in 2022.

need for a court order if at any point you breach any terms of this License Agreement. In no event will any delay or failure by Bentham Science Publishers in enforcing your compliance with this License Agreement constitute a waiver of any of its rights.

3. You acknowledge that you have read this License Agreement, and agree to be bound by its terms and conditions. To the extent that any other terms and conditions presented on any website of Bentham Science Publishers conflict with, or are inconsistent with, the terms and conditions set out in this License Agreement, you acknowledge that the terms and conditions set out in this License Agreement shall prevail.

Bentham Science Publishers Pte. Ltd.
80 Robinson Road #02-00
Singapore 068898
Singapore
Email: subscriptions@benthamscience.net

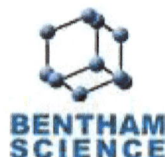

BENTHAM SCIENCE

CONTENTS

Yiming Wang, Yuqing Zhang and *Dingguo Zhang*

PREFACE

Despite major developments in the early diagnosis and understanding of underlying molecular mechanisms, cardiovascular diseases (CVDs) remain the leading cause of death (31% death globally), followed by cancers. The risk of developing CVDs is highest among all non-communicable diseases. It has increased multi-fold with the increase in prevalence of metabolic disorders, including obesity. CVDs affect people of all regions and all ages, and there are many socio-demographic risk factors. Despite major basic research in this area, translating laboratory discoveries into therapeutic interventions remains a major challenge, and only a handful of drugs have reached to clinical application. Thus drug development against cardiovascular diseases has many unique challenges which large pharmaceutical companies are often not willing to address. The 6th volume of the book series entitled, *"Frontiers in Cardiovascular Drug Discovery"* is a compilation of five reviews on diverse topics, including translational research towards improved drugs, various molecular pathways and biomarkers to be targeted for the drug discovery as well as challenges in cardiovascular drug development.

The review by Pratiti *et al* is focused on the piperazine-based drug ranolazine for the treatment of various cardiovascular diseases. Ranolazine was initially developed as an oral antianginal medicine, and later identified as a versatile cardiovascular drug against various indications. The authors have provided a detailed account of translational research work carried out on ranolazine for a whole range of other CVDs. In the second chapter Zhang *et al* have emphasized the importance of Rho/Rho kinase (ROCK) as an important drug target. Rho/Rho kinase is related to cardiovascular conditions such as coronary atherosclerosis, hypertension, and heart failure. Selective inhibitors of ROCK can treat many CVDs. This article presents the relationship between various CVDs and Rho/Rho kinase, and thus validates this as a legitimate drug target. Numerous examples of ROCK inhibitors with potential as drugs are also presented.

The review article of G. Mercanoglu and F. Mecanoglu provides a comprehensive account of major challenges and bottlenecks in CVD drug development, that have resulted in a huge vacuum in this drug pipeline. The authors have commented on reasons of a gradual shift of CVD drug development from large pharmaceutical companies to medium pharma industries, small biotech firms and research and development institutions. A field which was historically considered as a *"profitable"* area of therapeutic research and development now needs support from World Health Organizations and other NGOs. With this background, the authors have provided some logical solutions to overcome the existing problems. Platelet P2Y12 receptor (P2Y12R) for adenosine 5'diphosphate (ADP) plays a central role in platelet function, hemostasis, and thrombosis. Akaydin *et al* have discussed various approaches to inhibit P2Y12 receptors for the prevention of platelet aggregation and thrombosis. These inhibitors can also prevent and treat ischemic complications in patients with unstable angina, myocardial infarction and coronary intervention. Various classes of P2Y12 inhibiting drugs and their clinical outcomes are discussed. Kabir *et al* have contributed a comprehensive review on the nexus of diabetes and cardiovascular diseases such as atherosclerosis, hypertension and myocardial infarction. CVD is the most prevalent cause of mortality in the diabetic population. The authors have also provided a detailed account of the mechanisms of the onset of these diseases. Studies of the molecular mechanisms involved in the progression of CVDs in diabetes as well as biomarker identification can not only contribute to the early diagnosis and prevention of the disease, but it can also help in the novel target identification for anti-diabetic and anti-CVD drug development.

I would like to express our gratitude to all the authors for their scholarly contributions, and for the timely submissions of their reviews. The production team of Bentham Science Publishers also deserves our appreciation for the job very well done. Among them Ms. Mariam Mehdi (Assistant Manager Publications), and Mr. Mahmood Alam (Director Publications) have played a key role in the timely completion of the volume in hand. We sincerely hope that the efforts of authors and production team will help readers in a better understanding of the recent important developments in this key area of therapeutic intervention.

M. Iqbal Choudhary
H.E.J. Research Institute of Chemistry
International Center for Chemical and Biological Sciences
University of Karachi
Karachi
Pakistan

List of Contributors

Ankush Moza McLaren HealthCare, Premier, Medical Clinics, 1165 South Linden Road Flint, Michigan 48532, USA

Dingguo Zhang Department of Cardiology, The First Affiliated Hospital of Nanjing Medical University, Nanjing, China

Dolunay Merve Fakioğlu Department of Biochemistry, Faculty of Pharmacy, Gazi University, Ankara, Turkey

F. Mercanoglu Department of Cardiology, Istanbul Medical Faculty, Istanbul University, Istanbul, Turkey

G. Mercanoglu Department of Pharmacology, Hamidiye Faculty of Pharmacy, University of Health Sciences, Istanbul, Turkey

M.M. Towhidul Islam Department of Biochemistry and Molecular Biology, University of Dhaka, Dhaka-1000, Bangladesh

Mohammad Yousef McLaren HealthCare, G-3230 Beecher road, Suite 2, Flint, Michigan 48532, USA

Parul Sud McLaren HealthCare, G-3230 Beecher road, Suite 2, Flint, Michigan 48532, USA

Rebecca Pratiti McLaren HealthCare, G-3230 Beecher road, Suite 2, Flint, Michigan 48532, USA

Sevgi Akaydin Department of Biochemistry, Faculty of Pharmacy, Gazi University, Ankara, Turkey

Yearul Kabir Department of Biochemistry and Molecular Biology, University of Dhaka, Dhaka-1000, Bangladesh

Yiming Wang Department of Cardiology, Zhenjiang First People's Hospital, Zhenjiang, China

Yuqing Zhang Department of Cardiology, The Affiliated Jiangning Hospital of Nanjing Medical University, Nanjing, China

Cardiovascular Effects of Ranolazine and the Scope for Translational Research: A Current Review of Literature

Rebecca Pratiti[1,*], Parul Sud[1], Mohammad Yousef[1] and Ankush Moza[2]

[1] *McLaren HealthCare, G-3230 Beecher road, Suite 2, Flint, Michigan 48532, USA*

[2] *McLaren HealthCare, Premier Medical Clinics, 1165 South Linden Road Flint, Michigan 48532, USA*

Abstract: Ranolazine is approved for symptomatic stable angina patients on standard antianginal therapy. It inhibits myocardial late sodium current (INa) and partially inhibits fatty acid oxidation. INa is increased in the pathological conditions of ischemia and heart failure. Ranolazine changes myocardial fatty acid beta-oxidation to glucose oxidation, making the heart more oxygen efficient in ischemia. Thus, ranolazine improves myocardial desynchrony, mechanical dysfunction, diastolic depolarization, and action potential duration during ischemia. The book chapter focuses on salient features of ranolazine with emphasis on its indication in cardiovascular medicine, the knowledge gap in its translational research, and future scope. One of the important findings of the review is that ranolazine is a versatile cardiovascular medicine with effects on angina, heart failure, arrhythmia, and cardiomyopathy. Most animal studies of ranolazine had a correlation with human trials. Ranolazine, with its current cost and side effects profile, could be a second-line medication for angina, heart failure, and arrhythmia, specifically for patients having intolerance or side effects to first-line medications. Ranolazine as a pain modulator in angina, myotonia, and claudication needs to be further studied. Ranolazine may improve cardioversion rates in cardioversion and treatment-resistant patients with paroxysmal atrial fibrillation. Ranolazine is an option for preventing recurring shocks in patients with defibrillators who have recurrent ventricular tachycardias. Diabetes, hibernating myocardium and reperfusion injury are major modulators of ranolazine's treatment outcomes. Subsequently, better outcomes are seen in the presence of these pathologies. Ranolazine has similar efficacy as most oral hypoglycemics, and long-term studies are needed to evaluate its outcomes in diabetics with angina.

* **Corresponding author Rebecca Pratiti:** McLaren HealthCare, G-3230 Beecher road, Suite 2, Flint, Michigan 48532, USA; Tel: 8103422110; Fax: 8103425810; E-mail: rebeccapratiti@gmail.com

M. Iqbal Choudhary (Ed.)

Keywords: Angina Pectoris, Arrhythmias, Atrial Fibrillation, Angina Score, Antianginal Medications, Cardiomyopathy, Coronary Flow, Diastolic Dysfunction, Diabetes, Depression, Fatty Oxidation, Heart Failure, Hypoglycemic Agents, Myocardial Perfusion, Pulmonary Hypertension, QT Prolongation, Quality of Life, Ranolazine, Stable Angina, Sodium Current, Translational Research, Ventricular Function.

RANOLAZINE

Ranolazine is N-(2,6-dimethylphenyl)-4(2-hydroxy-3-[2-methoxyphenoxy]-pro pyl)-1-piperazine acetamide dihydrochloride. The drug was patented in 1986, and Food and Drug Administration (FDA) approved it in early 2006 for symptomatic patients on standard antianginal therapy under the tradename of Ranexa [1]. It has an empirical formula of $C_{24}H_{33}N_3O_4$ with a molecular weight of 427.54 g/mole [2]. Fig. (**1**) illustrates the chemical structure of ranolazine. Though the exact mechanism of action for ranolazine is unknown, some of its known effects in the cardiovascular system include partial inhibition of fatty acid oxidation and inhibition of late sodium current (I_{NA}) [3]. A typical cardiac cell action potential (AP) involves the following four phases [4]:

1. In Phase 0, the cell depolarizes due to the opening of fast sodium (Na^+) channels. When the voltage-gated fast sodium channels open and permit sodium to rapidly flow into the cell, the cell depolarizes, and the membrane potential reaches a maximum of +20 millivolts prior to sodium channel closure.
2. In phase 1, the fast sodium channels close, leading to cell repolarization. During this phase, the potassium (K^+) ions leave the cell through open potassium channels.
3. Phase 2 involves the opening of the voltage-gated calcium channels and the closure of fast potassium channels. As a result, after brief initial repolarization, the action potential plateau is observed because of increased calcium ion permeability and decreased potassium ion permeability. Consequently, the combination of decreased potassium efflux and increased calcium influx leads to the plateauing of the action potential.
4. During phase 3 rapid repolarization, the calcium channels close, and the slow potassium channels open, causing the plateau to end. As a result, the cell membrane potential returns to its resting level.
5. Phase 4 is the cell's resting membrane potential of -80 to -90 millivolts.

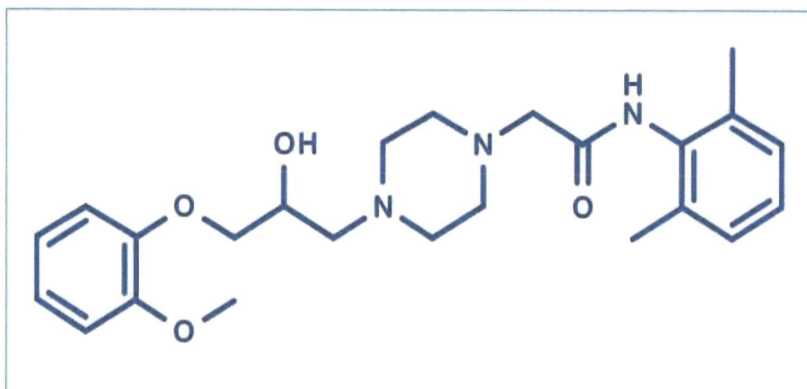

Fig. (1). Ranolazine chemical structure.

MECHANISM OF ACTION

Effects on Late Sodium Current

The cardiac cell action potential is changed under pathological conditions, including ischemia and arrhythmia. Ischemia is defined as inadequate blood flow leading to reduced oxygen delivery to the tissue. Ischemia leads to inefficient cell metabolism leading to extracellular accumulation of K^+. Ischemia-induced depolarization is slower, and it occurs because of ischemia-induced inactivation of some of the fast sodium channels. Thus, the number of fast Na^+ channels available for rapid action potential generation decreases [5]. Further, there is an important role played by late sodium current (INa) in the ischemic condition. Late INa is the inward current caused by the influx of Na^+ that is sustained throughout the plateau phase of the action potential. In this phase, the Na^+ that passes through voltage-gated Na channels fails to be inactivated completely and remains "open" for longer than it would normally be if the Na+ channels remained closed. Normally, late INa constitutes only 1% of the peak INa and is increased in pathological conditions of ischemia and heart failure [3].

Effect on Metabolism

Heart cells utilize fatty acid oxidation or glucose oxidation for energy production in the form of adenosine triphosphate (ATP). The fatty acid oxidation is more energy efficient for each mole utilized as compared to glucose. However, glucose oxidation is more oxygen efficient in the sense that less oxygen is utilized for glucose oxidation for each mole substrate. Normal myocardium prefers fatty acid oxidation under physiologic conditions and may switch to glucose oxidation under ischemia with oxygen deficiency. This step of energy change is important since fatty acid oxidation recovery is quicker with reperfusion. Further, fatty acids suppress glucose oxidation leading to an increase in glycolysis end-products, including lactate, pyruvate, and hydrogen within the cell. The accumulated hydrogen ions activate the Na^+/H^+ exchange system. This H^+ ion exchange with Na^+ causes cell swelling and subsequent exchange of Na^+ for Ca^{2+}, leading to intracellular calcium overloading with ultimate cell contracture and rupture [6]. Fig. (**2**) illustrates the molecular mechanism of ranolazine on cardiac metabolism.

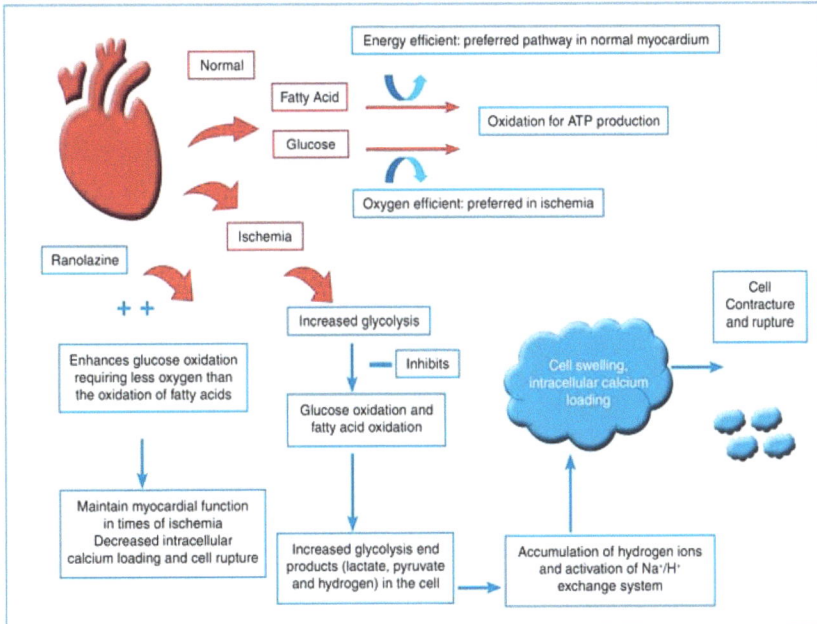

Fig. (2). Molecular mechanism of ranolazine on cardiac metabolism.

The exact mechanism of action of ranolazine for angina is still unknown though some mechanisms have been postulated. Ranolazine has an anti-ischemic effect *via* enhancing myocardial cellular glucose oxidation while inhibiting fatty acid beta-oxidation *via* pyruvate dehydrogenase. Higher doses of ranolazine (approximately equivalent to 100 µmol/L) are required to inhibit fatty acid oxidation by 12%. Furthermore, ranolazine, at a maximum, could only inhibit 60% of fatty acid beta-oxidation [3, 6]. Ranolazine also inhibits INa leading to a reduction in calcium overload in the ischemic myocyte [3]. This eventually improves the resting potential and decreases peak INa, late INa, myocardial desynchrony, mechanical dysfunction, diastolic depolarization (relaxation), and action potential duration [1, 7].

Fig. (**3**) gives the comparison of the action potential and sodium current (a) under physiological conditions, (b) during ischemia, and (c) with the effect of ranolazine.

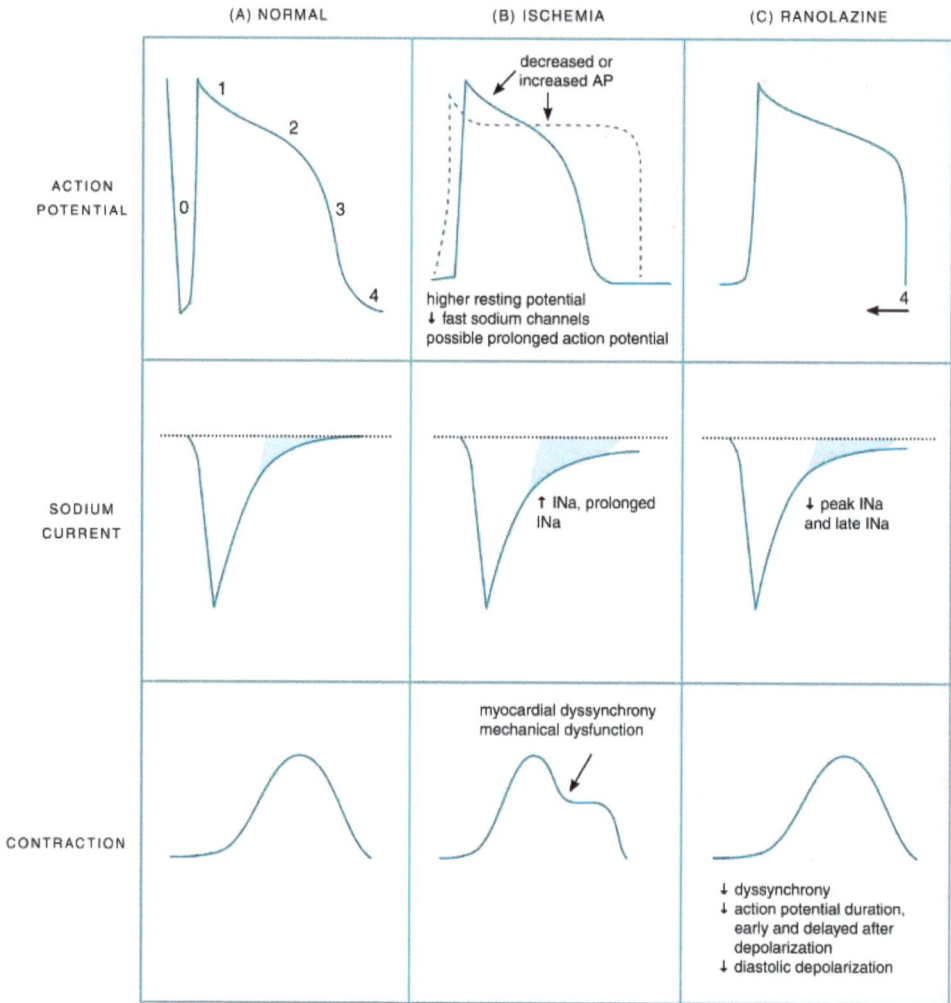

Fig. (3). Action potential and sodium current **(a)** under physiological conditions, **(b)** during ischemia, and **(c)** with the effect of ranolazine.

Dosage Formulations, Pharmacodynamics and Pharmacokinetics

Ranolazine has been studied in an immediate-release (IR) or extended-release (ER) formulation. ER ranolazine formulation is the only available formulation in the United States and is the most commonly used formulation. It is available in 500 mg and 1000 mg dosages and is taken twice a day for the indication of chronic angina [8]. Oral bioavailability varies from 30% to 55%, and peak concentration is achieved within 3-5 hours. Plasma protein binding is approximately 65%, and the majority of biotransformation is mediated by cytochrome P450 (CYP) 3A4 [3]. Multiple metabolites of ranolazine have been identified, though not studied in detail. Half-life is 7 h, and steady-state is mostly reached within 3 days with twice-daily dosing of ranolazine ER [2]. Age, gender, or food does not change the pharmacokinetics of ranolazine; however, ranolazine levels have been affected by CYP3A inhibitors/inducers, P glycoprotein inhibitors, and the presence of renal and hepatic impairment [9]. The estimated volume of distribution is 80 L, and almost 75% of the drug is excreted in urine as metabolites [6]. Maximum drug concentration increases by 30-40% in renal impairment and almost 70% in moderate liver impairment [9]. Ranolazine clearance by dialysis and the average plasma maximum concentration of ranolazine in dialysis patients is highly variable [10]. Ranolazine has multiple drug interactions with other heart medications, including digoxin and diltiazem [2]. There is an intravenous formulation of ranolazine that has not been used often in human studies.

Side Effects

General Side Effects

The most common side effects of ranolazine noted in early studies include dizziness, nausea, asthenia, and constipation. The incidence of side effects was dose-dependent, with higher doses of ranolazine (1000-1500 mg) causing more side effects. The prevalence of dizziness has remained around 11-12% in further clinical studies [8, 11]. Other side effects of ranolazine include dyspepsia and headache [9]. Ranolazine can also cause vomiting, vertigo, abnormal vision, confusion, postural hypotension, and syncope at plasma concentrations of more than 8000 ng/mL, clinically correlating with a ranolazine dose of 1000 mg two times a day or higher. Syncope has been reported in most ranolazine clinical studies with no evidence of ventricular arrhythmias [1, 3]. In a few patients, mild transient eosinophilia had occurred [3].

Tolerability of Ranolazine

Ranolazine has been well-tolerated in randomized control trials (RCT). In clinical practice, long-term treatment with ranolazine has also been well-tolerated, even in high-risk coronary artery disease patients. Survival analyses testing showed that symptomatic improvements attributable to ranolazine are not offset by increased mortality [11]. Ranolazine does not have any significant effects on heart rate or blood pressure at rest or during exercise, unlike most cardiac medication for ischemic heart disease or arrhythmia. Ranolazine could also be taken safely in the presence of most commonly used cardiac medications, including beta-blockers and calcium channel blockers, without any dose adjustment. Ranolazine with a

QT-prolonging effect and a theoretical risk of arrhythmia has been anti-arrhythmic in most studies. Discontinuation rates are higher in the elderly population, with adverse events being the most common cause of discontinuation and dizziness being the most common adverse event [11]. Discontinuation rates are lower in patients with chronic heart failure (CHF).

Drug-drug Interaction

A combination of ranolazine with flecainide could be pro-arrhythmic [12]. Ranolazine potentiates the effect of angiotensin-converting enzyme inhibitors (ACE-I) and angiotensin II receptor blockers (ARBs), leading to a higher prevalence of angioedema, dry cough, renal impairment, hypotension, anemia, and serum potassium > 5.5 mmol/L. Hence, patients on ranolazine should be monitored for these adverse effects [13]. In the Combination Assessment of Ranolazine in Stable Angina (CARISA) trial, the addition of ranolazine to standard treatment, including atenolol, amlodipine, and diltiazem, did not cause worsening of adverse events [14]. Ranolazine plasma levels are increased by CYP3A inhibitors, and hence the coadministration of other potent CYP3A inhibitors like ketoconazole, diltiazem, verapamil, *etc.,* should be avoided. Table 1 summarizes the potential ranolazine drug interactions.

Table 1. Ranolazine drug interactions.

Interaction	Medication Name
Medication levels that are increased by the addition of ranolazine	Digoxin, Aliskiren, Colchicine, Dabigatran, Dofetilide, Edoxaban, Everolimus, Lovastatin, Metformin, Midazolam, Morphine, Nadolol, Nimodipine, Red Yeast Rice, Sirolimus, Tacrolimus, Rimegepant
Medications that increase ranolazine levels	CYP 3A4 inhibitors (Ketoconazole, Diltiazem, Simvastatin, Macrolide Antibiotics, Protease Inhibitors, Grapefruit Juice, Alprazolam), P-glycoprotein Inhibitor (verapamil), P-glycoprotein/ABCB1 Inhibitors, Rifaximin
Medications that decrease ranolazine levels	CYP3A4 Inducers
Medication effects that are enhanced by ranolazine	ACE-I, ARB, Haloperidol, Risperidone
Abbreviations: CYP: cytochrome P450, ABCB1: ATP-binding cassette sub-family B member 1, ACE-I: Angiotensin-converting enzyme inhibitors, ARB: Angiotensin II receptor blockers	

QT-prolonging Effects

Ranolazine can increase the duration of action potential and cause QT prolongation. Although a rare side effect, many drugs with or without cardiac indication may induce electrophysiological changes of QT prolongation on electrocardiogram (ECG) [1]. This QT-prolonging effect could trigger a malignant form of polymorphic ventricular tachyarrhythmia called torsade de pointes [10]. The relationship between QT prolongation and the plasma concentration of ranolazine is linear. Ranolazine inhibits rapid delayed potassium rectifier current, late sodium current, and L-type calcium current with a net effect of a modest increase in the QT interval [6]. The mean QT prolongation is 6 msec with 1000 mg bid dosing, although almost 5% of the population may have QT prolongation by 15 msec with the highest plasma concentrations. The QT-prolonging effect is higher for patients with moderate to severe hepatic impairment [2]. Hence, preexisting QT prolongation, concomitant QT-prolonging drugs, or hepatic impairment are contraindications for ranolazine. Since most significant QT-prolonging effects were seen at 1500 mg dose, approval was sought for a maximal dose of 1000 mg formulation [6]. In the ranolazine clinical studies, including CARISA, Monotherapy Assessment of Ranolazine in Stable Angina trial (MARISA), Efficacy of Ranolazine in Chronic Angina (ERICA), and MERLIN-TIMI 36, the safety data did not show increased arrhythmia except for one case of torsade de pointes seen in both ranolazine and placebo groups in MERLIN-TIMI 36. In the Ranolazine Open-Label Experience (ROLE) study, the average increase in QTc interval was 2.4 msec, but 16 out of 746 patients had QTc of more than 500 msec. However, in the MERLIN TIMI-36 study, ranolazine showed decreased supraventricular tachycardia and a non-statistical trend for decreased new-onset atrial fibrillation (AF) [1].

Animal Studies

(I) Efficacy in Angina: Most animal studies show improvement in ischemia-reperfusion injury with ranolazine in the form of improved LV pressure, coronary flow, and infarct size [15]. Possible mechanisms for this effect include improved cytosolic and mitochondrial calcium overloading, reactive oxygen species, and Reperfusion Injury Salvage kinases (RISK) pathways [15, 16]. Multiple animal studies corroborate the prevention of calcium overloading by INa as the likely mechanism of ranolazine in ischemia. Most studies, though randomized, have not been longitudinal to evaluate the long-term effects of ranolazine in INa. The vasodilatory effect of ranolazine has been studied in some aortic preparations. This effect has been seen in aortic rings with endothelium contracted with phenylephrine [17]. This effect is attenuated by the inhibition of nitric oxide

synthase (NOS), suggesting NOS as the possible mechanism for vasodilation. This vasodilatory effect of ranolazine is also seen in the presence of nicardipine [18].

(II) Efficacy in Arrhythmia: Both *in vitro* and *in vivo* studies for the ranolazine effect on arrhythmias have been conducted in varied settings in different animal models. Most studies include action potential duration and arrhythmia mapping with no biochemical marker evaluation. Almost all studies have noted improvement with ranolazine. Ranolazine has a better anti-arrhythmic effect in atrial myocytes than in ventricular myocytes, which is an important caveat [19]. A low dose of ranolazine may cause more ventricular arrhythmias than a higher dose [20]. However, a contrary effect had been noted in human studies with higher doses of ranolazine predisposing to arrhythmias. Ranolazine may have more benefits in paroxysmal AF than persistent AF [21]. The antiarrhythmic effect of ranolazine seems to be dependent on the baseline steady-state ratio of activated/inactivated INa. This ratio may be affected by pathological conditions, including ischemia, heart failure, and diabetes mellitus (DM). Hence these factors, if not measured, could affect ranolazine study outcomes [19].

(III) Efficacy in Heart Failure: Studies about the effect of ranolazine on heart failure are positive except in studies wherein ranolazine was not given to the animals for at least 2-4 weeks prior to the outcome assessment [22]. Ranolazine, due to being a glycometabolic modulator, possibly needs chronic administration for improvement in heart failure. The most consistent improvement in heart failure is noted in LVEDP and a maximal rate of rise and fall in left ventricular pressure. Other effects include improving calcium alternans and pressure overload-induced cardiac hypertrophy [22, 23]. These changes are mediated by Ca^{2+}-dependent calmodulin (CaM)/CaMKII/MEF2 and CaM/ CaMKII/ calcineurin/ NFAT hypertrophy signaling pathways. Improvement is also noted in apoptotic pathways by TUNEL-positive cells and caspase-9 expression [23, 24].

(IV) Efficacy in Cardiomyopathy: Anthracyclines are a group of chemotherapeutic medications used in different forms of cancer. Anthracyclines inhibit the topoisomerase IIα enzyme that relaxes the topologically supercoiled DNA. Topoisomerase IIα facilitates DNA replication and transcription. Thus, anthracyclines interfere with cancer cell DNA synthesis and RNA transcription during mitosis, leading to cell cycle block at the G1 or G2 phases and then cell death [25, 26]. Anthracyclines induce ROS production that could hyperactivate the cardiac isoform of calmodulin-dependent protein kinase II δ. This further induces hyperactivation of the cardiac late sodium current with cytosolic calcium overload. Mitochondrial oxidative stress, NAD(P)H, and ATP depletion-induced energetic stress cause sustained ROS production, leading to cardiotoxicity and

cardiomyopathy [25].

Since some of the stressors were related to late sodium current, ranolazine was suggested as an intervention to prevent anthracycline-induced cardiomyopathy. In an animal study of 344 rats with cardiomyopathy caused by DOX, rats on placebo continued to have worsening progressive systolic and diastolic heart failure. Rats receiving ranolazine had improved diastolic function and stable systolic function with decreased mortality. Further molecular studies suggested that ranolazine decreased myocardial NADPH oxidase 2 expression, oxidative/nitrative stress, expression of the Na^+/Ca^{2+} exchanger 1, doxorubicin-induced hyper-phosphorylation, oxidation of Ca^{2+}/calmodulin-dependent protein kinase II, and decreased myocardial fibrosis [27].

(V) Efficacy in Metabolic Disorder: Most metabolic studies have been conducted for diabetes in rat models. Studies have shown improvement in biochemical tests, including fasting blood glucose level and glycated hemoglobin a1c (HbA1c) [28, 29]. Ranolazine also improves recruitment in muscle microvasculature and insulin-mediated whole-body glucose disposal [30]. It also improves inflammatory and oxidative stress markers, thus modulating glucose metabolism. Further, in diabetic cardiomyopathic rats, ranolazine improves caspase-3, Notch homolog 1 (NOTCH1), and neuregulin 1 (NRG1) expression [31]. Table **2** summarizes some of the animal studies related to ranolazine.

Table 2. Animal studies related to ranolazine.

Study	Animal model	Pre experiment ranolazine	During experiment ranolazine	Post experiment ranolazine	Biochemical outcomes	Ranolazine effect
I. Ischemia						
Calderon-Sanchez *et al.*, 2016 [32]	Rat	(+)	(+)	(+)	Intracellular Ca^{2+}, Diastolic Ca^{2+} concentration	Improvement
Ma *et al.*, 2014 [33]	Guinea pig isolated myocyte	(-)	(+)	(+)	Hypoxia and hydrogen peroxide-induced INa	Improvement
Aldakkak *et al.*, 2011 [15]	Guinea pig	(+)	(+)	(+)	Oxygen radical, Ca^{2+} overloading LV pressure, CF, VF, infarct size	Improvement. Did not affect mitochondrial permeability transition pore
Efentakis *et al.*, 2016 [16]	Rabbit heart	(+)	(+)	(+)	RISK pathway Infarct size	Improvement
II. Arrythmia						
Ogawa *et al.*, 2017 [34]	Rabbit	(-)	(-)	(+)	VT/VF post ischemia	Improvement

(Table 2) cont.....

Study	Animal model	Pre experiment ranolazine	During experiment ranolazine	Post experiment ranolazine	Biochemical outcomes	Ranolazine effect
Fumagalli *et al.*, 2014 [35]	Rat	(+)	(+)	(+)	Troponin VT/VF, LV systolic, diastolic function, neurological recovery post-resuscitation	Improvement
Bhimani *et al.*, 2014 [36]	Dog heart (closed or open)	(-)	(+)	(+)	Atrial flutter and AF cycle length, effective RP	Improvement
Moschovidis *et al.*, 2020 [20]	Rabbit Heart, post-MI	(-)	(+)	(-)	VA post-myocardial ischemia	Low dose worsened VA, and high dose improved VA
Hartmann *et al.*, 2016 [37]	Explanted human myocyte	(-)	(+)	(-)	Sarcoplasmic reticulum Ca$^+$ leak Atrial myocyte APD	Improvement in myocyte from AF heart, not from HF heart
Fromeyer *et al.*, 2016 [38]	Isolated rabbit hearts	(-)	(+)	(-)	QTc, effective RF, APD, prolongation of ventricular repolarization	Improvement
Ellerman *et al.*, 2018 [39]	Isolated rabbit hearts	(-)	(+)	(-)	Atrial APD, atrial effect RP	Improvement
Caves *et al.*, 2017 [19]	Isolated rabbit left atrial and right ventricular myocytes.	(-)	(+)	(-)	INa in atrial and ventricular myocytes depended on activated/inactivated state block.	Improvement was observed; Increased atrial effect than ventricular
Ramirez *et al.*, 2019 [21]	Isolated sheep heart	(-)	(+)	(+)	Dominant frequency, singularity point density	Improvement in PAF, not persistent AF
III. Vasodilation						
Malavaki *et al.*, 2015 [17]	Rabbit aorta	(-)	(-)	(+)	Vasodilatory effect with nicardipine	Improvement, time-dependent
Paredes-Carbajal *et al.*, 2013 [18]	Phenylephrine precontracted rat aortic rings	(-)	(+)	(+)	Aortic ring/ endothelium relaxation	Improvement was observed; Attenuated by nitric oxide synthase inhibitor
IV. Heart Failure						
Teng *et al.*, 2018 [40]	Rat heart	(-)	(-)	(+)	B-type natriuretic peptide-45, norepinephrine LV function	Improvement
Wang *et al.*, 2019 [23]	Rats	(+)	(+)	(-)	TUNEL-positive cells, caspase-9 expression, LVEDP, maximal rate of left ventricular pressure rise and fall	Improvement
Fukaya *et al.*, 2019 [41]	Dog hearts	(+)	(+)	(-)	Arrhythmogenic AP alternans APD and Ca^{2+} alternans in HF	Improvement

(Table 2) cont.....

Study	Animal model	Pre experiment ranolazine	During experiment ranolazine	Post experiment ranolazine	Biochemical outcomes	Ranolazine effect
Goldstein *et al.*, 2019 [22]	Swine hearts (advanced heart failure)	(-)	(+)	(-)	LVEDP, LV peak systolic pressure, maximal LV pressure rises	No improvement
Nie *et al.*, 2019 [24]	Mice	(+)	(+)	(-)	Ca^{2+}-dependent CaM/CaMKII/MEF2 and CaM/CaMKII/calcineurin/NFAT hypertrophy signaling pathways triggered by pressure overload, endoplasmic reticulum mediated apoptosis, pressure overload-induced cardiac hypertrophy, systolic and diastolic function	Improvement
V. Metabolic						
Tawfik *et al.*, 2019 [28]	Rats	(+)	(+)	(-)	Histopathological score, apoptotic markers, inflammatory and oxidative stress markers, fasting blood glucose, A1c	Improvement
Cassano *et al.* 2020 [29]	Rats (Diabetic)	(+)	(+)	(-)	Blood glucose levels, pro-inflammatory profile (interleukin-6) Lean body mass, learning, and long-term memory	Improvement
Chen *et al.*, 2020 [31]	Diabetic cardiomyopathy rats	(+)	(+)	(-)	Bcl-2, Bax, Caspase-3, NOTCH1, and NRG1 expression TUNEL staining (apoptosis), interventricular septum, LV internal diameter	Improved biochemical markers, apoptotic markers. No improvement in cardiac function and indices.
Fu *et al.*, 2013 [30]	Rats	(+)	(+)	(-)	Recruitment of muscle microvasculature, insulin-mediated whole-body glucose disposal, eNOS phosphorylation and cAMP production	Improvement

Abbreviations: AP: action potential, APD: action potential duration, AF: atrial fibrillation, Bcl-2: B-cell lymphoma 2, Bax: Bcl-2 associated X protein, Ca^{2+}: Calcium, CF: coronary flow, Caspase-3: cysteinyl aspartate specific proteinase-3, CaM: calmodulin, EDV: end-diastolic volume, ESV: end-systolic volume, HF: heart failure, INa: late sodium current, LV: left ventricle, LVEF: left ventricular ejection fraction, NO: nitric oxide, NOTCH 1: Notch homolog 1, NRG1: Neuregulin 1, PAF: paroxysmal atrial fibrillation, RV: right ventricle, RP: refractory period, RISK pathway: Reperfusion Injury Salvage Kinases pathway, VA: ventricular arrhythmias, VF: ventricular fibrillation, VT: ventricular tachycardia

E. Pharmacological Indication: Ranolazine ER tablets in the formulation of 500 mg or 1000 mg two times a day is FDA approved for chronic angina. It can be used with other anti-anginal medications, including beta-blockers (BB), nitrates, or calcium channel blockers (CCB), or could be substituted for these medications if they are not tolerated due to side effects [42]. Ranolazine has been used off-label for ventricular tachycardia (VT) [43 - 45].

CHRONIC STABLE ANGINA (CSA)

Chronic stable angina is the most common indication for ranolazine, especially refractory chronic angina, through which patients with ischemic heart disease (IHD) and ongoing angina benefit the most. Patients may be on maximized guideline-recommended first-line anti-anginal medications or may have an intolerance to some of the recommended medications. Multiple mechanisms have been researched to explain the antianginal effects of ranolazine. Most studied parameters include improved diastolic pressure [46], diastolic function [46, 47], ventricular dyssynchrony [48], endothelial function [49, 50] and myocardial perfusion [51]. The MARISA trial was the first to indicate that ranolazine monotherapy improved exercise duration, reduced angina frequency, and reduced the time before angina symptoms in patients with chronic angina. Later, the CARISA trial evaluated ranolazine in the presence of other antianginal medications and demonstrated similar benefits as in the MARISA trial. Additionally, there was a significant decrease in nitroglycerine (NTG) use in the ranolazine group [52, 53], though no mortality benefit was seen. Since patients in the previous trial were not on maximized doses of guideline-recommended antianginal medications, the ERICA trial enrolled patients taking amlodipine 10 mg daily and with ≥ 3 anginal attacks per week. Concomitant use of long-acting nitrates was allowed, and their percentage was similar in both ranolazine and placebo groups (between 40-45% in both groups). In this trial, ranolazine decreased angina frequency and NTG use per week and improved quality of life (QOL). These trials formed the major basis for the indication of ranolazine for chronic stable angina [52, 53]. We further explain the effect of ranolazine on angina below.

Improvement in Symptoms: MARISA trial enrolled 191 CSA patients with well-documented coronary artery disease (CAD) and at least a three-month history of effort angina responding to BB, CCB, and/or long-acting nitrates. All other antianginals were discontinued, and ranolazine monotherapy increased the total exercise duration, time to angina, and 1 mm ST-segment depression during exercise tolerance test (ETT) performed according to Bruce protocol at the end of one week of ranolazine in a dose-dependent manner compared to placebo [54]. It seemed that these benefits of ETT were independent of its effect on heart rate, blood pressure, and rate pressure product. However, ranolazine decreases heart rate (HR) and blood pressure (BP) during ETT, with the maximal effect seen at a dose of 1000 mg [55]. In a more recent study comparing ivabradine with ranolazine for changes in angina symptoms measured by Seattle Angina Questionnaire (SAQ), both ranolazine and ivabradine improved angina symptoms as compared to placebo. Additionally, ranolazine improved SAQ significantly higher than ivabradine [56]. Subset analysis showed that physical limitation, angina frequency, angina stability, treatment satisfaction, and disease perception of SAQ improved except for physical limitations of ranolazine as compared to ivabradine [56]. In a similar study in women, SAQ (all subsection), Duke Activity Score Index, and Women's Ischemia Symptom Questionnaire showed significant improvement after 4 weeks of ranolazine. In most of these studies, the prevalence of diabetes was around 29%, and the subgroup analysis for diabetics has not been reported [57]. The SAQ is a reliable and valid test and correlates with long-term survival and acute coronary syndrome (ACS) hospitalization among patients with chronic CAD [58]. A meta-analysis including seven studies has shown the net benefit of ranolazine in exercise stress test parameters. The studies included were scored as low risk for bias in 4 of the 7 domains of bias in the Cochrane Collaboration tool [59].

MERLIN TIMI 36 identified worsening angina as a requirement of additional therapy as defined by an increase in angina to a higher Canadian Cardiovascular Society classification requiring new or increasing doses of antianginal medications in response to symptom change. The study included hospitalized patients with non-ST elevation acute coronary syndromes (NSTE-ACS) as compared to previous studies, including patients with stable angina. In this study, similar to the previous study, compared to placebo, ranolazine reduced the incidence of recurrent ischemia (HR: 0.78; 95% CI: 0.67 to 0.91; $p < 0.002$), worsening angina (HR: 0.77; 95% CI: 0.59 to 1.00; $p < 0.048$), and intensification of antianginal therapy (HR: 0.77; 95% CI: 0.64 to 0.92, $p < 0.005$). This further led to decreased hospital stays and revascularization for worsening angina. However, all-cause mortality, cardiovascular death, or MI did not differ between the groups [60]. Consequently, this decreases the interaction of patients with health care systems [61]. Post-hoc analysis of MERLIN TIMI 36 study demonstrated consistent significant benefit of ranolazine in improving recurrent ischemia in diabetics, women, and patients with beta natriuretic peptide (BNP) >80 pg/ml [62].

Another study in patients with non-obstructive coronary artery disease (NOCAD) (<50% epicardial coronary stenosis) showed a direct correlation between changes in SAQ scores and myocardial perfusion reserve index (MPRI) (correlation 0.23; p=0.04). The improvement in SAQ scores with MPRI is more likely to be seen with lower coronary flow reserve (CFR <2) [63]. Zhu *et al.* compared ranolazine with ivabradine and nicorandil and found ranolazine to improve MPRI only if the patients had baseline CFR <2.5 or a global MPRI <2 [64]. In a Greek longitudinal observational study to evaluate ranolazine in routine clinical practice for 6 months, the symptoms of angina assessed by the Canadian Cardiovascular Society (CCS) grading system improved significantly. Adherence to medication was good, with only 7.9% discontinuing medication by three months. This improvement in angina symptoms was associated with improved function of daily life [65]. These benefits in angina frequency have also been noted in the veterans' population [66], shorter [67], or longer-term studies of 1-2 years in severe angina patients taking standard doses of atenolol, amlodipine, or diltiazem [14].

In a randomized control trial (RCT) of patients with chronic angina and incomplete revascularization following percutaneous coronary intervention (PCI), ranolazine, as compared to placebo, did not improve SAQ. Further analysis suggested improvement in SAQ scores with ranolazine at 6 months among diabetics (mean difference 3.3; 95% CI 0.6, 6.1; P=0.02) and patients with baseline SAQ angina frequency ≤60 (P=0.02), although the improvement was not sustained at 12 months [68]. Some of these patients may benefit from complete revascularization. One limitation of this trial was that it included a mixed group of patients with residual disease, including untreated chronic total occlusions and diffuse distal disease, and also the functional significance of untreated disease (stress, fractional flow reserve) was unknown.

Improvement in Heart Function: Despite multiple studies concluding that ranolazine improves clinical angina, few studies have studied the effect of ranolazine on human cardiac function. Studies have evaluated both right and left heart function. Most used tests include echocardiography and single-photon emission computerized tomography using nuclear imaging for myocardial perfusion. Most studies have shown improvement in diastolic function and myocardial perfusion imaging (MPI), with few studies showing improvement in systolic function.

Left Heart Function: A study evaluating both systolic and diastolic heart function after 2 months of ranolazine 1000 mg found a non-significant increase in left ventricular ejection fraction. Additionally, a significant increase was noted in deceleration time (DT), isovolumic contraction (ICT), isovolumic relaxation times (IRT), ejection time (ET), and myocardial performance index (MPI). The study postulated that shortened IRT, a diastolic parameter, as well as improvements in the systolic parameters of ICT and ET were the reasons for improved measured myocardial performance by MPI [69]. Murray *et al.* enrolled patients with systolic and diastolic heart failure to study the effect of ranolazine on left ventricular ejection fraction and autonomic measures. Follow-up was completed for an average of 24 months, and echo cardiac parameters were evaluated. LVEF was increased in 70% of ranolazine patients as compared to controls, with an average increase of 11.3 units. Being an open-label trial with unblinded echocardiographic evaluation, the study had a high risk for bias [70].

Hayashida *et al.* evaluated regional LV segments that were either normal (perfused by intact coronary vessels), ischemic (perfused by stenotic vessels but without ECG evidence suggesting myocardial necrosis), or infarcted (total coronary occlusion and with ECG evidence for necrosis). Ranolazine was administered as a single dose in the intravenous formulation. No change in peak filling rate was noted in the normal segments as compared to ischemic segments, leading to an improved regional diastolic function in ischemic segments. Thus, ranolazine may be beneficial in chronic under-perfused hibernating myocardium. The study also noted a significant decrease in HR as compared to placebo, and it is difficult to ascertain if the improvement in diastolic function is independent of the effect on heart rate and if similar results could be seen in echocardiographic evaluation [71]. A cohort study on diabetic, non-obstructive CAD patients found ranolazine treatment resulting in modest but significant improvement in diastolic function without any changes in CFR or exercise-stimulated myocardial blood flow. There was a significant inverse correlation whereby improvement following treatment with ranolazine was greater in patients with lower baseline-corrected CFR [47]. In contrast, a small pilot study of fifteen asymptomatic, moderate-severe aortic stenosis patients did not show a significant improvement in diastolic function or MPR with the use of ranolazine [72].

Two studies evaluating the effect of ranolazine on MPRI have shown positive results. One study observed an improvement in women with angina and NOCAD with at least 10% ischemic myocardium on stress cardiac magnetic resonance (CMR) imaging. The other study enrolled patients with a high probability of CAD and reversible perfusion defects on exercise treadmill gated single-photon CT MPI. In both studies, the images were read by experienced readers blinded to treatment assignment [51, 73]. However, in another study of 2 weeks duration in patients with NOCAD, there was no improvement in MPRI. In this study, the peak heart rate decreased significantly during pharmacological stress in the ranolazine group. The changes in MPRI predicted the change in SAQ and quality of life (QoL) score after adjustment for body mass index (BMI), prior myocardial infarction, and site (P = 0.0032). Consistent with other studies, low CFR<2.5 subjects had a better improved MPRI (P = 0.0137) [74].

Right Heart Function: Ranolazine has been studied for pulmonary hypertension (PH) with a pilot study conducted in 2015. The study enrolled 11 patients with Group 1 PH, with almost 90% of patients being on phosphodiesterase inhibitors. At the end of three months, patients' WHO class for PH, exercise tolerance, quality of life, echocardiographic and invasive hemodynamic parameters were evaluated. Though ranolazine in the dose of 1000 mg improved WHO PH class and echocardiographic features significantly, it did not improve invasive hemodynamic parameters. Major effects were seen in RV end-diastolic volume and right heart strain. Similar to left heart function, these changes were independent of changes in blood pressure and heart rate [75]. In a similar phase 1 placebo-controlled safety trial for Pulmonary Arterial Hypertension using ranolazine 500 mg dosing, there was no improvement in echocardiographic features, exercise testing, or hemodynamic monitoring. The study further showed that most patients did not reach therapeutic ranolazine blood levels with 500 mg dosing [76].

Further evaluation by Finch *et al.* found ranolazine in the dosage of 1000 mg two times a day given for an average of 6 -24 months improved ETT, functional class, echocardiographic and hemodynamic parameters in patients with PH related to heart failure with preserved ejection fraction. Most of the improvement was achieved in 6 months and remained stable over the 2 years of monitoring. A limitation of the study was the possible bias due to being an open labelled study type with an unblinded evaluation of outcomes. In this study, at day 180, mean pulmonary artery pressure (mPAP) decreased to 29.0 ± 9.2 mm Hg (p = 0.007), pulmonary capillary wedge pressure (PCWP) decreased to 13.1 ± 5.3 mm Hg (p = 0.004), and peripheral vascular resistance (PVR) did not change significantly [77]. Most of these studies enrolled a small number of stable patients from a specialty (PH clinic), which could lead to selection bias. Ranolazine is also not effective in improving New York Heart Association (NYHA) functional class, 6-minute walk distance, N-terminal pro-brain natriuretic peptide, or quality of life measures in patients with precapillary PH (groups I, III, and IV). A recent randomized placebo-controlled, double-blind study showed a significant increase in right ventricular ejection fraction (RVEF) at the end of 6 months compared with baseline in the ranolazine group after adjusting for baseline values, age, and sex. The absolute change in RVEF in ranolazine was an average of 7.6 with a standard error of 1.7 and a p-value of 0.005. There was also a significant increase in left ventricular end-diastolic volume index and LV and RV systolic volume [78].

Fig. (4) Illustration of the effect of ranolazine on hemodynamic and echocardiographic parameters of the heart.

Improvement in Quality of Life: Numerous quality of life (QoL) scores have been used to evaluate the QoL in CSA patients on ranolazine. Quality of life could be extrapolated from angina frequency, physical limitation, mental component, angina stability, and dyspnea scores. Studies have measured changes in QoL cross-sectionally or longitudinally over 1-12 months. Most of the QoL benefit for ranolazine is derived from the improvement in angina frequency, leading to better treatment satisfaction without improvement in physical limitation. Few studies have shown benefits in SAQ QoL in angina patients, although similar benefits were not seen in PH.

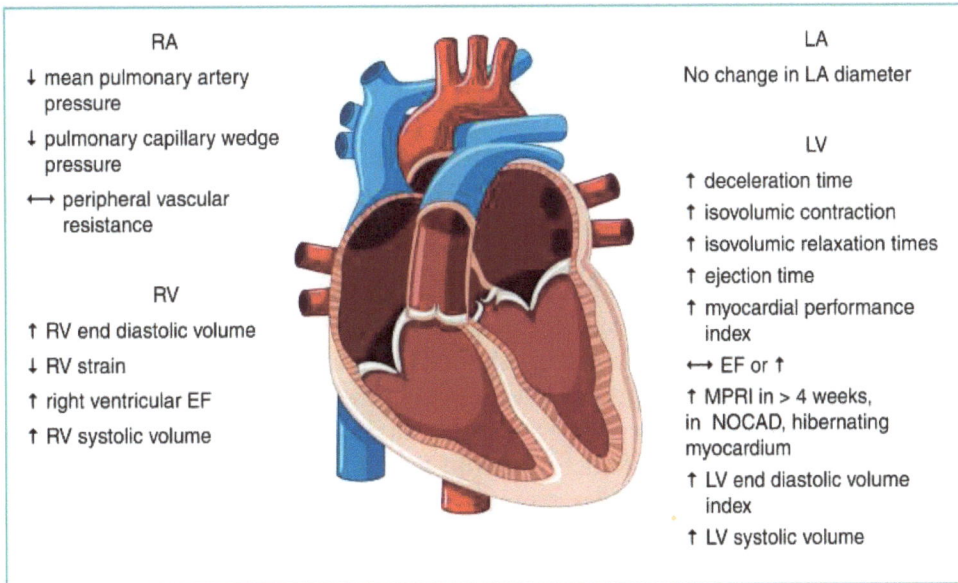

RA
↓ mean pulmonary artery pressure
↓ pulmonary capillary wedge pressure
⟷ peripheral vascular resistance

RV
↑ RV end diastolic volume
↓ RV strain
↑ right ventricular EF
↑ RV systolic volume

LA
No change in LA diameter

LV
↑ deceleration time
↑ isovolumic contraction
↑ isovolumic relaxation times
↑ ejection time
↑ myocardial performance index
⟷ EF or ↑
↑ MPRI in > 4 weeks, in NOCAD, hibernating myocardium
↑ LV end diastolic volume index
↑ LV systolic volume

Fig. (4). Ranolazine effect on heart hemodynamic and echocardiographic parameters.

Willis *et al.* studied the effects of a 12-week exercise training program with and without ranolazine on ETT, daily physical activity, and QoL in CSA patients. In this study, a 12-week exercise program itself improved aerobic fitness, physical activity, and health-related QoL (HRQoL) in both ranolazine and placebo groups. There was no significant difference in primary outcomes between these groups. Also, measured outcomes including physical activity, non-exercise physical activity, and sedentary time tracked *via* accelerometers increased similarly in both groups. It is difficult to ascertain the barriers to translating improved angina scores to improving quality of life, especially since ranolazine had improved ETT in multiple other studies [79]. In Type 2 Diabetes Evaluation of Ranolazine in Subjects With Chronic Stable Angina (TERISA) trial, the physical component of Medical Outcomes Short Form-36 (SF-36) improved significantly with ranolazine though the mental component remained the same. Patients with CAD are at higher risk of developing depression, and its presence affects outcomes of CAD. Hence it may be important to control depression and anxiety in quality-of-life studies for ranolazine [80]. Optimism also plays a role in the self-perception of quality of life and leads to better health outcomes [81]. In TERISA trial of patients with DM and chronic stable angina, both SAQ QoL and Rose dyspnea scores improved more in the ranolazine group, though it was not statistically significant (p= 0.08). Further, the number needed to treat for ranolazine to achieve a clinically significant improvement in angina was 11, indicating low efficacy. This efficacy increases if the baseline anginal symptoms are severe [80]. Contrarily, in the MERLIN TIMI study of ACS patients, the QoL and Medical Outcomes Study 12-item Short Form (SF-12) mental component significantly improved as compared to SAQ physical limitations and SF-12 physical component. Longitudinal analyses showed female sex, DM, and lack of early revascularization therapy were independently associated with significantly worse outcomes in health status and QOL scores. However, no differential treatment effects (i.e., treatment X subgroup interaction) related to any of these clinical or demographic factors were seen [58].

An Epistemonikos database-based meta-analysis of 16 studies suggested ranolazine probably results in little or no difference in the quality of life. Ranolazine might decrease the frequency of anginal events, but the certainty of the evidence is low, with a probable increase in the incidence of adverse effects. The meta-analysis included ranolazine from 500 to 1000 mg dosage formulation; the lower doses being less efficacious could have affected the overall results [82]. On the other hand, the Cochrane review summarized that there is moderate-quality evidence that people with stable angina who received ranolazine as an add-on therapy to standard of care medication had fewer angina episodes but increased risk of presenting non-serious adverse events compared to those given placebo. Further, there was moderate evidence for ranolazine on quality of life, though the effect per se was uncertain [83]. In this review, meta-analysis for ranolazine 1000 mg dosing was significant in reducing angina frequency, while including studies with all dosing led to a non-significant effect on angina frequency [83].

D. Cost-effectiveness: Various cost-effectiveness models for ranolazine have been studied in different populations. Most studies have shown a modest cost-benefit for ranolazine in patients with at least daily to weekly angina. Studies varied in factors leading to benefits. In a Markov model, ranolazine patients lived a mean of 0.700 quality-adjusted life years (QALYs) at the cost of $15,661 as compared to standard of care (SoC) patients of 0.659 QALYs at the cost of $14,321. The incremental cost-effectiveness ratio (ICER) for the addition of ranolazine was $32,682/QALY. Monte Carlo simulation found that at a $50,000/QALY willingness-to-pay threshold, ranolazine was cost-effective in 97% of 10,000 iterations [84]. In a decision tree model adapted to the Greek setting, ranolazine plus SoC resulted in an ICER equal to €4620 per QALY gained. In the probabilistic sensitivity analysis, the likelihood was 100% for ranolazine plus SoC being cost-effective at the threshold of €34,000 per QALY gained. This model considered patient compliance, angina frequency, hospitalization, procedures [PCI, coronary artery bypass graft (CABG)], routine monitoring of medications, and medication acquisition. However, the analysis was conducted according to the third-party payer perspective, and hence only direct costs were considered. The indirect cost to patients may be higher than the cost considered in the analysis [85]. In a UK study that included direct and indirect costs, ranolazine was cost-effective [86]. Meta-analysis of cost-effectiveness studies on ranolazine had also shown benefits [87].

In a Markov-based Unites States societal perspective model, the incremental cost-effectiveness ratio for the addition of ranolazine to SoC for diabetics and chronic stable angina patients was \$45,308/QALY. Most of the benefit in this model was contributed by patients' bodily pain improvement-based gain in QALYs (2.73 versus 3.96, p = 0.01) [88]. On the other hand, in a Spanish study, ANCOVA model results showed that 41.47% of the variability of the ICER was due to the utility level associated with moderate angina frequency for non-hospitalized patients [89]. Monte Carlo stimulation had demonstrated ranolazine to be cost-effective in 71-100% of 10,000 iterations in different studies [85, 88]. Most models extrapolated results for one year since few studies are long-term. Further, most models did not include adverse events or productivity losses which may further increase or decrease the cost per QALY gained [86]. In a three-year follow-up study on refractory angina patients, cardiac hospitalization (p = 0.003), followed by PCI and myocardial infarction, continued to be lower in patients on ranolazine as compared to patients not on ranolazine. Mortality was also low, at only 3% overall for 3-year follow-up [90].

In a study of real-world data, ranolazine treatment in patients with stable ischemic heart disease (IHD) was associated with fewer revascularization procedures, shorter length of stay if hospitalized, and lower associated healthcare costs compared with patients initiating BB or long-acting nitrates, though the procedure rates and healthcare costs were similar to patients initiating CCBs. CCBs though less expensive, have additional effects on BP and heart rate, and hence ranolazine may be a good option in patients who have side effects or contraindication to CCBs to decrease inpatient resource utilization [91]. Clinical Outcomes Utilizing Revascularization and Aggressive Drug Evaluation (COURAGE) trial found that delaying revascularization through guideline-directed medical therapy did not increase irreversible ischemic events or 1- year mortality. However, patients were more likely to undergo subsequent revascularization for continued angina and dissatisfaction with their current treatment regimen [91]. Health utility estimates for CSA patients change by angina frequency, and hence angina frequency should be considered for cost-effectiveness studies [92]. A Veterans based cohort study of 37,060 patients showed PCI [Hazards ration (HR) 1.16; confidence interval (CI) 1.08 - 1.25,p <0.00] and ACS hospitalization (HR 1.13; 95% CI 1.00 to 1.27, p <0.042) occurred more often in ranolazine patients while CABG (HR0.82; 95% CI 0.68 to 1.00, p <0.046) and atrial fibrillation related hospitalization (HR 0.74; 95% CI 0.67 to 0.82, p <0.001) occurred more often in conventional treatment group without ranolazine. Adjusted one-year costs were similar in both groups (p=0.71). Although the total cost and outpatient cost remained similar in both groups, pharmacy costs were higher for ranolazine, and inpatient costs were higher for the conventional group [93].

ACUTE CORONARY SYNDROME (ACS)

Because of the efficacy of ranolazine in CSA, studies have evaluated ranolazine in ACS. Ranolazine has been used as an antianginal medication [94], a metabolic modulator during ischemia [95], medication improving reperfusion injury after PCI [96], cardiac dysfunction [97], and as an antiarrhythmic during ACS or post ACS period [98]. Though some of these studies have shown a positive effect, ranolazine has little benefit in the immediate post ACS period. In a pilot RCT of patients with stable effort angina and positive stress test undergoing elective PCI, ranolazine given as 1000 mg two times a day for seven days prior to PCI resulted in a significant decrease in peri-procedural MI with no effect on the major adverse cardiac event (MACE) [96]. In patients presenting with chest pain due to cardiac microvascular dysfunction, CFR <2 (diagnosed by cardiac Rb-82 positron emission tomography and computed tomography imaging) ranolazine may improve CFR [99]. Ranolazine, given as intravenous formulation followed by oral formulation in ACS, significantly decreased non-sustained ventricular tachycardia (VT), supraventricular tachycardia, ventricular pauses ≥ 3 seconds, and a trend for reduction in new-onset AF during the seven days post-ACS period [45]. No improvement has been noted in sustained monomorphic or polymorphic VT. These anti-arrhythmic effects of ranolazine are independent of TIMI risk, prior heart failure, reduced EF, and prolonged QT interval [45]. The median AF burden in Holter monitoring, *i.e.*, the proportion of recorded time patients spent in AF, tends to be lower with ranolazine, 5.1% in ranolazine recipients versus 14.1% in placebo recipients (p = 0.056) [100]. Ranolazine has a lesser effect than amlodipine on clopidogrel-induced inhibition of platelet reactivity in CAD patients, especially with high platelet reactivity at baseline [101]. Thus, ranolazine may be a better anti-anginal treatment for CAD patients on clopidogrel with high platelet reactivity.

In a translational study by Schemer *et al.*, ACS patients were randomized to ranolazine or placebo in addition to SoC for 6 weeks. Nitric oxide synthesis can be decreased by asymmetric (ADMA) and symmetric dimethylarginine (SDMA), two methylation products of arginine protein residues by protein arginine methyltransferase 1 (PRMT-1) and PRMT-2. The nitric oxide pathway is involved in oxidative stress. In the ranolazine group, plasma arginine levels were significantly higher at the end of the study than at baseline. However, ADMA and SDMA levels did not differ. Urine levels of the oxidative stress marker 8-is--PGF2α tended to be lower in ranolazine-treated patients indicating lower oxidative stress in this group of ACS patients [95]. A similar small hypothesis-generating study with 6 weeks of ranolazine showed a trend in improving the global strain rate assessed by speckle-tracking echocardiography in patients with unstable angina [97].

In MERLIN TIMI 36 study, adding ranolazine to standard treatment for ACS was not effective in reducing MACE. Additionally, ranolazine did not adversely affect the risk of all-cause death or symptomatic documented arrhythmia [98]. In a subgroup analysis of MERLIN TIMI 36 study that enrolled 3565 patients with a history of prior angina presenting with ACS in the form of unstable angina or non-ST elevated myocardial infarction (NSTEMI), the sub-study evaluated patients who had PCI within 30 days of the index event. Ranolazine significantly decreased the primary composite endpoint events (CV death, MI, or recurrent ischemia) at 1 year (HR, 0.71; 95% CI, 0.55- 0.91; P =0.01) in this group of patients. Similar benefits were not noted in patients on medical management after ACS. This is contrary to the opinion that anti-anginal medication has more benefits in medical management [94]. In another analysis of the same study, ranolazine, similar to CSA, improved rates of worsening angina and the requirement for anti-anginal treatment 30 days post-ACS. This improvement in ischemia was not associated with decreased hospitalization, revascularization, or electrocardiographic changes in ischemia. The MACE rates showed improvement though it was not significant (P=0.055) [98]. In a subgroup analysis at 1-year, patients with baseline beta type natriuretic peptide >80 pg/ml benefitted the most with a significant reduction in primary endpoint including CV death, MI, and recurrent ischemia. This may be explained by ranolazine's effect on improving ventricular wall stress [102]. Thus, BNP may be a good biomarker to identify high-risk ACS patients who would benefit from ranolazine. It could further be used as a cardiac biomarker in ranolazine studies. A similar subgroup analysis showed a decrease in recurrent ischemia in women and diabetics [100, 103].

ATRIAL FIBRILLATION

Ranolazine's inhibitory potential on different cardiac ion channels is differential with major action on peak and late INa, with minor effects on rapidly activating delayed-rectifier K^+ current (IKr) and L-type Ca^{2+} (ICa-L) channels. Likewise, ranolazine has a lower threshold for atrial effect as compared to ventricles.

Ranolazine decreases conduction velocity and enhances post-repolarization refractoriness [7]. Ranolazine has shown benefits in early and late atrial depolarization in animal studies that have been translated to human studies. Ranolazine decreases the incidence of AF in ACS, decreases the time spent in AF in post ACS period, time to cardioversion, the incidence of perioperative AF during open-heart surgeries, and AF recurrence rate after successful cardioversion [7].

Prevention of Chronic Atrial Fibrillation: AF could occur in the setting of structural heart disease, perioperatively, or during ACS. AF may be paroxysmal or permanent, wherein the patient is in irregular heart rhythm permanently. AF could be managed by rate control or rhythm control with a goal to change the rhythm to normal sinus. Rhythm control strategies could be invasive, including cardioversion, ablation, or non-invasive, in the form of medical management. Anti-arrhythmic medications, though mostly safe, have considerable side effects, thus limiting their long-term use. Ranolazine has been studied for rhythm control in AF undergoing cardioversion or receiving other antiarrhythmic medications. Ranolazine has some efficacy in doses of 500-750 mg to prevent recurrence of AF after successful cardioversion. In a study on patients after successful cardioversion from AF, a divergence was noted around 10-20 days between ranolazine and placebo groups, indicating the ineffectiveness of ranolazine in preventing early recurrence of AF after cardioversion which is usually caused by electrical remodeling and systemic inflammation. After this early phase, ranolazine has a better effect in preventing AF, especially from pulmonary vein triggers [104].

Murdock *et al.* have conducted a retrospective case series and cohort study to evaluate the impact of ranolazine on increasing successful cardioversion rates in treatment-resistant and cardioversion-resistant AF patients. Though these studies did not have a placebo arm, the successful cardioversion rates were 59-76% in this high-risk group [105].

This data is further confirmed in a metanalysis of 10 studies that showed ranolazine was effective in reducing the risk of AF (p=0.003), especially post-operative AF when compared to non-post-operative AF (odds ratio [OR] 0.70; 95% CI 0.54–0.83; p = 0.005). Moreover, improved successful cardioversion rates and time to cardioversion were noted [106]. Another meta-analysis with similar results showed significant heterogeneity in the studies that improved when ranolazine data were pooled by drug dosage results. Ranolazine <1000 mg had lower heterogeneity. However, the weighted mean difference for AF conversion was greater for the higher dose of ranolazine. Statistical testing also showed publication bias. One salient limitation of these studies is a short-term follow-up, and they lack data about efficacy in subgroups including diabetes, low EF, and history of CAD since these are known risk factors for AF [107, 108].

Rhythm Control for Atrial Fibrillation in the Presence and Absence of other Medications

In an RCT enrolling new-onset AF, starting iv amiodarone with one oral dose of ranolazine 1500 mg non significantly improved conversion rate to normal sinus rhythm (p=0.056) as compared to amiodarone only. Further median time to conversion and the cumulative conversion rates were higher in the combined treatment group. This finding was associated with a significant increase in QTc, though the increase did not lead to increased arrhythmia or treatment discontinuation. The study postulated the combination of ranolazine and amiodarone to be synergistic. Other adverse events included episodes of hypotension <90 mm Hg that were seen in both groups [109]. A one-time high dose of ranolazine with amiodarone significantly improved cardioversion success rates. Another related study testing ranolazine 750 mg combined with reduced dronedarone dosages also found that the combination had good efficacy in reducing the burden of AF. This combination was synergistic, and most of the AF burden reduction was achieved within 4 weeks and was sustained till the end of the study at 12 weeks. This study enrolled a distinct group of patients with dual-chamber programmable pacemakers implanted for standard clinical indications so that the AF burden could be continuously monitored. Ranolazine has not been studied in comparison to other standard antiarrhythmics and in permanent AF patients [110].

In addition to the effect on ion channels, additional restoration of mitochondrial function (oxidative stress) in atrial tissue and activation of Akt/mammalian target of rapamycin signaling pathway may contribute to the anti-AF effects of ranolazine [111]. Another study showed increased refractoriness and fibrillation inducibility threshold without significantly altering mean arterial blood pressure with ranolazine [112]. Analysis of atrial fibrillatory wave (f-wave) provides qualitative and quantitative insight into atrial-specific effects of antiarrhythmic drugs. Antiarrhythmic drugs, including dofetilide, amiodarone, sotalol, and flecainide, used in preventing AF reproducibly reduce the f-wave dominant frequency (DF) in ECG. Ranolazine could possibly lower AF DF but could not change fibrillatory wave amplitude in a small cohort study [113]. Thus, for AF, animal studies have translated to human clinical studies with good efficacy. Further RCTs are needed to substantiate the findings from the initial studies.

Post-operative Atrial Fibrillation (POAF) in Patients Undergoing Cardiac Surgery

POAF is a complication of cardiac surgeries that occurs in almost 20% to 50% of patients. It increases the risk for embolism, cardiac-related deaths, duration of hospitalization, and costs. BB and amiodarone are efficacious, though they may have some hemodynamic side effects [114]. After on-pump surgery, patients developing POAF had significantly reduced time to conversion after treatment with amiodarone combined with ranolazine, then with amiodarone alone in a randomized trial with 41 patients. There was no significant correlation between time to conversion of POAF, age, surgical time, heart-lung machine time, and aortic cross-clamp time [115]. In another retrospective cohort study, ranolazine was independently associated with a significant reduction of AF compared to amiodarone after CABG, with no difference in adverse events [116]. Amiodarone, being a medication with a long half-life, requires multiple dosing up to 7 days pre-op for POAF prevention. Contrarily, pre-operative ranolazine for 1-3 days prevents POAF [116, 117]. However, large-scale randomized control trials are warranted before any strong conclusions can be made regarding the role of ranolazine in post CABG AF.

CARDIOMYOPATHY

Cardiomyopathy could be caused by multiple risk factors, including IHD, non-ischemic idiopathic, drug-induced, stress, *etc.*

Chemotherapy-induced Cardiomyopathy

Anthracyclines are a group of chemotherapeutic medications with effective anti-tumor cytotoxic activity on breast cancers, soft tissue sarcomas, non-Hodgkin's lymphomas, acute lymphoblastic, myeloblastic and myelogenous leukemias. Doxorubicin [(DOX), or Adriamycin] and daunorubicin are the most commonly used anthracyclines. Anthracyclines are cardiotoxic and lead to cardiomyopathy. Late sodium current-induced stressor is one of the suggested mechanisms for cardiomyopathy. Common cardiovascular drugs, including BB, ACE-I, ARB, and CCB, have prevented chemotherapy-induced reduced LVEF in some limited studies. But these effects are associated with hemodynamic effects, including heart rate-pressure products, rather than their ability to prevent an earlier diastolic dysfunction [118]. These findings led to Ranolazine to Treat Early Cardiotoxicity Induced by Antitumor Drugs (INTERACT) study, a phase 2b study comparing single-agent ranolazine with common cardiovascular drugs to treat early diastolic dysfunction induced by cancer drugs. In this pilot study, 3 patients had treatment failure with standard meds as compared to none in the ranolazine group. Treatment failure was defined as failure to normalize or improve impaired relaxation or biomarker elevations at the end of five weeks. The patients in the standard group had a trend for lower blood pressure and pulse. Thus, ranolazine added to standard treatment or for patients not tolerating standard treatment may improve diastolic dysfunction caused by anthracyclines [118]. Some data show that ranolazine is protective in diabetic cardiomyopathy-induced apoptosis by activating the NOTCH1/NRG1 signaling pathway. Consequently, ranolazine may have additive benefits in diabetic patients requiring chemotherapy [31].

Hypertrophic Cardiomyopathy

Hypertrophic cardiomyopathy (HCM) is a commonly inherited cardiomyopathy with mavacamten as the only disease-modifying therapeutic option. Common symptoms include LV outflow tract obstruction, diastolic dysfunction, and arrhythmias that require management with BB, CCB, and disopyramide [119]. With more genetic testing identifying carriers of the HCM gene without phenotypic symptoms or cardiac dysfunction, the focus is increasing on finding therapeutic options delaying or preventing the phenotypic features of HCM. Diltiazem studied in this setting delayed the onset of cardiac dysfunction in HCM [119]. In a younger population, a medication with an effect on heart rate may be limited by its side effects of hypotension or exercise intolerance. Ranolazine, preventing calcium overload and having a neutral effect on heart rate, may be appropriate for clinical use in HCM. In an HCM mutation mice model, phenotypic effects of inotropic insufficiency, increased diastolic tension, and premature contractions were observed. Ranolazine treatment impeded these effects to prevent the development of myocardial mechanical abnormalities [119].

Ranolazine has also been studied in clinical HCM patients with unsuccessful results. In this cohort of nonobstructive HCM patients with LV thickness ≥ 15 mm and exertional symptoms (angina, dyspnea), ranolazine reduced PVC burden; however, it showed no overall effect on exercise performance, plasma prohormone brain natriuretic peptide levels, diastolic function, or QoL [120]. Another similar study reported improvement in SAQ and QoL, but it was limited by small sample size, lack of blinding and short-term follow-up [120, 121].

ARRHYTHMIAS

Ranolazine's effect as an antiarrhythmic agent has been more of an incidental finding. Most animal studies conducted for ranolazine pharmacology showed QTc prolongation, and hence monitoring for arrhythmia has been common for most ranolazine animal studies and clinical trials. Even though the rates of torsade de pointes were rare, ranolazine decreased the prevalence of both atrial and ventricular arrhythmia. The atrial effects are achieved at lower doses as compared to the ventricular antiarrhythmic effects. Ranolazine effect in atrial fibrillation is discussed separately in the atrial fibrillation section. Ranolazine does not have any effects on the resting membrane potential of either atrial or ventricular myocytes. Multiple animal studies have confirmed the ventricular antiarrhythmic effect of ranolazine in the setting of ischemic-reperfusion injury and heart failure [122]. In clinical translation, some of these benefits have been noticed in the setting of NSTEMI [60].

Studies trying to evaluate these benefits further in preventing VA, including VT and ventricular fibrillation (VF) in implantable cardioverter-defibrillator (ICD) patients, did not show benefits. In a small prospective observational study conducted in 2017, including 17 patients with ICD and worsening ventricular arrhythmia burden and 12 ICD patients with angina, ranolazine significantly decreased the median number of ventricular tachycardia episodes per patient, anti-tachycardia pacing and shock delivery, and fewer patients had episodes of non-sustained VT and VT. Specifically, none of the patients in the angina group developed VA while on ranolazine treatment [123]. However, larger RCT with ranolazine did not support this benefit. In summary, ranolazine does not improve time to ICD placement for primary or secondary prevention and does not decrease VT rates, ICD shocks, or deaths. There was a trend for improvement; however, it was statistically non-significant. In the prespecified secondary analysis, ranolazine significantly lowered the risk of ICD therapies for recurrent VT or VF requiring anti-tachycardic pacing or shock (hazard ratio: 0.70; 95% confidence interval: 0.51 to 0.96; p = 0.028) [124]. There was an almost 50% study drug discontinuation rate, reducing the study power to detect a significant positive treatment effect. On the other hand, the side effect profile of ranolazine could have been greater than what was documented in this study of high-risk patients [125]. Ranolazine decreases the PVC burden and may even alleviate PVC-induced cardiomyopathy [126]. Ranolazine may be considered as a second or third-line treatment for multiple drug-refractory VA in ICD patients without mortality benefit. Ranolazine also has some benefits related to VA prevention in long QT syndrome that is discussed separately in the next section.

LONG QT SYNDROMES (LQTS 3)

LQT3 is the third most common type of LQTS, and it differs significantly from its other variants LQTS1 and 2, in its clinical and electrophysiological characteristics. Arrhythmias, though less prevalent, are more lethal in LQTS3, occurring mostly at rest or sleep or with bradycardic events without any stressors. Consequently, BB or pacemakers are not beneficial in preventing bradycardia or arrhythmia in these patients. Flecainide is efficacious in LQTS3 though it could cause a Brugada-like pattern in the presence of D1790G mutation. This same mutation is found in spontaneous type 1 Brugada [127].

Pathophysiology

In a cellular model with induced LQTS-related arrhythmias by anemone toxin II, ranolazine neutralized the arrhythmias induced by INa to a similar extent in both endocardial and epicardial cells [128]. Further, the magnitude of INa is higher in patients with D1790G mutation LQTS3 [127]. Ranolazine attenuates increased monophasic action potential duration at 90% repolarization and reduces episodes of early after-depolarization and VT produced by anemone toxin II [129].

Efficacy

Ranolazine decreases QTc in LQTS3 caused by ΔKPQ and D1790G mutation [127, 130]. There is some indirect data available to suggest that ranolazine decreases QT interval in LQTS 3 with similar efficacy as flecainide and mexiletine. The QT shortening effect of ranolazine is sustained and significant except for substantial nocturnal bradycardia (<40 beats/min) and a heart rate of 60-70 beats/min [127]. Echocardiographically, patients have improved diastolic function [130]. Not many studies have been conducted for ranolazine in other types of LQTS. Ranolazine in LQTS 2 causes QT prolongation, T wave flatness with asymmetry, and decreases the maximum magnitude of the T vector. It also increases the early and late repolarization duration of the T wave loop by almost 30% without any changes in the QRS-T angle [131].

HEART FAILURE (HF)

The incidence and prevalence of HF are increasing because of the increase in life expectancy and improved therapeutic options for CAD patients. HF has a significant effect on morbidity and mortality. HF could be right or left-sided, with both sides being involved in rare cases. Left-sided HF could lead to pulmonary congestion with pulmonary hypertension. Left-sided HF is classified as heart failure with preserved ejection fraction (HFpEF) or heart failure with reduced ejection fraction (HFrEF). These subtypes of HF have unique pathophysiology, treatment, and prognosis. HFrEF is mostly caused by ischemic events. Most common etiologies for HF include CAD, smoking, hypertension, obesity, diabetes, and valvular heart disease. Less prevalent causes are myocarditis, idiopathic and infiltrative disease, peripartum state, HIV infection, connective tissue disease, substance use, and chemotherapeutic medications [132].

Pathophysiology

HF is associated with a progressive pathology wherein abnormal heart pumping leads to the activation of neurohormonal systems, neuroendocrine system, sympathetic nervous system, renin-angiotensin system, leading to LV remodeling, changes in excitation-contraction coupling, increased and persistent late sodium current with calcium overloading [132]. These changes involve multiple systems and regulatory proteins. Patients with LV heart failure may be asymptomatic or symptomatic. In the early phases of HF, if the compensatory homeostatic mechanism counteracts the abnormal heart function, patients remain asymptomatic. However, as the disease progresses, most patients become symptomatic in a subacute form (chronic heart failure) or in an acute form (acute exacerbation of HF). The precipitating events could be related to the stress caused to the heart, including ischemia, infection, fluid intake, salt intake, uncontrolled comorbidities, *etc.*

Heart Failure with Preserved Ejection Fraction (Diastolic)

In HFpEF, acute infusion of ranolazine decreases LVEDP, pulmonary capillary wedge pressure, mean pulmonary artery pressure, and cardiac output. There is no effect on relaxation parameters, including tau or rate of decline of left ventricular pressure per minute [dP/dtmin]. Ranolazine administration for 2 weeks does not affect echocardiographic or cardiopulmonary exercise test parameters and has no significant effect on N-terminal pro–B-type natriuretic peptide (NT-pro-BNP) levels [133]. Similarly, ranolazine with amiodarone was more efficacious in converting POAF in HFrEF than HFpEF [115]. Another study postulated that ranolazine improves diastolic function only in chronic ischemic myocardium segments supplied by stenotic vessels without the presence of necrosis or myocardial infarction [71]. Ranolazine seems to have a mild benefit in improving diastolic relaxation in chemotherapy-associated cardiomyopathy and hereditary long QT-syndrome, LQT3-ΔKPQ induced abnormal diastolic relaxation [118, 130].

Heart Failure With Reduced Ejection Fraction (Systolic)

Studies are lacking on the effect of ranolazine in HFrEF. Ranolazine mitigated right ventricular strain and exercise tolerance in patients with right ventricular ischemia and PAH [75, 124]. In patients with ischemic or non-ischemic cardiomyopathy with reduced EF and implantable cardioverter-defibrillator placement, ranolazine decreases recurrent events of VT or VF requiring ICD therapy without evidence for increased mortality [124].

Further studies are lacking on ranolazine's effect on ejection fraction and quality of life in heart failure patients. The effect on heart failure by ranolazine is through its glucometabolic mechanism. Thus, possibly long-term administration of ranolazine may be needed to achieve its benefits, especially in patients with abnormal glucose metabolism.

GLYCEMIC EFFECTS

Glycometabolic effects of medications are being increasingly noticed. Though diabetes and CAD are two distinct diseases, they share similar pathophysiology causing endothelial dysfunction, impaired vascular smooth muscle function, and hypercoagulability [134]. Hyperglycemia worsens myocardial perfusion by impairing coronary vasomotor function, causing greater platelet aggregation, inflammation, and oxidative stress [135]. The increasing prevalence of diabetes and its association with CAD and heart failure has led to FDA's recommendation to evaluate all diabetic drugs for their cardiovascular effects. Recently, sodium-glucose transport protein 2 inhibitors have shown a decrease in myocardial infarction, stroke, and cardiovascular mortality [136]. Despite the increased use of medications for diabetes and CAD to prevent secondary and tertiary complications, CAD is the most common cause of death in DM. Nearly 50% of adults with both DM and CAD have chronic angina, with the angina being more severe with poorer glucose control [137]. Diabetes is also associated with worse outcomes in stable and unstable angina [138]. This association has a vicious cycle with poorer glycemic control leading to CAD and ACS events, causing dysregulation of glucose metabolism. Unexpectedly, ranolazine was found to improve glycemic control in both diabetics and non-diabetics in clinical studies [137].

Mechanism of Action

The mechanism by which ranolazine improves glycemia remains incompletely understood. Preclinical studies have shown that mice with type 1 or type 2 diabetes exhibit increased persistent sodium current in their cardiac myocytes that may be mitigated by the INa inhibition of ranolazine [135]. Studies from isolated rat and human pancreatic islets suggest ranolazine may promote glucose-stimulated insulin secretion [139]. Other suggested mechanisms are inhibition of sodium channels in pancreatic alpha cells (analogous to the myocardial action), resulting in reduced glucagon release and a decrease in fatty acid oxygenation in the liver, thus shifting the liver's energy source from fatty acids to glucose [137]. Hyperglycemia increases phosphorylation of kinase CaMKII in the heart, which increases INa [135].

Effect on Glycated Hemoglobin A1c (HbA1c)

The earliest data on the glycemic effects of ranolazine is from a post-study subgroup analysis of MERLIN TIMI 36. In 4918 enrolled patients, ranolazine significantly reduced absolute HbA1c levels at 4 months compared with placebo (5.9% versus 6.2%; P<0.001). In diabetics treated with ranolazine, the mean absolute decrease in HbA1c is about -0.64, comparable to most antidiabetic oral medications, which decrease HbA1c by 0.5 on average [136]. In non-diabetics, it seemed that ranolazine prevented the incidence of new-onset HbA1c of ≥ 6%; however, the incidence of new-onset diabetes was similar to placebo at one year [140]. These findings have been substantiated in RCTs with similar benefits [134]. Additionally, ranolazine decreases fasting glucose, fasting glucagon, and postprandial glucagon levels [134]. Decreased fasting and postprandial glucagon levels are associated with improved hyperglycemia and HbA1c levels. The improved glycemic effects in diabetics with CAD also lead to decreased recurrent ischemia, angina episodes requiring sublingual nitroglycerine, improved quality of life, and treatment satisfaction [135]. However, the effect of ranolazine on SAQ angina frequency neutralizes at one year of treatment [137]. Embase and PubMed meta-analysis have observed the improvement in HbA1c with placebo-corrected change in A1C ranging from −0.28 to −0.7 [141, 142]. The weighted mean difference in HbA1c of −0.49%. Ranolazine is not associated with serious hypoglycemia [142]. The HbA1c lowering effect of ranolazine does not seem to be modulated by concurrent diabetic medications [139]. Most of the HbA1c lowering effect of ranolazine is seen at a dose of at least 1000 mg two times a day. At lower doses ranging from 500 to 1000 mg, the studies are equivocal, with most showing benefits. Ranolazine has similar efficacy as trimetazidine, another glycometabolic modulator [140]. Ranolazine does not have any effect on lipid profile and body weight [138].

Modifier effect of Metformin

Ranolazine has multiple mechanisms to decrease glucose, one being increasing the effect of metformin. Ranolazine increases metformin absorption and steady-state metformin concentrations and potentiates the effect of metformin [137]. Ranolazine decreases metformin excretion and thus contributes to its higher steady-state concentration. Metformin dose should not exceed >1700 mg when administered concomitantly with ranolazine at a dose of 1000 mg two times a day [143]. Hence, some of the ranolazine's effects on HbA1c could be modified by metformin. Consequently, in some studies, the metformin dose in the ranolazine arm was reduced to <1000 mg, with its confounding effect on HbA1c [137]. In the clinical trials, ranolazine had a higher HbA1c lowering effect than placebo in the presence of other oral hypoglycemic medications. Most RCTs had a similar proportion of patients on metformin [139]. Ranolazine, in combination with a sulfonylurea, has improved glycemic control as compared to glimepiride alone [144].

OTHER ADDITIONAL EFFECTS OF RANOLAZINE

Ranolazine has been evaluated in non-cardiovascular settings for claudication [145], myotonia congenita [146], and non-dystrophic myotonia [147]. It has also been studied as an anti-inflammatory [148] and anti-metastatic drug [149]. These effects have been studied in small pilot studies with sample sizes of around 15 in either animal models or human studies with statistically significant improved outcomes with ranolazine.

FUTURE IMPLICATIONS

2012 American College of Cardiology guidelines on stable ischemic heart disease (SIDH) recommended ranolazine as a substitute for beta-blockers for the relief of symptoms in patients with SIHD if initial treatment with beta-blockers leads to unacceptable side effects or is ineffective or if initial treatment with beta-blockers is contraindicated. Ranolazine could also be used in combination with beta-blockers for the relief of symptoms when initial treatment with beta-blockers is not successful in patients with SIHD [42]. Table **3** summarizes the cardiovascular effects of ranolazine.

Table 3. Summary of cardiovascular effects of ranolazine.

Disease	Evidence of Benefit	RCTs/Meta-analysis	Presence of Other Medications	Outcome Assessed
CSA Symptoms	(+++)	MARISA, MERLIN TIMI 36, Meta-analysis+ benefit	BB, CCB, and/or long-acting nitrates, ivabradine	ETT, SAQ9, Duke Activity Score Index and Women's Ischemia Symptom Questionnaire, recurrent ischemia, improved function of daily life.

(Table 3) cont.....

Disease	Evidence of Benefit	RCTs/Meta-analysis	Presence of Other Medications	Outcome Assessed
CSA heart function	(+) (-)	small sample sized RCTs, pre-post studies		DT, ICT, IRT, ET, MPI, LVEF, diastolic function, MPRI, RV end diastolic volume (EDV), right heart strain, mPAP, PCWP, PVR, 6-minute walk distance, NTproBNP, RVEF, LVEDV index, LV and RV systolic volume
CSA quality of life	(+) (-)	TERISA, MERLIN TIMI, meta-analysis + (mild or low benefit)		SAQ QoL, daily physical activity, health related QoL, SF-36, Rose dyspnea scores, SF-12
CSA Cost-effectiveness	(+) (-)	meta-analysis benefit +	BB, CCB, and/or long-acting nitrates	QALYs, ICER, Monte Carlo simulation, decision tree model, third-party payer perspective, direct and indirect cost, societal perspective, total cost, outpatient cost, inpatient cost, repeat ischemic event, repeat revascularization
ACS	(++) (-)	MERLIN TIMI 36 study, RCTs ++	SoC	Peri-procedural MI, MACE, CFR (by cardiac Rb-82 positron emission tomography), NSVT, SVT, ventricular pauses ≥ 3 seconds , new onset AF, AF burden, clopidogrel's inhibition of platelet reactivity, oxidative stress, global strain rate (by speckle-tracking echocardiography), worsening angina, requirement for anti-anginal treatment, decreased hospitalization, revascularization, electrocardiographic changes of ischemia, recurrent ischemia

(Table 3) cont.....

Disease	Evidence of Benefit	RCTs/Meta-analysis	Presence of Other Medications	Outcome Assessed
Chronic paroxysmal AF	(++)	RCTs, cohort/case series studies, Meta-analysis + benefit	Amiodarone, dronedarone	Cardioversion rates, recurrent AF after cardioversion, time to cardioversion, median time to conversion, cumulative conversion rate, QTc, refractoriness and fibrillation inducibility threshold, DF
Post-operative atrial fibrillation	(+)	Few studies	Amiodarone	reduced time to conversion
Chemotherapy induced cardiomyopathy	(+)	(-), Pre post studies	SoC	LVEF, diastolic dysfunction
Hypertrophic cardiomyopathy	(-)	(-)		exercise performance, plasma prohormone BNP levels, diastolic function, QoL PVC burden
Arrhythmia	(+)	(-)	SoC	QTc prolongation, AF, VT, VF, ICD therapies for recurrent VT or VF, anti-tachycardia pacing, shock delivery, episodes of NSVT and VT, PVC burden
Long QT syndrome type 3	(+)	(-)		QT interval, diastolic function, T wave flatness, maximum magnitude T vector
Heart failure	(+)	(-)		LVEDP, PCWP, mPAP, cardiac output, rate of decline of LV pressure per minute, NT-pro-BNP
Glycemic effects	(++)	RCTs, Meta-analysis+	SoC	HbA1c, fasting glucose, fasting glucagon, post prandial glucagon levels.

(Table 3) cont.....

Disease	Evidence of Benefit	RCTs/Meta-analysis	Presence of Other Medications	Outcome Assessed
Abbreviations: AF Atrial fibrillation, BB beta blocker, CCB calcium channel blocker, CFR Coronary flow reserve, DT Deceleration time, DF f-wave dominant frequency, ETT Exercise tolerance test, ET Ejection time, EDV end diastolic volume, HbA1c Glycated hemoglobin a1c, ICT Isovolumic contraction , IRT Isovolumic relaxation times, ICER Incremental cost-effectiveness ratio, ICD implantable cardioverter defibrillator, LVEF left ventricular ejection fraction, LVEDV Left ventricular end diastolic volume, LVEDP Left ventricular end diastolic pressure, MARISA Monotherapy Assessment of Ranolazine In Stable Angina trial, MERLIN TIMI Metabolic Efficiency with Ranolazine for Less Ischemia in Non-ST- Elevation ACS Thrombolysis in Myocardial Infarction 36, MPI Myocardial performance index, MPRI Myocardial perfusion reserve index, MI Myocardial infarction, MACE Major adverse cardiac event, mPAP Mean pulmonary artery pressure, NTproBNP N-terminal pro–B-type natriuretic peptide, NSVT Non sustained ventricular tachycardia, PCWP Pulmonary capillary wedge pressure, PVR Peripheral vascular resistance, PVC Premature ventricular complexes, QALYs Quality-adjusted life years, QoL Quality of life, RCT randomized control trials, RV right ventricle, RVEF Right ventricular ejection fraction, SAQ9 Seattle angina questionnaire, SF Medical Outcomes Short Form, SoC Standard of care, SVT Supra-ventricular tachycardia, TERISA Type 2 Diabetes Evaluation of Ranolazine in Subjects With Chronic Stable Angina trial, VF ventricular fibrillation, VT ventricular tachycardia, 6MWT minute walk test. (+) improvement, (-) no improvement.				

Gaps in Translational Research

Ranolazine with proven efficacy in animal studies for heart disease and arrhythmia had not shown similar efficacy and benefits in human studies. Some of these animal studies have been conducted *in vivo* with isolated cells or cell cultures. Human physiology differs from animal models and may contribute to inefficacy. A considerable amount of animal studies have been conducted with injectable or immediate-release formulations of ranolazine, with the outcome measured immediately. In comparison, most effects in humans are seen after an average of 2-6 weeks of treatment. Some of the effects of ranolazine may be immediate, but most of them seem to be gradual onset, especially the ones on the heart. Moreover, the most used formulation in clinical trials was oral sustained release ranolazine; hence there may be some differences in the effects of immediate or sustained release ranolazine.

Further, very few animal studies have been done with the administration of ranolazine prior to the experiment, and few have protocols for continuing ranolazine after the experiment. Most results of ranolazine were in the acute setting in animal studies. Studies on the effect of ranolazine in INa overtime prior to the experiment, along with acute administration during the experiment, are lacking. How this affects INa and the ratio of activated/inactivated INa steady state in the myocyte over time is not studied well [19]. The antiarrhythmic effect of ranolazine seems to be dependent on the baseline steady-state ratio of activated/inactivated INa. These ratios may be affected by pathological conditions, including ischemia, heart failure, and diabetes. Hence this factor, if not measured, maybe a major confounder for ranolazine studies under different pathology [19]. Studies for ranolazine's effect on heart failure were positive except in studies wherein ranolazine was not given to the animals for at least 2-4 weeks prior to the outcome assessment. Ranolazine being a glycometabolic modulator, needs chronic administration for improvement in heart failure.

Within the spectrum of CAD, multiple pathophysiologies play a key role in precipitating angina, including the slow progressive formation of atherosclerotic thrombus, acute formation of embolus, and unpredictable vasospastic phenomenon. This is further complicated by how the different heart muscles cope and function in the setting of stunning hibernation, chronic ischemia, acute ischemia, reperfusion, toxic metabolites, *etc.* To mimic a similar spectrum of CAD in animal models is difficult. Different methodologies are employed in animal models to mimic recurrent ischemia with reperfusion, cardiotoxic effects, and vasospasms. Hence, when translated to clinical trials, angina frequency is decreased by ranolazine in obstructive CAD but not in non-obstructive CAD with coronary microvascular dysfunction. MPRI studies may be conducted concurrently in animal models to see if it could be a marker that has a higher correlation with clinical trial outcomes. This approach may be cost-effective.

The underlying presence of diabetes also plays an important role in how much benefit could be derived from ranolazine in a particular trial. Most RCTs with proper randomization and a similar proportion of diabetics may seem to neutralize the confounding effect of diabetes. Also, the proportion of diabetics itself may be important (*e.g.,* 15% of diabetics vs. 30%). Mostly, it seems diabetics derive more benefit from ranolazine as compared to non-diabetics. Some studies may have to specify the inclusion or exclusion of diabetes or perform sub-analysis for diabetics separately. This confounding effect may be related to diabetes per se with its pathogenesis or may be related to the effect of hyperglycemia on cardiac cells or diabetic medications. For example, *in vitro*, sulfonylureas such as glibenclamide diminish the electrical activity of the heart muscle preparations, while chlorpropamide stimulates it, whereas glimepiride does not seem to affect it markedly [150]. *In vivo*, glibenclamide and glimepiride decrease, while gliclazide and tolbutamide increase, the amount of strophanthidin- and ischemia-induced ventricular ectopic beats and the duration of ventricular fibrillation. This effect of glimepiride was dependent on the metabolic state of the animal model. The different actions of sulfonylureas on the electrophysiological properties of the heart cannot be explained solely by their ATP-dependent potassium channel blocking potencies [150]. Fig. (**5**) elucidates the barriers in translational research, and Fig. (**6**) summarizes the therapeutic effects of ranolazine.

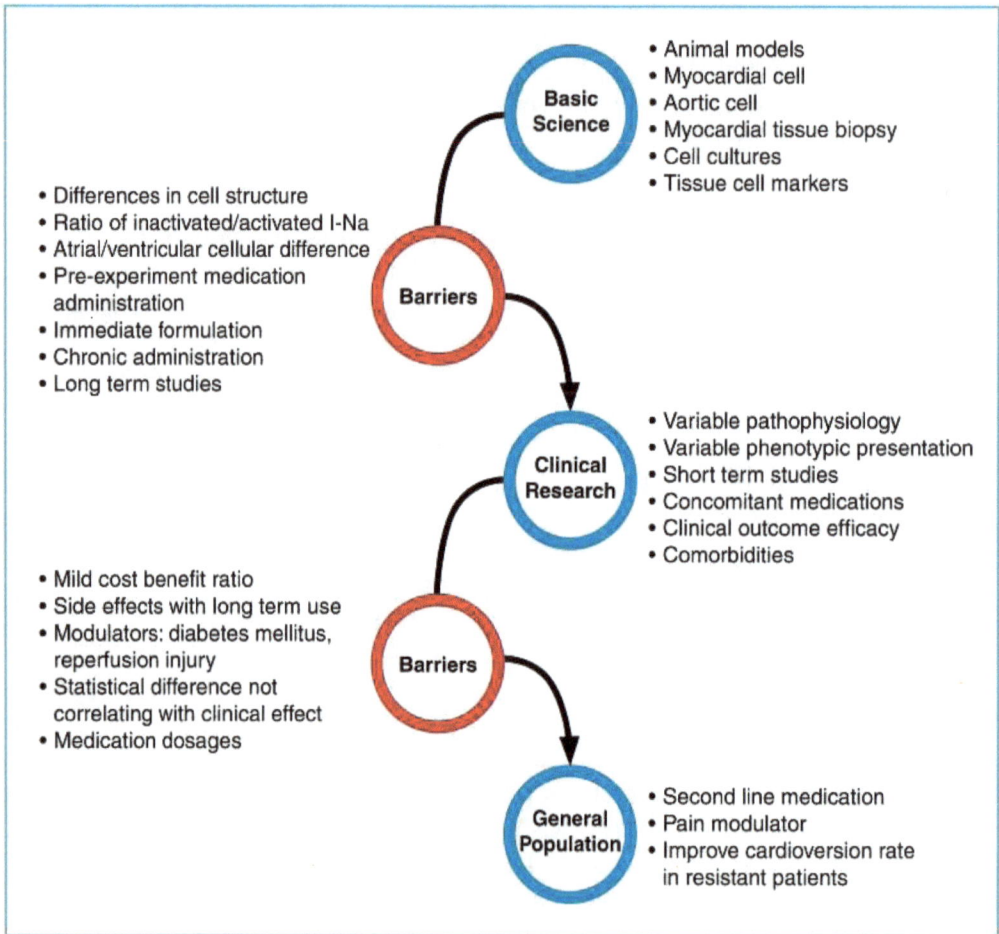

Fig. (5). Translational research-related barriers.

Quality of life and angina	Heart function	Antiarrhythmic	Ancillary effects
No or minimal effects on heart rate and blood pressure	Diastolic function in systolic and diastolic heart failure	Median atrial fibrillation burden post ACS	Glycometabolic deceases HbA1c
Non obstructive CAD with CFR<2	Regional diastolic function in ischemic segment	Peri-operative, open heart surgery related atrial fibrillation	Micro vascular dysfunction
Chronic stable angina	Diastolic function in diabetic non obstructive CAD	Decrease QT interval in LQT3 syndrome	Myotonia congenita
ACS in diabetics, women and elevated BNP	Diastolic function in women with non obstructive CAD	Decrease reoccurrence of AF after cardioversion, improve cardioversion rates	
	Right heart function in Group 1 Pulmonary arterial hypertension	Decrease PVC burden	
		Lower risk for ICD therapies for recurrent VT VF	

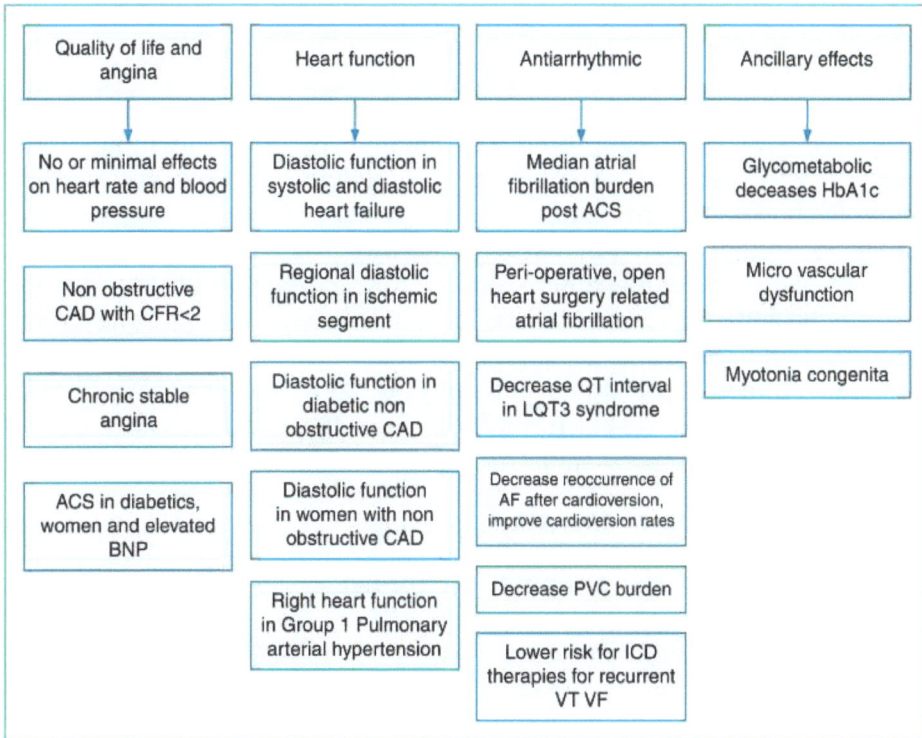

Fig. (6). Summary of ranolazine effects.

Possible Causes of Inefficacy in Studies

Ranolazine had consistently shown improvement in angina scores and ETT in multiple studies with no benefit in quality of life, MACE, or mortality. The role of depression in stable angina is an important factor to be considered. This confounding factor would be neutralized in RCTs, though it still may affect the quality of life studies. In the TERISA trial, the physical component of Medical Outcomes Short Form-36 (SF-36) improved significantly with ranolazine though the mental component remained the same. Patients with CAD are at higher risk for developing depression, and the presence of depression affects the outcomes of CAD. Hence, it may be important to control depression and anxiety in quality-of-life studies for ranolazine. Benefit is seen more with higher baseline angina, with the number needed to treat being 11 for a clinically significant benefit. On the other hand, though angina and ETT parameters improved, few studies have documented a decrease in ischemia on continuous monitoring. It could be postulated that ranolazine is a cardiac pain (angina) modulator with minimal physiological effect. Although being a pain modulator, this benefit may still lead to decreased recurrent hospitalization and resource utilization.

In preclinical and some clinical studies, ranolazine had shown an increase in QTc by 2-6 msec with the possibility of worsening arrhythmias, including torsade de pointes. When evaluated in the setting of angina, ranolazine is more anti-arrhythmic and Brady arrhythmic with rare ventricular tachyarrhythmias. Further research examining the effects of ranolazine on pacemaker activity and atrioventricular nodal conduction is needed to explain these effects of ranolazine. Ranolazine's anti-arrhythmic effect in ischemia-reperfusion injury and heart failure is shown in both animal and human studies. However, these effects are not substantiated under other similar pathophysiological settings [122, 124]. Hence, complete knowledge of the electrophysiological state of the myocardium in CAD, ACS, NOCAD, and HF is essential for further evaluation of ranolazine.

CONCLUSION AND SUMMARY

- Ranolazine is a versatile cardiovascular medicine with effects on angina, heart failure, arrhythmia, and cardiomyopathy.
- Most animal studies of ranolazine have been correlated with human trials.
- Ranolazine, with its current cost and side effects profile, could be a second line of medication for angina, heart failure, and arrhythmia patients who cannot tolerate or have side effects to first-line medications. This is in concordance with the 2012 guidelines for SIDH by the American College of Cardiology.
- Ranolazine's effect as a pain modulator in angina, myotonia, and claudication needs further studies.
- Ranolazine may improve cardioversion rates in cardioversion and treatment-resistant patients with paroxysmal atrial fibrillation. Ranolazine may also be considered as an option in patients with defibrillators with recurrent ventricular tachycardias on antiarrhythmics to prevent recurrent shocks.
- The presence of diabetes, hibernating myocardium from a chronic stenotic vessel, and reperfusion injury are major modulators of treatment outcomes of ranolazine, with better outcomes being seen in the presence of these pathologies. Hence, these factors should be taken into consideration for ranolazine studies.
- Ranolazine has similar efficacy as most oral hypoglycemics, and long-term studies are needed to evaluate outcomes in diabetics with chronic stable angina.

LIST OF ABBREVIATIONS

ATP	Adenosine triphosphate
ABCB1	ATP-binding cassette sub-family B member 1
ACE-I	Angiotensin-converting enzyme inhibitors
ARB	Angiotensin II receptor blockers

AF	Atrial fibrillation
ACS	Acute coronary syndrome
AP	Action potential
Bid	Two times a day
BB	Beta blockers
BNP	Beta natriuretic peptide
Ca^{2+}	Calcium
CYP	Cytochrome P450
CARISA	Combination Assessment of Ranolazine in Stable Angina
CCB	Calcium channel blockers
CAD	Coronary artery disease
CFR	Coronary flow reserve
CMR	Cardiac magnetic resonance
CSA	Chronic stable angina
CI	Confidence interval
CABG	Coronary artery bypass graft
DF	f-wave dominant frequency
DM	Diabetes Mellitus
DT	Deceleration time
DOX	Doxorubicin
ER	Extended release
ECG	Electrocardiogram
ERICA	Efficacy of Ranolazine in Chronic Angina
ET	Ejection time
ETT	Exercise tolerance test
FDA	Food and Drug Administration
H$^+$	Hydrogen
HbA1c	Glycated hemoglobin a1c
HR	Hazards ratio
HCM	Hypertrophic cardiomyopathy
HFpEF	Heart failure with preserved ejection fraction
HFrEF	Heart failure with reduced ejection fraction
HF	Heart failure
INA	Late sodium current
IR	Immediate release

ICD	Implantable cardioverter defibrillator
ICT	Isovolumic contraction
IRT	Isovolumic relaxation times
ICER	Incremental cost-effectiveness ratio
IHD	Ischemic heart disease
K$^+$	Potassium
LVEDP	Left ventricular end-diastolic pressure
LVEF	Left ventricular ejection fraction
LQTS3	Long QT syndrome type 3
MARISA	Monotherapy Assessment of Ranolazine In Stable Angina trial
MERLIN TIMI 36	Metabolic Efficiency with Ranolazine for Less Ischemia in Non-ST- Elevation ACS Thrombolysis in Myocardial Infarction 36
MI	Myocardial infarction
MPRI	Myocardial perfusion reserve index
MPI	Myocardial performance index
MACE	Major adverse cardiac event
mPAP	Mean pulmonary artery pressure
Na$^+$	Sodium
NOS	Nitrogen oxide synthase
NOTCH1	Notch homolog 1
NRG1	Neuregulin 1
NTG	Nitroglycerine
NOCAD	Non-obstructive CAD
NYHA	New York Heart Association
NSTEMI	Non-ST elevated myocardial infarction
NT-pro BNP	N-terminal pro–B-type natriuretic peptide
NSVT	Non sustained ventricular tachycardia
OR	Odds ratio
PH	Pulmonary hypertension
PCWP	Pulmonary capillary wedge pressure
PVR	Peripheral vascular resistance
PCI	Percutaneous coronary intervention
POAF	Post-operative atrial fibrillation
PVC	Premature ventricular complexes
QOL	Quality of life

QALY	Quality-adjusted life years
ROS	Reactive oxygen species
ROLE	Ranolazine Open-Label Experience
RVEF	Right ventricular ejection fraction
RCT	Randomized control trial
SAQ	Seattle angina questionnaire
SF	Medical Outcomes Short Form
SoC	Standard of care
SVT	Supraventricular tachycardia
SIHD	Stable ischemic heart disease
TERISA	Type 2 Diabetes Evaluation of Ranolazine in Subjects With Chronic Stable Angina
VA	Ventricular arrhythmia
VT	Ventricular tachycardia
VF	Ventricular fibrillation
6MWT	6-minute walk test

CONSENT FOR PUBLICATION

Not applicable.

CONFLICT OF INTEREST

The authors declare no conflict of interest, financial or otherwise.

ACKNOWLEDGEMENTS

The authors are thankful to the librarian Ms. Diane Gardner for her help in collecting the articles for the review and Mr. William Joy for providing graphical diagrams.

REFERENCES

[1]   Nash DT, Nash SD. Ranolazine for chronic stable angina. Lancet 2008; 372(9646): 1335-41.
       [http://dx.doi.org/10.1016/S0140-6736(08)61554-8] [PMID: 18929905]

[2]   Thadani U. Should ranolazine be used for all patients with ischemic heart disease or only for symptomatic patients with stable angina or for those with refractory angina pectoris? A critical appraisal. Expert Opin Pharmacother 2012; 13(17): 2555-63
       [http://dx.doi.org/10.1517/14656566.2012.740458] [PMID: 23121448]

[3]   Chaitman BR. Ranolazine for the treatment of chronic angina and potential use in other cardiovascular conditions. Circulation 2006; 113(20): 2462-72.
       [http://dx.doi.org/10.1161/CIRCULATIONAHA.105.597500] [PMID: 16717165]

[4]   Hall J. Cardiac muscle; the heart as a pump and function of the heart valves. Guyton and Hall Textbook of Medical Physiology 2011; p. 12.

[5]   Klabunde RE. Cardiac electrophysiology: normal and ischemic ionic currents and the ECG. Adv Physiol Educ 2017; 41(1): 29-37.
[http://dx.doi.org/10.1152/advan.00105.2016] [PMID: 28143820]

[6]   Anderson JR, Nawarskas JJ. Ranolazine. A metabolic modulator for the treatment of chronic stable angina. Cardiol Rev 2005; 13(4): 202-10.
[http://dx.doi.org/10.1097/01.crd.0000161979.62749.e7] [PMID: 15949056]

[7]   Saad M, Mahmoud A, Elgendy IY, Richard Conti C. Ranolazine in cardiac arrhythmia. Clin Cardiol 2016; 39(3): 170-8.
[http://dx.doi.org/10.1002/clc.22476] [PMID: 26459200]

[8]   Jerling M. Clinical pharmacokinetics of ranolazine. Clin Pharmacokinet 2006; 45(5): 469-91.
[http://dx.doi.org/10.2165/00003088-200645050-00003] [PMID: 16640453]

[9]   Cheng JW. Ranolazine for the management of coronary artery disease. Clin Ther 2006; 28(12): 1996-2007.
[http://dx.doi.org/10.1016/j.clinthera.2006.12.009] [PMID: 17296457]

[10]   Scoville BA, Segal JH, Salama NN, *et al.* Single dose oral ranolazine pharmacokinetics in patients receiving maintenance hemodialysis. Ren Fail 2019; 41(1): 118-25.
[http://dx.doi.org/10.1080/0886022X.2019.1585371] [PMID: 30909832]

[11]   Koren MJ, Crager MR, Sweeney M. Long-term safety of a novel antianginal agent in patients with severe chronic stable angina: the Ranolazine Open Label Experience (ROLE). J Am Coll Cardiol 2007; 49(10): 1027-34.
[http://dx.doi.org/10.1016/j.jacc.2006.10.067] [PMID: 17349881]

[12]   Ellermann C, Wolfes J, Puckhaber D, *et al.* Digitalis promotes ventricular arrhythmias in flecainide- and ranolazine-pretreated hearts. Cardiovasc Toxicol 2019; 19(3): 237-43.
[http://dx.doi.org/10.1007/s12012-018-9494-7] [PMID: 30515668]

[13]   Marciniak TA, Serebruany V. Ranolazine, ACE Inhibitors, and Angiotensin Receptor Blockers. Am J Med 2019; 132(12): e844-5.
[http://dx.doi.org/10.1016/j.amjmed.2019.02.032] [PMID: 30871921]

[14]   Chaitman BR, Pepine CJ, Parker JO, *et al.* Effects of ranolazine with atenolol, amlodipine, or diltiazem on exercise tolerance and angina frequency in patients with severe chronic angina: a randomized controlled trial. JAMA 2004; 291(3): 309-16.
[http://dx.doi.org/10.1001/jama.291.3.309] [PMID: 14734593]

[15]   Aldakkak M, Camara AK, Heisner JS, Yang M, Stowe DF. Ranolazine reduces Ca^{2+} overload and oxidative stress and improves mitochondrial integrity to protect against ischemia reperfusion injury in isolated hearts. Pharmacol Res 2011; 64(4): 381-92.
[http://dx.doi.org/10.1016/j.phrs.2011.06.018] [PMID: 21741479]

[16]   Efentakis P, Andreadou I, Bibli S-I, *et al.* Ranolazine triggers pharmacological preconditioning and postconditioning in anesthetized rabbits through activation of RISK pathway. Eur J Pharmacol 2016; 789: 431-8.
[http://dx.doi.org/10.1016/j.ejphar.2016.08.001] [PMID: 27492365]

[17]   Malavaki C, Hatziefthimiou A, Daskalopoulou SS, Stefanidis I, Karatzaferi C, Aidonidis I. Ranolazine enhances nicardipine-induced relaxation of alpha1-adrenoceptor-mediated contraction on isolated rabbit aorta. Acta Cardiol 2015; 70(2): 157-62.
[http://dx.doi.org/10.1080/AC.70.2.3073506] [PMID: 26148375]

[18]   Paredes-Carbajal MC, Monsalvo I, Hernández-Díaz C, Regla I, Demare P, Mascher D. Effects of ranolazine on vasomotor responses of rat aortic rings. Arch Med Res 2013; 44(1): 8-12.
[http://dx.doi.org/10.1016/j.arcmed.2012.11.002] [PMID: 23149158]

[19]   Caves RE, Cheng H, Choisy SC, *et al.* Atrial-ventricular differences in rabbit cardiac voltage-gated Na^+ currents: Basis for atrial-selective block by ranolazine. Heart Rhythm 2017; 14(11): 1657-64.

[http://dx.doi.org/10.1016/j.hrthm.2017.06.012] [PMID: 28610990]

[20] Moschovidis V, Simopoulos V, Stravela S, *et al.* Dose-Dependent Effects of Ranolazine on Reentrant Ventricular Arrhythmias Induced After Subacute Myocardial Infarction in Rabbits. J Cardiovasc Pharmacol Ther 2020; 25(1): 65-71.
[http://dx.doi.org/10.1177/1074248419858113] [PMID: 31242756]

[21] Ramirez RJ, Takemoto Y, Martins RP, *et al.* Mechanisms by which ranolazine terminates paroxysmal but not persistent atrial fibrillation. Circ Arrhythm Electrophysiol 2019; 12(10): e005557.
[http://dx.doi.org/10.1161/CIRCEP.117.005557] [PMID: 31594392]

[22] Goldstein RE, Klein MG, Ouimet SP, *et al.* Hemodynamic effects of late sodium current inhibitors in a swine model of heart failure. J Card Fail 2019; 25(10): 828-36.
[http://dx.doi.org/10.1016/j.cardfail.2019.08.015] [PMID: 31461671]

[23] Wang GT, Li H, Yu ZQ, He XN. Effects of ranolazine on cardiac function in rats with heart failure. Eur Rev Med Pharmacol Sci 2019; 23(21): 9625-32.
[PMID: 31773713]

[24] Nie J, Duan Q, He M, *et al.* Ranolazine prevents pressure overload-induced cardiac hypertrophy and heart failure by restoring aberrant Na^+ and Ca^{2+} handling. J Cell Physiol 2019; 234(7): 11587-601.
[http://dx.doi.org/10.1002/jcp.27791] [PMID: 30488495]

[25] Corradi F, Paolini L, De Caterina R. Ranolazine in the prevention of anthracycline cardiotoxicity. Pharmacol Res 2014; 79: 88-102.
[http://dx.doi.org/10.1016/j.phrs.2013.11.001] [PMID: 24269342]

[26] Minotti G, Menna P, Salvatorelli E, Cairo G, Gianni L. Anthracyclines: molecular advances and pharmacologic developments in antitumor activity and cardiotoxicity. Pharmacol Rev 2004; 56(2): 185-229.
[http://dx.doi.org/10.1124/pr.56.2.6] [PMID: 15169927]

[27] Cappetta D, Esposito G, Coppini R, *et al.* Effects of ranolazine in a model of doxorubicin-induced left ventricle diastolic dysfunction. Br J Pharmacol 2017; 174(21): 3696-712.
[http://dx.doi.org/10.1111/bph.13791] [PMID: 28320043]

[28] Tawfik MK, Ameen AM. Cardioprotective effect of ranolazine in nondiabetic and diabetic male rats subjected to isoprenaline-induced acute myocardial infarction involves modulation of AMPK and inhibition of apoptosis. Can J Physiol Pharmacol 2019; 97(7): 661-74.
[http://dx.doi.org/10.1139/cjpp-2018-0571] [PMID: 31157553]

[29] Cassano V, Leo A, Tallarico M, *et al.* Metabolic and cognitive effects of ranolazine in Type 2 Diabetes Mellitus: Data from an in vivo Model. Nutrients 2020; 12(2): 382.
[http://dx.doi.org/10.3390/nu12020382] [PMID: 32023991]

[30] Fu Z, Zhao L, Chai W, Dong Z, Cao W, Liu Z. Ranolazine recruits muscle microvasculature and enhances insulin action in rats. J Physiol 2013; 591(20): 5235-49.
[http://dx.doi.org/10.1113/jphysiol.2013.257246] [PMID: 23798495]

[31] Chen X, Ren L, Liu X, *et al.* Ranolazine protects against diabetic cardiomyopathy by activating the NOTCH1/NRG1 pathway. Life Sci 2020; 261: 118306.
[http://dx.doi.org/10.1016/j.lfs.2020.118306] [PMID: 32828943]

[32] Calderón-Sánchez EM, Domínguez-Rodríguez A, López-Haldón J, *et al.* Cardioprotective effect of ranolazine in the process of ischemia-reperfusion in adult rat cardiomyocytes. Rev Esp Cardiol (Engl Ed) 2016; 69(1): 45-53.
[http://dx.doi.org/10.1016/j.rec.2015.02.027] [PMID: 26183665]

[33] Ma J, Song Y, Shryock JC, *et al.* Ranolazine attenuates hypoxia- and hydrogen peroxide-induced increases in sodium channel late openings in ventricular myocytes. J Cardiovasc Pharmacol 2014; 64(1): 60-8.
[http://dx.doi.org/10.1097/FJC.0000000000000090] [PMID: 24705174]

[34]   Ogawa T, Honjo H, Yamazaki M, *et al.* Ranolazine facilitates termination of ventricular tachyarrhythmia associated with acute myocardial ischemia through suppression of late INa-mediated focal activity. Circ J 2017; 81(10): 1411-28.
[http://dx.doi.org/10.1253/circj.CJ-17-0128] [PMID: 28552884]

[35]   Fumagalli F, Russo I, Staszewsky L, *et al.* Ranolazine ameliorates postresuscitation electrical instability and myocardial dysfunction and improves survival with good neurologic recovery in a rat model of cardiac arrest. Heart Rhythm 2014; 11(9): 1641-7.
[http://dx.doi.org/10.1016/j.hrthm.2014.05.023] [PMID: 24858811]

[36]   Bhimani AA, Yasuda T, Sadrpour SA, *et al.* Ranolazine terminates atrial flutter and fibrillation in a canine model. Heart Rhythm 2014; 11(9): 1592-9.
[http://dx.doi.org/10.1016/j.hrthm.2014.05.038] [PMID: 25066042]

[37]   Hartmann N, Mason FE, Braun I, *et al.* The combined effects of ranolazine and dronedarone on human atrial and ventricular electrophysiology. J Mol Cell Cardiol 2016; 94: 95-106.
[http://dx.doi.org/10.1016/j.yjmcc.2016.03.012] [PMID: 27056421]

[38]   Frommeyer G, Ellermann C, Dechering DG, *et al.* Ranolazine and vernakalant prevent ventricular arrhythmias in an experimental whole-heart model of short QT syndrome. J Cardiovasc Electrophysiol 2016; 27(10): 1214-9.
[http://dx.doi.org/10.1111/jce.13029] [PMID: 27283775]

[39]   Ellermann C, Kohnke A, Dechering DG, *et al.* Ranolazine prevents levosimendan-induced atrial fibrillation. Pharmacology 2018; 102(3-4): 138-41.
[http://dx.doi.org/10.1159/000490572] [PMID: 29982246]

[40]   Teng S, Ren Z, Zhao K. Vagal stimulation facilitates improving effects of ranolazine on cardiac function in rats with chronic ischemic heart failure. Curr Mol Med 2018; 18(1): 36-43.
[http://dx.doi.org/10.2174/1566524018666180608085330] [PMID: 29879885]

[41]   Fukaya H, Plummer BN, Piktel JS, *et al.* Arrhythmogenic cardiac alternans in heart failure is suppressed by late sodium current blockade by ranolazine. Heart Rhythm 2019; 16(2): 281-9.
[http://dx.doi.org/10.1016/j.hrthm.2018.08.033] [PMID: 30193854]

[42]   Fihn SD, Gardin JM, Abrams J, *et al.* 2012 ACCF/AHA/ACP/AATS/PCNA/SCAI/STS guideline for the diagnosis and management of patients with stable ischemic heart disease: executive summary: a report of the American College of Cardiology Foundation/American Heart Association task force on practice guidelines, and the American College of Physicians, American Association for Thoracic Surgery, Preventive Cardiovascular Nurses Association, Society for Cardiovascular Angiography and Interventions, and Society of Thoracic Surgeons. Circulation 2012; 126(25): 3097-137.
[http://dx.doi.org/10.1161/CIR.0b013e3182776f83] [PMID: 23166210]

[43]   Al-Khatib SM, Stevenson WG, Ackerman MJ, *et al.* 2017 AHA/ACC/HRS guideline for management of patients with ventricular arrhythmias and the prevention of sudden cardiac death: a report of the American College of Cardiology/American Heart Association Task Force on Clinical Practice Guidelines and the Heart Rhythm Society. J Am Coll Cardiol 2018; 72(14): e91-e220.
[http://dx.doi.org/10.1016/j.jacc.2017.10.054] [PMID: 29097296]

[44]   Bunch TJ, Mahapatra S, Murdock D, *et al.* Ranolazine reduces ventricular tachycardia burden and ICD shocks in patients with drug-refractory ICD shocks. Pacing Clin Electrophysiol 2011; 34(12): 1600-6.
[http://dx.doi.org/10.1111/j.1540-8159.2011.03208.x] [PMID: 21895727]

[45]   Scirica BM, Morrow DA, Hod H, Murphy SA, Belardinelli L, Hedgepeth CM, *et al.* CLINICAL PERSPECTIVE. Circulation 2007; 116(15): 1647-52.
[http://dx.doi.org/10.1161/CIRCULATIONAHA.107.724880] [PMID: 17804441]

[46]   Babalis D, Tritakis V, Floros G, *et al.* Effects of ranolazine on left ventricular diastolic and systolic function in patients with chronic coronary disease and stable angina. Hellenic J Cardiol 2015; 56(3): 237-41.
[PMID: 26021246]

[47]   Shah NR, Cheezum MK, Veeranna V, *et al*. Ranolazine in symptomatic diabetic patients without obstructive coronary artery disease: impact on microvascular and diastolic function. J Am Heart Assoc 2017; 6(5): e005027.
[http://dx.doi.org/10.1161/JAHA.116.005027] [PMID: 28473401]

[48]   Venkataraman R, Chen J, Garcia EV, *et al*. Effect of ranolazine on left ventricular dyssynchrony in patients with coronary artery disease. Am J Cardiol 2012; 110(10): 1440-5.
[http://dx.doi.org/10.1016/j.amjcard.2012.06.055] [PMID: 22884560]

[49]   Lamendola P, Nerla R, Pitocco D, *et al*. Effect of ranolazine on arterial endothelial function in patients with type 2 diabetes mellitus. Atherosclerosis 2013; 226(1): 157-60.
[http://dx.doi.org/10.1016/j.atherosclerosis.2012.10.051] [PMID: 23146293]

[50]   Deshmukh SH, Patel SR, Pinassi E, *et al*. Ranolazine improves endothelial function in patients with stable coronary artery disease. Coron Artery Dis 2009; 20(5): 343-7.
[http://dx.doi.org/10.1097/MCA.0b013e32832a198b] [PMID: 19444092]

[51]   Venkataraman R, Belardinelli L, Blackburn B, Heo J, Iskandrian AE. A study of the effects of ranolazine using automated quantitative analysis of serial myocardial perfusion images. JACC Cardiovasc Imaging 2009; 2(11): 1301-9.
[http://dx.doi.org/10.1016/j.jcmg.2009.09.006] [PMID: 19909934]

[52]   Mezincescu A, Karthikeyan VJ, Nadar SK. Ranolazine: A true pluripotent cardiovascular drug or jack of all trades, master of none? Sultan Qaboos Univ Med J 2018; 18(1): e13-23.
[http://dx.doi.org/10.18295/squmj.2018.18.01.003] [PMID: 29666676]

[53]   Rayner-Hartley E, Sedlak T. Ranolazine: a contemporary review. J Am Heart Assoc 2016; 5(3): e003196.
[http://dx.doi.org/10.1161/JAHA.116.003196] [PMID: 26979079]

[54]   Chaitman BR, Skettino SL, Parker JO, *et al*. Anti-ischemic effects and long-term survival during ranolazine monotherapy in patients with chronic severe angina. J Am Coll Cardiol 2004; 43(8): 1375-82.
[http://dx.doi.org/10.1016/j.jacc.2003.11.045] [PMID: 15093870]

[55]   Stone PH, Chaitman BR, Stocke K, Sano J, DeVault A, Koch GG. The anti-ischemic mechanism of action of ranolazine in stable ischemic heart disease. J Am Coll Cardiol 2010; 56(12): 934-42.
[http://dx.doi.org/10.1016/j.jacc.2010.04.042] [PMID: 20828645]

[56]   Villano A, Di Franco A, Nerla R, *et al*. Effects of ivabradine and ranolazine in patients with microvascular angina pectoris. Am J Cardiol 2013; 112(1): 8-13.
[http://dx.doi.org/10.1016/j.amjcard.2013.02.045] [PMID: 23558043]

[57]   Mehta PK, Sharma S, Minissian M, *et al*. Ranolazine reduces angina in women with ischemic heart disease: results of an open-label, multicenter trial. J Womens Health (Larchmt) 2019; 28(5): 573-82.
[http://dx.doi.org/10.1089/jwh.2018.7019] [PMID: 30888919]

[58]   Arnold SV, Morrow DA, Wang K, *et al*. Effects of ranolazine on disease-specific health status and quality of life among patients with acute coronary syndromes: results from the MERLIN-TIMI 36 randomized trial. Circ Cardiovasc Qual Outcomes 2008; 1(2): 107-15.
[http://dx.doi.org/10.1161/CIRCOUTCOMES.108.798009] [PMID: 20031797]

[59]   Banon D, Filion KB, Budlovsky T, Franck C, Eisenberg MJ. The usefulness of ranolazine for the treatment of refractory chronic stable angina pectoris as determined from a systematic review of randomized controlled trials. Am J Cardiol 2014; 113(6): 1075-82.
[http://dx.doi.org/10.1016/j.amjcard.2013.11.070] [PMID: 24462341]

[60]   Wilson SR, Scirica BM, Braunwald E, *et al*. Efficacy of ranolazine in patients with chronic angina observations from the randomized, double-blind, placebo-controlled MERLIN-TIMI (Metabolic Efficiency With Ranolazine for Less Ischemia in Non-ST-Segment Elevation Acute Coronary Syndromes) 36 Trial. J Am Coll Cardiol 2009; 53(17): 1510-6.

[http://dx.doi.org/10.1016/j.jacc.2009.01.037] [PMID: 19389561]

[61]   Rayner-Hartley E, Parvand M, Humphries KH, Starovoytov A, Park JE, Sedlak T. Ranolazine for symptomatic management of microvascular angina. Am J Ther 2020; 27(2): e151-8.
[http://dx.doi.org/10.1097/MJT.0000000000000779] [PMID: 29746286]

[62]   Cavallino C, Facchini M, Veia A, Bacchni S, Rognoni A, Rametta F, *et al.* New anti-anginal drugs: ranolazine 2015.
[http://dx.doi.org/10.2174/1871525713666141219112841]

[63]   Rambarat CA, Elgendy IY, Handberg EM, *et al.* Late sodium channel blockade improves angina and myocardial perfusion in patients with severe coronary microvascular dysfunction: Women's Ischemia Syndrome Evaluation-Coronary Vascular Dysfunction ancillary study. Int J Cardiol 2019; 276: 8-13.
[http://dx.doi.org/10.1016/j.ijcard.2018.09.081] [PMID: 30293664]

[64]   Zhu H, Xu X, Fang X, Zheng J, Zhao Q, Chen T, *et al.* Effects of the antianginal drugs ranolazine, nicorandil, and ivabradine on coronary microvascular function in patients with nonobstructive coronary artery disease: a meta-analysis of randomized controlled trials 2019.
[http://dx.doi.org/10.1016/j.clinthera.2019.08.008] [PMID: 31548105]

[65]   Alexopoulos D, Kochiadakis G, Afthonidis D, *et al.* Ranolazine reduces angina frequency and severity and improves quality of life: Observational study in patients with chronic angina under ranolazine treatment in Greece (OSCAR-GR). Int J Cardiol 2016; 205: 111-6.
[http://dx.doi.org/10.1016/j.ijcard.2015.10.180] [PMID: 26730841]

[66]   Greene RS, Rangel RM, Edwards KL, Chastain LM, Brouse SD, Alvarez CA, *et al.* Ranolazine for the treatment of refractory angina in a veterans population 2012.
[http://dx.doi.org/10.1016/j.carrev.2011.06.001] [PMID: 21856249]

[67]   Rousseau MF, Pouleur H, Cocco G, Wolff AA. Comparative efficacy of ranolazine versus atenolol for chronic angina pectoris. Am J Cardiol 2005; 95(3): 311-6.
[http://dx.doi.org/10.1016/j.amjcard.2004.09.025] [PMID: 15670536]

[68]   Alexander KP, Weisz G, Prather K, *et al.* Effects of ranolazine on angina and quality of life after percutaneous coronary intervention with incomplete revascularization: results from the ranolazine for incomplete vessel revascularization (RIVER-PCI) trial. Circulation 2016; 133(1): 39-47.
[http://dx.doi.org/10.1161/CIRCULATIONAHA.115.019768] [PMID: 26555329]

[69]   Figueredo VM, Pressman GS, Romero-Corral A, Murdock E, Holderbach P, Morris DL. Improvement in left ventricular systolic and diastolic performance during ranolazine treatment in patients with stable angina. J Cardiovasc Pharmacol Ther 2011; 16(2): 168-72.
[http://dx.doi.org/10.1177/1074248410382105] [PMID: 20924097]

[70]   Murray GL, Colombo J. Ranolazine preserves and improves left ventricular ejection fraction and autonomic measures when added to guideline-driven therapy in chronic heart failure 2014.
[http://dx.doi.org/10.5301/heartint.5000219] [PMID: 27004101]

[71]   Hayashida W, van Eyll C, Rousseau MF, Pouleur H. Effects of ranolazine on left ventricular regional diastolic function in patients with ischemic heart disease. Cardiovasc Drugs Ther 1994; 8(5): 741-7.
[http://dx.doi.org/10.1007/BF00877121] [PMID: 7873471]

[72]   Singh A, Steadman CD, Khan JN, Reggiardo G, McCann GP. Effect of late sodium current inhibition on MRI measured diastolic dysfunction in aortic stenosis: a pilot study. BMC Res Notes 2016; 9(1): 64.
[http://dx.doi.org/10.1186/s13104-016-1874-0] [PMID: 26847571]

[73]   Mehta PK, Goykhman P, Thomson LE, *et al.* Ranolazine improves angina in women with evidence of myocardial ischemia but no obstructive coronary artery disease. JACC Cardiovasc Imaging 2011; 4(5): 514-22.
[http://dx.doi.org/10.1016/j.jcmg.2011.03.007] [PMID: 21565740]

[74]   Bairey Merz CN, Handberg EM, Shufelt CL, *et al.* A randomized, placebo-controlled trial of late Na

current inhibition (ranolazine) in coronary microvascular dysfunction (CMD): impact on angina and myocardial perfusion reserve. Eur Heart J 2016; 37(19): 1504-13.
[http://dx.doi.org/10.1093/eurheartj/ehv647] [PMID: 26614823]

[75] Khan SS, Cuttica MJ, Beussink-Nelson L, *et al.* Effects of ranolazine on exercise capacity, right ventricular indices, and hemodynamic characteristics in pulmonary arterial hypertension: a pilot study. Pulm Circ 2015; 5(3): 547-56.
[http://dx.doi.org/10.1086/682427] [PMID: 26401256]

[76] Gomberg-Maitland M, Schilz R, Mediratta A, *et al.* Phase I safety study of ranolazine in pulmonary arterial hypertension. Pulm Circ 2015; 5(4): 691-700.
[http://dx.doi.org/10.1086/683813] [PMID: 26697176]

[77] Finch KT, Stratton EA, Farber HW. Ranolazine for the treatment of pulmonary hypertension associated with heart failure with preserved ejection fraction: A pilot study. J Heart Lung Transplant 2016; 35(11): 1370-3.
[http://dx.doi.org/10.1016/j.healun.2016.07.015] [PMID: 27623099]

[78] Han Y, Forfia P, Vaidya A, *et al.* Ranolazine improves right ventricular function in patients with precapillary pulmonary hypertension: results from a double-blind, randomized, placebo-controlled trial. J Card Fail 2021; 27(2): 253-7.
[http://dx.doi.org/10.1016/j.cardfail.2020.10.006] [PMID: 33223140]

[79] Willis LH, Slentz CA, Johnson JL, *et al.* Effects of exercise training with and without ranolazine on peak oxygen consumption, daily physical activity, and quality of life in patients with chronic stable angina pectoris. Am J Cardiol 2019; 124(5): 655-60.
[http://dx.doi.org/10.1016/j.amjcard.2019.05.063] [PMID: 31296368]

[80] Arnold SV, Kosiborod M, McGuire DK, *et al.* Effects of ranolazine on quality of life among patients with diabetes mellitus and stable angina. JAMA Intern Med 2014; 174(8): 1403-5.
[http://dx.doi.org/10.1001/jamainternmed.2014.2120] [PMID: 24887304]

[81] Fanaroff AC, Prather K, Brucker A, *et al.* Relationship between optimism and outcomes in patients with chronic angina pectoris. Am J Cardiol 2019; 123(9): 1399-405.
[http://dx.doi.org/10.1016/j.amjcard.2019.01.036] [PMID: 30771861]

[82] Ranolazine for ischemic heart disease. Available from: https://www.epistemonikos.org/en/matrixes/5a902f6b7db23a68c27e9da9

[83] Salazar CA, Basilio Flores JE, Veramendi Espinoza LE, Mejia Dolores JW, Rey Rodriguez DE, Loza Munarriz C. Ranolazine for stable angina pectoris. Cochrane Database Syst Rev 2017; 2(2): CD011747.
[http://dx.doi.org/10.1002/14651858.CD011747.pub2] [PMID: 28178363]

[84] Kohn CG, Parker MW, Limone BL, Coleman CI. Cost-effectiveness of ranolazine added to standard-of-care treatment in patients with chronic stable angina pectoris. Am J Cardiol 2014; 113(8): 1306-11.
[http://dx.doi.org/10.1016/j.amjcard.2014.01.407] [PMID: 24560062]

[85] Kourlaba G, Vlachopoulos C, Parissis J, Kanakakis J, Gourzoulidis G, Maniadakis N. Ranolazine for the symptomatic treatment of patients with chronic angina pectoris in Greece: a cost-utility study. BMC Health Serv Res 2015; 15(1): 566.
[http://dx.doi.org/10.1186/s12913-015-1228-y] [PMID: 26684327]

[86] Coleman CI, Freemantle N, Kohn CG. Ranolazine for the treatment of chronic stable angina: a cost-effectiveness analysis from the UK perspective. BMJ Open 2015; 5(11): e008861.
[http://dx.doi.org/10.1136/bmjopen-2015-008861] [PMID: 26546142]

[87] Vellopoulou K, Kourlaba G, Maniadakis N, Vardas P. A literature review to evaluate the economic value of ranolazine for the symptomatic treatment of chronic angina pectoris. Int J Cardiol 2016; 211: 105-11.
[http://dx.doi.org/10.1016/j.ijcard.2016.02.140] [PMID: 26994453]

[88]   Nguyen E, Coleman CI, Kohn CG, Weeda ER. Ranolazine in patients with type 2 diabetes and chronic angina: A cost-effectiveness analysis and assessment of health-related quality-of-life. Int J Cardiol 2018; 273: 34-8.
[http://dx.doi.org/10.1016/j.ijcard.2018.09.060] [PMID: 30266352]

[89]   Hidalgo-Vega A, Ramos-Goñi JM, Villoro R. Cost-utility of ranolazine for the symptomatic treatment of patients with chronic angina pectoris in Spain. Eur J Health Econ 2014; 15(9): 917-25.
[http://dx.doi.org/10.1007/s10198-013-0534-8] [PMID: 24122303]

[90]   Storey KM, Wang J, Garberich RF, *et al.* Long-term (3 years) outcomes of ranolazine therapy for refractory angina pectoris (from the Ranolazine Refractory Registry). Am J Cardiol 2020; 129: 1-4.
[http://dx.doi.org/10.1016/j.amjcard.2020.05.020] [PMID: 32540170]

[91]   Meyer N, Tran O, Hartsfield C, Nguyen L, Kazi DS, Koch B. Revascularization rates and associated costs in patients with stable ischemic heart disease initiating ranolazine versus traditional antianginals as add-on therapy. Am J Cardiol 2019; 123(10): 1602-9.
[http://dx.doi.org/10.1016/j.amjcard.2019.02.014] [PMID: 30832963]

[92]   Kohn CG, Parker MW, Limone BL, Coleman CI. Impact of angina frequency on health utility values of patients with chronic stable angina. Health Qual Life Outcomes 2014; 12(1): 39.
[http://dx.doi.org/10.1186/1477-7525-12-39] [PMID: 24628859]

[93]   Bress AP, Dodson JA, King JB, *et al.* Clinical and economic outcomes of ranolazine versus conventional antianginals users among veterans with chronic stable angina pectoris. Am J Cardiol 2018; 122(11): 1809-16.
[http://dx.doi.org/10.1016/j.amjcard.2018.08.027] [PMID: 30292334]

[94]   Gutierrez JA, Karwatowska-Prokopczuk E, Murphy SA, *et al.* Effects of ranolazine in patients with chronic angina in patients with and without percutaneous coronary intervention for acute coronary syndrome: observations from the MERLIN-TIMI 36 trial. Clin Cardiol 2015; 38(8): 469-75.
[http://dx.doi.org/10.1002/clc.22425] [PMID: 26059896]

[95]   Schwemer TF, Deutscher N, Diermann N, *et al.* Effect of ranolazine on plasma arginine derivatives and urinary isoprostane 8-iso-PGF 2α in patients with myocardial infarction in the randomized RIMINI-Trial. Sci Rep 2019; 9(1): 1-6.
[http://dx.doi.org/10.1038/s41598-019-42239-1] [PMID: 30626917]

[96]   Pelliccia F, Pasceri V, Marazzi G, Rosano G, Greco C, Gaudio C. A pilot randomized study of ranolazine for reduction of myocardial damage during elective percutaneous coronary intervention. Am Heart J 2012; 163(6): 1019-23.
[http://dx.doi.org/10.1016/j.ahj.2012.03.018] [PMID: 22709755]

[97]   Schwemer TF, Radziwolek L, Deutscher N, *et al.* Effect of ranolazine on ischemic myocardium IN patients with acute cardiac ischemia (RIMINI-Trial): a randomized controlled pilot trial. J Cardiovasc Pharmacol Ther 2019; 24(1): 62-9.
[http://dx.doi.org/10.1177/1074248418784290] [PMID: 29938533]

[98]   Morrow DA, Scirica BM, Karwatowska-Prokopczuk E, *et al.* Effects of ranolazine on recurrent cardiovascular events in patients with non-ST-elevation acute coronary syndromes: the MERLIN-TIMI 36 randomized trial. JAMA 2007; 297(16): 1775-83.
[http://dx.doi.org/10.1001/jama.297.16.1775] [PMID: 17456819]

[99]   Safdar B, D'Onofrio G, Dziura J, Russell RR, Johnson C, Sinusas AJ. Ranolazine and microvascular angina by PET in the emergency department: results from a pilot randomized controlled trial. Clin Ther 2017; 39(1): 55-63.
[http://dx.doi.org/10.1016/j.clinthera.2016.12.002] [PMID: 28081848]

[100] Keating GM. Ranolazine: a review of its use as add-on therapy in patients with chronic stable angina pectoris. Drugs 2013; 73(1): 55-73.
[http://dx.doi.org/10.1007/s40265-012-0005-z] [PMID: 23329466]

[101] Pelliccia F, Greco C, Gaudio C, *et al*. Comparison of the pharmacodynamic effects of ranolazine versus amlodipine on platelet reactivity in stable patients with coronary artery disease treated with dual antiplatelet therapy : The ROMAN (RanOlazine vs. aMlodipine on platelet reactivity in stable patients with CAD treated with dual ANtiplatelet therapy) study. J Thromb Thrombolysis 2015; 40(3): 331-9.
[http://dx.doi.org/10.1007/s11239-015-1203-9] [PMID: 25761430]

[102] Morrow DA, Scirica BM, Sabatine MS, *et al*. B-type natriuretic peptide and the effect of ranolazine in patients with non-ST-segment elevation acute coronary syndromes: observations from the MERLIN-TIMI 36 (Metabolic Efficiency With Ranolazine for Less Ischemia in Non-ST Elevation Acute Coronary-Thrombolysis In Myocardial Infarction 36) trial. J Am Coll Cardiol 2010; 55(12): 1189-96.
[http://dx.doi.org/10.1016/j.jacc.2009.09.068] [PMID: 20298924]

[103] Mega JL, Hochman JS, Scirica BM, Murphy SA, Sloan S, McCabe CH, *et al*. Clinical perspective. Circulation 2010; 121(16): 1809-17.
[http://dx.doi.org/10.1161/CIRCULATIONAHA.109.897231] [PMID: 20385930]

[104] De Ferrari GM, Maier LS, Mont L, *et al*. Ranolazine in the treatment of atrial fibrillation: results of the dose-ranging raffaello (ranolazine in atrial fibrillation following an electrical cardioversion) study. Heart Rhythm 2015; 12(5): 872-8.
[http://dx.doi.org/10.1016/j.hrthm.2015.01.021] [PMID: 25602175]

[105] Dagres N, Iliodromitis EK, Lekakis JP, *et al*. Ranolazine for the prevention or treatment of atrial fibrillation: a systematic review. J Cardiovasc Med (Hagerstown) 2014; 15(3): 254-9.
[http://dx.doi.org/10.2459/JCM.0b013e328365b554] [PMID: 24662415]

[106] Guerra F, Romandini A, Barbarossa A, Belardinelli L, Capucci A. Ranolazine for rhythm control in atrial fibrillation: A systematic review and meta-analysis. Int J Cardiol 2017; 227: 284-91.
[http://dx.doi.org/10.1016/j.ijcard.2016.11.103] [PMID: 27839812]

[107] Gong M, Zhang Z, Fragakis N, *et al*. Role of ranolazine in the prevention and treatment of atrial fibrillation: A meta-analysis of randomized clinical trials. Heart Rhythm 2017; 14(1): 3-11.
[http://dx.doi.org/10.1016/j.hrthm.2016.10.008] [PMID: 27746384]

[108] Scirica BM, Belardinelli L, Chaitman BR, *et al*. Effect of ranolazine on atrial fibrillation in patients with non-ST elevation acute coronary syndromes: observations from the MERLIN-TIMI 36 trial. Europace 2015; 17(1): 32-7.
[http://dx.doi.org/10.1093/europace/euu217] [PMID: 25210025]

[109] Fragakis N, Koskinas KC, Katritsis DG, Pagourelias ED, Zografos T, Geleris P. Comparison of effectiveness of ranolazine plus amiodarone versus amiodarone alone for conversion of recent-onset atrial fibrillation. Am J Cardiol 2012; 110(5): 673-7.
[http://dx.doi.org/10.1016/j.amjcard.2012.04.044] [PMID: 22621799]

[110] Reiffel JA, Camm AJ, Belardinelli L, *et al*. The HARMONY trial: combined ranolazine and dronedarone in the management of paroxysmal atrial fibrillation: mechanistic and therapeutic synergism. Circ Arrhythm Electrophysiol 2015; 8(5): 1048-56.
[http://dx.doi.org/10.1161/CIRCEP.115.002856] [PMID: 26226999]

[111] Zou D, Geng N, Chen Y, *et al*. Ranolazine improves oxidative stress and mitochondrial function in the atrium of acetylcholine-CaCl2 induced atrial fibrillation rats. Life Sci 2016; 156: 7-14.
[http://dx.doi.org/10.1016/j.lfs.2016.05.026] [PMID: 27208652]

[112] Carvas M, Nascimento BC, Acar M, Nearing BD, Belardinelli L, Verrier RL. Intrapericardial ranolazine prolongs atrial refractory period and markedly reduces atrial fibrillation inducibility in the intact porcine heart. J Cardiovasc Pharmacol 2010; 55(3): 286-91.
[http://dx.doi.org/10.1097/FJC.0b013e3181d26416] [PMID: 20075744]

[113] Black-Maier EW, Pokorney SD, Barnett AS, *et al*. Ranolazine reduces atrial fibrillatory wave frequency. Europace 2017; 19(7): 1096-100.
[http://dx.doi.org/10.1093/europace/euw200] [PMID: 27756767]

[114]   Tsu LV, Lee S. Use of ranolazine in the prevention and treatment of postoperative atrial fibrillation in patients undergoing cardiac surgery. Ann Pharmacother 2014; 48(5): 633-7.
[http://dx.doi.org/10.1177/1060028014523257] [PMID: 24523397]

[115]   Simopoulos V, Tagarakis GI, Daskalopoulou SS, *et al.* Ranolazine enhances the antiarrhythmic activity of amiodarone by accelerating conversion of new-onset atrial fibrillation after cardiac surgery. Angiology 2014; 65(4): 294-7.
[http://dx.doi.org/10.1177/0003319713477911] [PMID: 23427280]

[116]   Miles RH, Passman R, Murdock DK. Comparison of effectiveness and safety of ranolazine versus amiodarone for preventing atrial fibrillation after coronary artery bypass grafting. Am J Cardiol 2011; 108(5): 673-6.
[http://dx.doi.org/10.1016/j.amjcard.2011.04.017] [PMID: 21726841]

[117]   Tagarakis GI, Aidonidis I, Daskalopoulou SS, *et al.* Effect of ranolazine in preventing postoperative atrial fibrillation in patients undergoing coronary revascularization surgery. Curr Vasc Pharmacol 2013; 11(6): 988-91.
[http://dx.doi.org/10.2174/1570161111106140128123506] [PMID: 23140547]

[118]   Minotti G, Menna P, Calabrese V, *et al.* Pharmacology of ranolazine versus common cardiovascular drugs in patients with early diastolic dysfunction induced by anthracyclines or nonanthracycline chemotherapeutics: A phase 2b minitrial. J Pharmacol Exp Ther 2019; 370(2): 197-205.
[http://dx.doi.org/10.1124/jpet.119.258178] [PMID: 31101682]

[119]   Coppini R, Mazzoni L, Ferrantini C, *et al.* Ranolazine prevents phenotype development in a mouse model of hypertrophic cardiomyopathy. Circ Heart Fail 2017; 10(3): e003565.
[http://dx.doi.org/10.1161/CIRCHEARTFAILURE.116.003565] [PMID: 28255011]

[120]   Olivotto I, Camici PG, Merlini PA, *et al.* Efficacy of ranolazine in patients with symptomatic hypertrophic cardiomyopathy: the RESTYLE-HCM randomized, double-blind, placebo-controlled study. Circ Heart Fail 2018; 11(1): e004124.
[http://dx.doi.org/10.1161/CIRCHEARTFAILURE.117.004124] [PMID: 29321131]

[121]   Gentry JL III, Mentz RJ, Hurdle M, Wang A. Ranolazine for treatment of angina or dyspnea in hypertrophic cardiomyopathy patients (RHYME). J Am Coll Cardiol 2016; 68(16): 1815-7.
[http://dx.doi.org/10.1016/j.jacc.2016.07.758] [PMID: 27737749]

[122]   Gupta T, Khera S, Kolte D, Aronow WS, Iwai S. Antiarrhythmic properties of ranolazine: A review of the current evidence. Int J Cardiol 2015; 187: 66-74.
[http://dx.doi.org/10.1016/j.ijcard.2015.03.324] [PMID: 25828315]

[123]   Curnis A, Salghetti F, Cerini M, *et al.* Ranolazine therapy in drug-refractory ventricular arrhythmias. J Cardiovasc Med (Hagerstown) 2017; 18(7): 534-8.
[http://dx.doi.org/10.2459/JCM.0000000000000521] [PMID: 28368882]

[124]   Zareba W, Daubert JP, Beck CA, *et al.* Ranolazine in high-risk patients with implanted cardioverter-defibrillators: the RAID trial. J Am Coll Cardiol 2018; 72(6): 636-45.
[http://dx.doi.org/10.1016/j.jacc.2018.04.086] [PMID: 30071993]

[125]   Albert CM. Ranolazine in Patients With Implantable Cardioverter-Defibrillators: Ready for Prime Time?. DC: American College of Cardiology Foundation Washington 2018.
[http://dx.doi.org/10.1016/j.jacc.2018.06.008]

[126]   Yeung E, Krantz MJ, Schuller JL, Dale RA, Haigney MC. Ranolazine for the suppression of ventricular arrhythmia: a case series. Ann Noninvasive Electrocardiol 2014; 19(4): 345-50.
[http://dx.doi.org/10.1111/anec.12137] [PMID: 24533675]

[127]   Chorin E, Hu D, Antzelevitch C, *et al.* Ranolazine for congenital long-QT syndrome type III: experimental and long-term clinical data. Circ Arrhythm Electrophysiol 2016; 9(10): e004370.
[http://dx.doi.org/10.1161/CIRCEP.116.004370] [PMID: 27733495]

[128]   Miranda VM, Beserra SS, Campos DR. Inotropic and antiarrhythmic transmural actions of ranolazine

in a cellular model of type 3 long QT syndrome. Arq Bras Cardiol 2020; 114(4): 732-5.
[http://dx.doi.org/10.36660/abc.20190220] [PMID: 32491007]

[129]   Wu L, Shryock JC, Song Y, Li Y, Antzelevitch C, Belardinelli L. Antiarrhythmic effects of ranolazine in a guinea pig *in vitro* model of long-QT syndrome. J Pharmacol Exp Ther 2004; 310(2): 599-605.
[http://dx.doi.org/10.1124/jpet.104.066100] [PMID: 15031300]

[130]   Moss AJ, Zareba W, Schwarz KQ, Rosero S, McNitt S, Robinson JL. Ranolazine shortens repolarization in patients with sustained inward sodium current due to type-3 long-QT syndrome. J Cardiovasc Electrophysiol 2008; 19(12): 1289-93.
[http://dx.doi.org/10.1111/j.1540-8167.2008.01246.x] [PMID: 18662191]

[131]   Vicente J, Johannesen L, Mason JW, *et al.* Comprehensive T wave morphology assessment in a randomized clinical study of dofetilide, quinidine, ranolazine, and verapamil. J Am Heart Assoc 2015; 4(4): e001615.
[http://dx.doi.org/10.1161/JAHA.114.001615] [PMID: 25870186]

[132]   Braunwald E, Zipes D, Libby P, Bonow R, Mann D, Tomaselli GF. Braunwald's heart disease: a textbook of cardiovascular medicine. 2019.47: 913-32.

[133]   Maier LS, Layug B, Karwatowska-Prokopczuk E, *et al.* Ranolazine for the treatment of diastolic heart failure in patients with preserved ejection fraction: the RALI-DHF proof-of-concept study. JACC Heart Fail 2013; 1(2): 115-22.
[http://dx.doi.org/10.1016/j.jchf.2012.12.002] [PMID: 24621836]

[134]   Eckel RH, Henry RR, Yue P, *et al.* Effect of ranolazine monotherapy on glycemic control in subjects with type 2 diabetes. Diabetes Care 2015; 38(7): 1189-96.
[http://dx.doi.org/10.2337/dc14-2629] [PMID: 26049552]

[135]   Arnold SV, McGuire DK, Spertus JA, Li Y, Yue P, Ben-Yehuda O, *et al.* Effectiveness of ranolazine in patients with type 2 diabetes mellitus and chronic stable angina according to baseline hemoglobin A1c 2014.
[http://dx.doi.org/10.1016/j.ahj.2014.06.020] [PMID: 25262254]

[136]   Association AD. 10. Cardiovascular disease and risk management: Standards of Medical Care in Diabetes—2019. Diabetes Care 2019; 42 (Suppl. 1): S103-23.
[http://dx.doi.org/10.2337/dc19-S010] [PMID: 30559236]

[137]   Fanaroff AC, James SK, Weisz G, Prather K, Anstrom KJ, Mark DB, *et al.* Glycometabolic effects of ranolazine in patients with and without diabetes mellitus in the ranolazine in patients with incomplete revascularization after percutaneous coronary intervention (river-pci) trial. J Am Coll Cardiol 2017; 69(18): 2304.
[http://dx.doi.org/10.1016/j.jacc.2017.02.056] [PMID: 28473136]

[138]   Morrow DA, Scirica BM, Chaitman BR, McGuire DK, Murphy SA, Karwatowska-Prokopczuk E, *et al.* Clinical perspective. Circulation 2009; 119(15): 2032-9.
[http://dx.doi.org/10.1161/CIRCULATIONAHA.107.763912] [PMID: 19349325]

[139]   Chisholm JW, Goldfine AB, Dhalla AK, *et al.* Effect of ranolazine on A1C and glucose levels in hyperglycemic patients with non-ST elevation acute coronary syndrome. Diabetes Care 2010; 33(6): 1163-8.
[http://dx.doi.org/10.2337/dc09-2334] [PMID: 20357382]

[140]   Lisi D, Andrews E, Parry C, Hill C, Ombengi D, Ling H. The effect of ranolazine on glycemic control: a narrative review to define the target population. Cardiovasc Drugs Ther 2019; 33(6): 755-61.
[http://dx.doi.org/10.1007/s10557-019-06917-6] [PMID: 31802311]

[141]   Greiner L, Hurren K, Brenner M. Ranolazine and its effects on hemoglobin A1C. Ann Pharmacother 2016; 50(5): 410-5.
[http://dx.doi.org/10.1177/1060028016631757] [PMID: 26917816]

[142]   Zeng X, Zhang Y, Lin J, Zheng H, Peng J, Huang W. Efficacy and safety of ranolazine in diabetic

patients: a systematic review and meta-analysis. Ann Pharmacother 2017; 52(5): 1060028017747901.
[http://dx.doi.org/10.1177/1060028017747901] [PMID: 29231052]

[143] Zack J, Berg J, Juan A, *et al.* Pharmacokinetic drug-drug interaction study of ranolazine and metformin in subjects with type 2 diabetes mellitus. Clin Pharmacol Drug Dev 2015; 4(2): 121-9.
[http://dx.doi.org/10.1002/cpdd.174] [PMID: 27128216]

[144] Pettus J, McNabb B, Eckel RH, *et al.* Effect of ranolazine on glycaemic control in patients with type 2 diabetes treated with either glimepiride or metformin. Diabetes Obes Metab 2016; 18(5): 463-74.
[http://dx.doi.org/10.1111/dom.12629] [PMID: 26749407]

[145] Ma A, Garland WT, Smith WB, *et al.* A pilot study of ranolazine in patients with intermittent claudication. Int Angiol 2006; 25(4): 361-9.
[PMID: 17164742]

[146] Arnold WD, Kline D, Sanderson A, *et al.* Open-label trial of ranolazine for the treatment of myotonia congenita. Neurology 2017; 89(7): 710-3.
[http://dx.doi.org/10.1212/WNL.0000000000004229] [PMID: 28710329]

[147] Stunnenberg BC, LoRusso S, Arnold WD, *et al.* Guidelines on clinical presentation and management of nondystrophic myotonias. Muscle Nerve 2020; 62(4): 430-44.
[http://dx.doi.org/10.1002/mus.26887] [PMID: 32270509]

[148] Naveena R, Hashilkar NK, Davangeri R, Majagi SI. Effect of anti-inflammatory activity of ranolazine in rat model of inflammation. Indian J Med Res 2018; 148(6): 743-7.
[http://dx.doi.org/10.4103/ijmr.IJMR_1504_16] [PMID: 30778009]

[149] Driffort V, Gillet L, Bon E, *et al.* Ranolazine inhibits NaV1.5-mediated breast cancer cell invasiveness and lung colonization. Mol Cancer 2014; 13(1): 264.
[http://dx.doi.org/10.1186/1476-4598-13-264] [PMID: 25496128]

[150] Koltai MZ. Influence of hypoglycaemic sulphonylureas on the electrophysiological parameters of the heart. Diabetes Res Clin Pract 1996; 31 (Suppl.): S15-20.
[http://dx.doi.org/10.1016/0168-8227(96)01225-9] [PMID: 8864636]

CHAPTER 2

Rho/Rho Kinase Signaling Pathway and Disease: from Bed to Bench

Yiming Wang[1,#], **Yuqing Zhang**[2,#] and **Dingguo Zhang**[3,*]

[1] *Department of Cardiology, Zhenjiang First People's Hospital, Zhenjiang, China*

[2] *Department of Cardiology, The Affiliated Jiangning Hospital of Nanjing Medical University, Nanjing, China*

[3] *Department of Cardiology, The First Affiliated Hospital of Nanjing Medical University, Nanjing, China*

Abstract: Since Madaule and Axel first discovered Rho gene in 1985, Rho and its signal transduction pathway have been extensively studied. Rho protein family belongs to the small GTP binding protein of Ras super-family, whose molecular weight is between 20kd-30kd. As a molecular switch, Rho protein family controls many signal transduction pathways in eukaryotic cells. There are two states of Rho protein, one is the inactivation state bound to GDP (GDP Rho), the other is the activation state bound to GTP (GTP Rho). In the resting state, the GDP Rho dissociation inhibitor (rho GDI) is bound to the GDP Rho and located in the cytoplasm. GTP was substituted for GDP to activate Rho protein by guanosine exchange factor (GEFs). GTP Rho interacts with the downstream effector Rho kinase (ROCK). There are two types of ROCK: ROCK1 and ROCK2. The activation of ROCK can inhibit the activity of myosin phosphorylated light chain phosphatase (MYPT1), thus increasing the level of myosin phosphorylated light chain (MLC) in cells, leading to increased sensitivity of vascular smooth muscle cells to Ca^{2+} and vasoconstriction. Previous studies have shown that Rho/ROCK signaling pathway not only plays an important role in vasoconstriction, but also regulates cell movement, proliferation, adhesion, activation of cytokines and migration of inflammatory cells. At the molecular level, the expression of ROCK up-regulates various factors that promote oxidative stress, inflammation, thrombosis and fibrosis, and down-regulates endothelial nitric oxide synthetase. At the cellular level, it is involved in many cell functions such as gene expression, cytokinesis, cell adhesion and migration. It has been found that Rho/Rho kinase is related to cardiovascular diseases, such as coronary atherosclerotic heart disease, hypertension, heart failure and so on. Fasudil, a potent and selective inhibitor of ROCK, can treat many cardiovascular diseases and has been used in clinical practice. This article reviews the relationship between Rho/Rho kinase and many system diseases.

[*] **Corresponding author Dingguo Zhang**: Department of Cardiology, The First Affiliated Hospital of Nanjing Medical University, Nanjing, China; E-mail: zhdg0223@126.com
[#] Yiming Wang and Yuqing Zhang have equal contribution

M. Iqbal Choudhary (Ed.)

Keywords: Atherosclerosis, Cardiovascular disease, Cerebrovascular disease, Fasudil, Ischemia heart disease, Renal injury, Rho, ROCK, Stroke.

INTRODUCTION

In 1985, rho, as a ras homologue, was first cloned as a Ras related monomer GTPase. Rho GTPase is a member of Ras protein superfamily, including more than 20 intracellular signal proteins, such as RhoA, RAC, Cdc42 and so on [1]. Rho GTPase is a kind of small molecule GTP binding protein widely existing in eukaryotes and plays an important role in cytoskeleton construction [2]. The protein family can be anchored to cell membrane by lipid modification. Under the regulation of Rho GDIs, Rho-GRFs and Rho-GAPs, it can switch between the active state of GTP-binding and the inactive state of binding to GDP, thus realizing the function of molecular switch. Rho kinases (ROCKs) [3] are important effector molecules downstream of Rho GTPase, and are serine/threonine protein kinases, which form cytoskeleton and play an important regulatory role in cell movement, migration and gene expression. At present, studies have confirmed that ROCKs participate in the activation of many signaling pathways and play an important role in many pathological states, such as coronary atherosclerosis [4], adriamycin-induced heart injury [5], pulmonary hypertension [6], pulmonary interstitial fibrosis [7] and acute kidney injury [8]. In this chapter, we focus on the role of Rho/Rho kinase in cardiovascular diseases, such as coronary atherosclerotic heart disease, hypertension, heart failure and other system diseases.

BIOLOGICAL EFFECTS OF RHO PROTEIN

Rho Protein Classification

Rho protein is a small molecule guanosine triphosphate (GTP) binding protein. It is a subgroup of Ras superfamily with a molecular weight of 20-30 kDa. It is a signal polypeptide with only one subunit composed of about 200-300 amino acids. Mammalian Rho GTPase family has at least 10 members, including Rho, Rac, Cdc42, Rnd1/Rho6, Rnd2/Rho7, Rnd3/RhoE, RhoD, RhoG, TC10, and TTF [9]. Rho GTPase family is an intracellular signal sensor which connects signal chains on cell surface to multiple intracellular reactions. In addition to controlling intercellular adhesion, polarization, vesicular transport and cell cycle, they are best known for their role in regulating actin dynamics required for cell migration [10].

Rho Protein Structure and Activity Regulation

Rho protein, like other small G proteins, has a conserved GTPase domain, GTP/GDP binding domain and effector binding domain. In addition, Rho protein has a post-translational modified C-terminal, which interacts with some regulatory factors and membrane structures, such as cell membrane, inclusion body and Golgi apparatus. In cells, Rho protein has GTP enzyme activity, which performs its molecular switching function through the conversion between GTP-binding activated type and GDP binding inactivated type. Rho protein can induce or terminate the cascade activation reaction through the mutual transformation between GTP and GDP, and therefore produce many biological effects. The balance between GTP and GDP is mainly regulated by three upstream regulatory factors: (1) guanosine nucleoside exchange factors (GEFs), a positive regulator of Rho protein, promote the exchange of the hydrolyzed GDP and the active GTP, and activate Rho protein as well. There are more than 80 species, such as VAV, LBC and DBL families; Bioinformatics analysis of the human Rho-GEFs shows that approximately 40% contain a putative PDZ-binding motif at the C-terminus. PDZ domains are protein-protein interaction domains that act as scaffolds to concentrate signaling molecules at specialized regions in the cell. (2) GTPase activating proteins (GAPs), a negative regulator of Rho protein, is responsible for catalyzing the hydrolysis of GTP to GDP, which subsequently inactivates the Ras GTPases, while GEFs facilitate the replacement of Ras-bound GDP with GTP in order to activate Ras GTPases; (3) GDP dissociation inhibitors (GDIs), that inhibit the conversion of GDP/GTP and the hydrolysis of GTP, thus inhibiting the activation of Rho protein. Whereas the number of GEFs and GAPs greatly outnumber the GTPases, there are only three conventional GDIs, immediately implying that many GTPases can bind to a single GDI [11].

Downstream Effector Molecules of Rho

The functional diversity of Rho family is related to the diversity of downstream effector molecules. The known downstream effector molecules of RhoA include [12] ROCK, p21 activated kinase, Protein kinase N (PKN), citron, PI3K, *etc.*, which mediate the role of RhoA. Rho related coil forming protein kinase (ROCK), a member of serine/threonine protein kinase family, is the clearest downstream target effector molecule of RhoA. Rock is the main effector molecule of Rho/Rock signal transduction pathway. Rho/ROCK pathway mediates cytoskeleton recombination, tension filament and adhesion plaque formation, vascular remodeling, cell differentiation, gene expression, apoptosis and calcium sensitivity [13].

RHO KINASE

Structure and Classification of Rho Kinases

Up to now, more than 50 downstream effectors and target proteins of Rac, Rho and Cdc42 have been identified by yeast two hybrid system and affinity chromatography. A representative class of effectors is Rho kinase family. Among them, Rho kinase, also known as Rho associated coil forming protein serine/threonine kinase (ROCK), is a serine/threonine protein kinase. Its primary structure contains kinase domain/catalytic domain (CD) and Rho binding domain (RBD) from N-terminal (Fig. **1A**). The crystal structure of ROCK has been clarified. ROCK exists in the form of homodimer and has no activity under the resting state. The formation of dimer is realized by the winding of PH domain (Figs. **1B** and **C**).

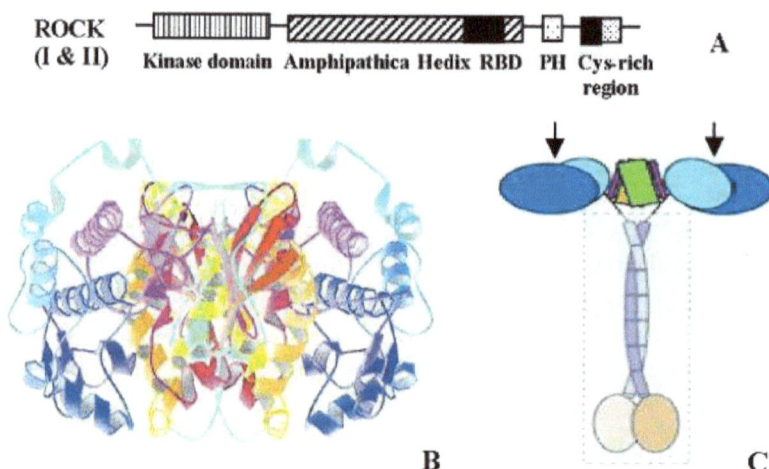

Fig. (1). **A**: Primary functional structure of ROCK; **B**: Crystal structure of ROCK; **C**: Overall structure diagram of ROCK. Arrows indicate the active sites of the kinase domains, which are facing toward the kinase domains dimerized by the capped helix-bundle (CHB) domain(top). Gray box includes coiled-coil region and the PH domain.

Rho kinase has two isomers: ROCK1 (also called ROCK I, ROKβ, rho-kinase β, or p160 ROCK) and ROCK2 (also known as ROCK II, ROKα, or rho kinase α); human ROCK1 and ROCK2 genes are located on chromosome 18 and chromosome 2, respectively [14]. The expression of the two genes in amino acid sequence is 65% similar, and that in their expressed kinase domain is 92%. ROCK1 and ROCK2 are widely distributed and widely expressed in various tissues. ROCK2 is mainly expressed in the heart, lungs, brain and skeletal muscle, and Rock1 is mainly expressed in liver, spleen, kidney and testis [15]. Both proteins are expressed in vascular smooth muscle and heart. Most Rho kinases were found in the cytoplasm by biochemical separation technology, and Rho kinase could be found throughout the cytosol by immunocytochemistry. When Rho GTP was transfected or stimulated with growth factor, some Rho kinases were translocated to the cell membrane [16].

ROCK deletion mouse model has been developed to discriminate specific and nonredundant functions of ROCK1 and ROCK2 *in vivo* [17]. However, a high rate of lethality of total homozygous deletion of ROCK1 or ROCK2 during embryonic and perinatal time were found, unfortunately [18]. This indicates the redundant roles of ROCK isoforms during embryonic development. Nevertheless, the genetic background influences the phenotype of both $Rock1^{-/-}$ and $Rock2^{-/-}$ mice notably [19]. In $ROCK1^{-/-}$ and $ROCK2^{-/-}$ mice with the C57BL/6 mice background, open eyelids at birth and presence of the omphalocele phenotype were observed, which suggested that both Rock1 and Rock2 are necessary for eyelids and ventricular body wall closure, and each isoform does not compensate for the absence of the other [18]. Most $ROCK1^{-/-}$ mice died soon after birth as a result of cannibalization of the omphalocele by the mother; however, most of the surviving $ROCK1^{-/-}$ mice, both male and female, subsequently developed normally [20]. Interestingly, mice expressing mutated MYPT1 that cannot be phosphorylated by ROCK exhibit a similar omphalocele phenotype, thus supporting a role of ROCK in signaling cascades that regulate closure of the ventral body wall at the umbilical ring [21]. This indicates that the correlation between the phenotype of mice carrying genetic manipulation of known ROCK targets, as well as upstream ROCK regulators, and ROCK knockout phenotypes can provide useful data to identify ROCK signaling pathway components and to understand their biologic functions. Unfortunately, available data required to establish such phenotypic correlations are still limited. Because of the high number and diversity of ROCK substrates and upstream ROCK regulators (membrane receptors/ligands; more than 30 RhoA exchange factors), each having numerous different targets in addition to ROCK and different expression profiles according to cell/tissue types, such a correlation is difficult to make and can potentially lead to misinterpretation from what we currently know. The cardiomyocyte -specific deletion of ROCK2 suppressed the cardiac hypertrophy [22], while the ROCK1 haploinsufficiency did not prevent cardiac hypertrophy but reduced fibrosis [23].

Regulation Mechanism of Rho Kinase Activity

Rho kinase is an important effector molecule of GTP binding protein, which can participate in many physiological functions and cell processes through Rho/Rho kinase signaling pathway. In resting state, ROCK has no enzyme activity, because there is a "self-inhibition" mechanism of ROCK kinase activity. The C-terminal is the negative regulation region of kinase activity, because the C-terminal reverses its catalytic domain and forms an automatic inhibition ring, making ROCK achieve an inactive state [21]. In other words, Ras binding domain(RBD), plant homeodomain (PHD) and Cysteine rich domain (CRD) domains of ROCK can cover the catalytic active sites of Rock through a mechanism of refolding, which makes rock unable to bind to ATP and its downstream substrate macromolecular polypeptides/proteins. Under physiological conditions, when Rho binding to GTP binds to RBD, it changes the spatial structure of Rock, destroys the negative regulatory interaction between catalytic domain and C-terminal, and exposes the active center, thus showing catalytic activity, activating kinase and reacting to extracellular signals. Research has shown that the 160-kDa protein kinase ROCKI employs only 10 residues of a 13 amino acid stretch at the C-terminal part of the coiled-coil to bind a predominantly hydrophobic patch assembled by the switch regions of RhoA [24]. At the same time, the overall structure of the ROCKI-RBD parallel coiled-coil is distinct from the structure of unbound ROCKII-RBD, the C-terminal part where the interaction with RhoA takes place shares high structural similarity. Besides, other substances, such as arachidonic acid (AA) and sphingosine phosphorylcholine (SPC), can activate rock directly without relying on Rho [7]. In addition, caspase-2,3 (caspase-2,3-containing cysteine aspartate specific protein) can also partially hydrolyze the reversion of rock, and then activate Rho A [25, 26].

Rho Kinase Inhibitor

Fasudil hydrochloride and Y27632 are the main Rho kinase inhibitors found [27]. The former was first used in Japan to prevent cerebral vasospasm after subarachnoid hemorrhage (SAH) in 1995. It is the first and only Rho kinase inhibitor used in the clinic. Y27632 is a non-selective ROCK inhibitor, which can inhibit vascular smooth muscle proliferation, control blood pressure and intraocular pressure only in animal models. Y39983 optimized by Y27632 has a stronger effect on Rock [28]. It is especially effective in the treatment of glaucoma [29]. In recent years, some new ROCK inhibitors have been found, such as sr-1459, sr-899, 6-fluindazole, dimethyl fasudil (h-1152p), rki1342, rki1447, *etc.* [28]. And AR-13324 has recently passed the clinical trials, whereas AMA0076, K115, PG324, Y39983 and RKI-983 are still under trial [28]·

As the only Rho kinase inhibitor that is used in the clinic, fasudil was initially used to treat subarachnoid hemorrhage in Japan. At present, it has been used in angina pectoris [30], heart failure [31], hypertension [32] and other aspects in foreign countries. Clinical practice shows that human body has a good response to this drug. Clinical application confirmed that fasudil has good therapeutic effect on cardiovascular diseases, including angina pectoris, hypertension, coronary vasospasm, restenosis after coronary recanalization and atherosclerosis [31]. Fasudil can also play a potential role in anti-fibrosis of heart and kidney by inhibiting aldosterone and renin. This research result has been confirmed in the diabetic rat model [33]. As a protein kinase inhibitor, fasudil also regulates cell proliferation, migration and adhesion, bone scaffold rearrangement, cytoplasmic movement and inflammatory cell movement at the cellular level and regulates inflammation and thrombosis at the molecular gene level [34].

RHO/RHO KINASE AND CARDIOVASCULAR DISEASE

Rho/Rho Kinase and Hypertension

Arterial hypertension is a major risk factor and one of the most common cardiovascular diseases [35]. It was reported that over 1 billion people have elevated blood pressure and about 45% of adults are affected by the disease. In 2016 the global health study report on patients from 67 countries was released in Lancet, which identified hypertension as the world's leading cause for death and disability-adjusted years since 1990 [36]. Increased peripheral vascular resistance due to increased vasoconstriction and arterial wall remodeling results in high arterial pressure levels. In addition, increased cardiac output, reduced renal sodium/water excretion and a distorted CNS for blood pressure regulation are key components of the pathogenesis of hypertension. Many factors, especially renin angiotensin aldosterone system and reactive oxygen species (ROS) are implicated in the pathophysiology of hypertension [37]. On the other hand, cardiovascular cells produce ROS under the influence of various pressures, such as stretch, hypoxia and angiotensin II, leading to changes in the redox state of blood vessels. These changes in turn activate specific signaling pathways, leading to smooth muscle contraction and proliferation, and induce inflammatory response and damage to endothelium-dependent relaxation [38].

The contractile state of vascular smooth muscle determines the size of vascular lumen. The abnormal increase of vascular smooth muscle tension is involved in the pathogenesis of vascular diseases. A better understanding of the molecular mechanisms regulating vascular tension is essential for the prevention and treatment of vascular diseases. The most important pathogenesis of hypertension is the increase of vascular resistance, but its molecular mechanism has not been fully elucidated. Rho/Rho kinase signaling pathway can mediate the change of vascular tension, regulate vascular resistance and even participate in the occurrence and development of hypertension through various effects on vascular smooth muscle cells (VSMC) [13]. The role of rock signaling in arterial hypertension has been widely studied. Studies with gene deletion mice showed that [39, 40] normal hemodynamic parameters, normal blood pressure and normal heart rate values were observed under basal conditions in $Rock1^{-/-}$, $Rock1^{+/-}$, and $Rock2^{+/-}$ mice when compared with those of control mice. Studies with Ang II induced hypertension model in $ROCK1^{+/-}$ mice also found that [41] ROCK1 does not participate in the regulation of blood pressure and high blood pressure, although perivascular fibrosis is reduced in the heart of $Rock1^{+/-}$ mice compared with controls. Besides, Yao *et al* demonstrated that [42] the basal systolic blood pressure in $Rock1^{+/-}$ and $Rock2^{+/-}$ mice was approximately 15 mmHg lower than that of control mice, thus raising the possibility that both ROCK1 and ROCK2 can control blood pressure. ROCK inhibitors such as Y27632 and fasudil have significant antihypertensive effects on various hypertensive rats, with no effect on normal rats' blood pressure [43]. The activity of Rho/ ROCK pathway was significantly increased in spontaneous hypertension [44], DOCA salt induced hypertension [45], renal hypertension [46] and other hypertensive rat models [13]. Therefore, Rho/ ROCK pathway may be involved in the occurrence and development of hypertension.

Case control studies of Chinese Han population indicated that [47] ROCK1 and ROCK2 contribute to the genetic susceptibility of hypertension and stroke. A genetic analysis showed that the Thr431Asn ROCK2 variant (rs2230774, C/A) influences blood pressure [48]. The AA genotype (Asn/Asn ROCK2) is associated with high basal blood pressure and increased systemic vascular resistance. The association of ROCK2 with hypertension was also evaluated in the HYPGENE study [49], which has a large prospective cohort of hypertensive patients and healthy, normotensive controls. Data strongly suggest that a major haplotype block at the ROCK2 locus is recessively associated with a lower risk of hypertension.

Rho/Rho Kinase and Pulmonary Hypertension

Pulmonary hypertension (PH) is an incurable disease characterized by persistent vasoconstriction, progressive vascular remodeling and irreversible right ventricular dysfunction [50] and eventually leads to death [51]. However, hypoxic pulmonary vasoconstriction (HPV) is known to be the main pathophysiological factor leading to the rise of pulmonary arterial pressure, and the biological mechanism leading to multiple HPV and vascular remodeling [52].

Rho/Rho kinase signaling pathway plays an important role in pulmonary vasoconstriction and remodeling. Most studies have shown that Rho/RhoA pathway and its downstream effectors, Rho kinase (Rock-1 and rock-2) signaling pathway play an important role in different experimental models of pulmonary hypertension, including chronic hypoxia [53], monocrotaline [54], bleomycin [55], shunt and vascular endothelial growth factor receptor inhibition [56]. Pulmonary hypertension is associated with hypoxia, endothelial dysfunction, vascular smooth muscle cells and excessive contraction related proliferation, which enhances ROS production and inflammatory cell migration, among which Rho kinase is basically involved. Acute vasodilator effects of inhaled fasudil as a more feasible option to locally deliver the drug for PH has been tested in 15 patients [57]. Animal data has shown that [58] fasudil significantly improved PH, to a greater degree than did bosentan (an endothelin receptor blocker) and sildenafil (a phosphodiesterase 5 inhibitor). In addition, studies have shown that long-term use of fasudil can inhibit monocrotaline induced pulmonary arterial pressure in rats [59] and hypoxia induced pulmonary hypertension in mice [60]. However, up till now, no clinical trial has assessed the long-term efficacy of fasudil in the treatment of PH and limited data suggest that the mid-term use of fasudil could improve exercise capacity and reduce in-hospital mortality [61].

Rho/Rho Kinase and Atherosclerosis

Atherosclerosis (AS) is characterized by chronic inflammation, lipid accumulation and arterial wall fibrosis, which leads to the accumulation of plaques, leading to the decline of smooth muscle contractile function and endothelial relaxation. The commonly accepted pathogenesis of atherosclerosis is "injury response theory" [62]. The damage of endothelium is the starting factor of AS [63]. The proliferation and migration of vascular smooth muscle cells play an important role in AS. Many animal studies have proved that ROCK is the key to the multiple inflammatory steps of atherosclerosis. The respective role of ROCK1 and ROCK2 in the development of atherosclerosis has been characterized by transplantation of the *Rock1* $^{/}$ and *Rock2* $^{-/-}$ bone marrow into the irradiated *Ldlr−/−* mice. Limited atherosclerosis and decreased inflammatory cells (macrophages, T cells) in the atherosclerotic lesions of *Ldlr−/−* mice was found when bone marrow–derived cells lack of ROCK1 replaced the bone marrows of *Ldlr−/−* mice [64]. Moreover, bone marrow–derived cells of *Rock2* deletion or haploinsufficiency transplantation into *Ldlr−/−* mice also protects from atherosclerosis and reduces lipid deposition in atherosclerotic plaques [65, 66]. Selective inhibitors can increase the expression of eNOS (endothelial nitric oxide synthase), reduce vascular inflammation, and reduce the formation of atherosclerotic plaques. In mouse models of accelerated atherosclerosis, such as apolipoprotein E deficient mice [67], Rock- dependent smooth muscle contraction was observed in the early stage of atherosclerosis in the aorta (without changing the expression of ROCK). In the formation of atherosclerotic lesions, ROCK activity, as indicated by the extent of phosphorylation of the Ezrin/Radixin/Moesin (ERM) family, a substrate of Rho-kinase, can be inhibited by Y27632 treatment, which increases in some regions and cell types including endothelial cells, adipocytes and peripheral macrophages [68]. In addition, in apolipoprotein E-knockout mice model [69], the treatment of fasudil caused arterial thickness, maximum flow rate and macrophage aggregation in the decreased atherosclerotic lesions. In clinical settings, the elevated ROCK activity and impaired endothelial function in CAD patients has been found [70]. Furthermore, treatment with fasudil reduced the overactivity of ROCK in patients with atherosclerosis and improved endothelium-dependent vasodilation as well as flow-mediated, endothelium-dependent dilation [71]. However, a presumably not "overactive" phenomenon was found in healthy individuals but not in patients with CAD. A negative feedback loop with increased transcription of Rho might be induced when ROCK was inhibited in healthy individuals. This would in turn lead to a compensatory increase in the downstream effects of Rho, including suppression of eNOS production. At the same time, an excess of NO production might be induced when ROCK was inhibited in healthy individuals, which resulted into the formation of peroxynitrite, and then leading to eNOS uncoupling and worsening endothelial function [72]. Therefore, some basal ROCK activity is probably required for the maintenance of vascular homeostasis and emphasizes the importance of selective ROCK inhibitors for clinical usage.

Rho/Rho Kinase and Myocardial Ischemia Reperfusion Injury

Rock has been found to play an important role in myocardial ischemia/reperfusion (I/R) injury, in which blood flow is limited or cut off, and then introduced into the region [73]. I/R leads to oxidative stress, mitochondrial dysfunction, inflammation and tissue damage. The Rho /ROCK activities were increased in I/R injuries. However, the Rho /ROCK signal has harmful effects on several *in vivo* models of I/R injury, including mice [74], rats [75] and swine [76]. In these models, ROCK inhibitors such as fasudil or Y27632 can significantly inhibit rock activity after ischemia-reperfusion, reduce infarct size and inflammatory factor levels, reduce apoptosis and enhance contractile function. The mechanism of Rho /ROCK signal contributing to I/R injury includes inhibition of rescue kinase pathway of reperfusion injury, such as PI-3K/Akt/eNOS signal [73]. Evidence has shown that inhibition of ROCK by Y-27632 leads to reduced myocardial infarction size and cardiomyocyte apoptosis *via* the PARP/ERK signaling pathway [77]. Moreover, Y27632 increase lactate dehydrogenase and glyceraldehyde-3-phosphate dehydrogenase in I/R model [78]. Therefore, cardioprotective effect of Y27632 involves increased energy production. The possible mechanisms of fasudil action against myocardial I/R injury are improvement in coronary vasodilation, inhibition of apoptosis and oxidative stress, relieving inflammation, and reduction in endoplasmic reticulum stress and metabolism [79]. In addition, fasudil protects the heart against I/R injury by attenuating endoplasmic reticulum stress and modulating SERCA activity, mainly due to JAK2/STAT3 activation and less due to PI3K/Akt signaling [80]. Pharmacological inhibition of arginase and remote ischemic preconditioning are known to protect the heart against I/R injury. Arginase is activated by peroxynitrite/ROCK signaling cascade in myocardial I/R [81]. In addition, evidence has demonstrated that remote ischemic post-conditioning could attenuate I/R injury and the underlying mechanisms might be associated with a reduction in myocardial apoptosis and the suppression of the Rho-kinase signaling pathway [82]. Ischemic postconditioning may also reduce myocardial necrosis and apoptosis during ischemia/reperfusion. A synergistic protective effect of fasudil pretreatment and ischemic postconditioning on myocardial ischemia/reperfusion injury has been demonstrated in rats model [83], which was mediated *via* upregulating the PI3K/Akt/eNOS pathway, increasing expression of antiapoptotic Bcl-2, and decreasing expression of proapoptotic Bax. In clinical settings, evidence demonstrated that [84] Rho kinase is involved in the pathogenesis of heart I/R injury in patients (38 patients with acute ST-segment elevation myocardial infarction, 26 patients with atherosclerosis and 22 normal subjects.). Therefore, inhibition of Rho kinase may be an additional therapeutic intervention for the treatment of I/R.

Rho/Rho Kinase and Adriamycin-induced Heart Injury

The anthracycline antibiotic adriamycin (ADR) is one of the most effective clinical anticancer drugs, which has been widely used for the treatment on a wide range of human neoplasms, such as acute leukemia, lymphoma, breast cancer and a number of solid tumors [85]. Yet its multiple side effects limited the clinical use of ADR in chemotherapy, and the severe cumulative cardiac toxicity is most common [86]. Evidence indicated that the occurrence of cardiac events associated with ADR therapy in cancer patients is estimated between 10% to 25%. Still now, the mechanism of ADR-induced cardiac toxicity seems to be distinct from the mechanism for anticancer action,and appears to be related with oxidative stress, cardiac cell apoptosis and mitochondrial dysfunction in the heart. We previously found evident cardiac damage in mouse administrated with Adriamycin [5], including cardiac functions (decreased left ventricular EF, the left ventricular FS, increased left vetricular volume), cardiac injury marker (increased creatine kinase, lactate dehydrogenase), plasma antioxidant enzymes activity (decreased superoxide dismutase) and lipid peroxidation (elevated malondialdehyde). However, fasudil treatment notably ameliorated adriamycin induced cardiac damage (Fig. **2**), restored heart function, suppressed cell apoptosis and senescence, ameliorated redox imbalance and DNA damage. Therefore, the RhoA/ROCK signaling pathway plays an important role in the progression of chronic heart failure induced by ADR, which needs clinical evidence in future.

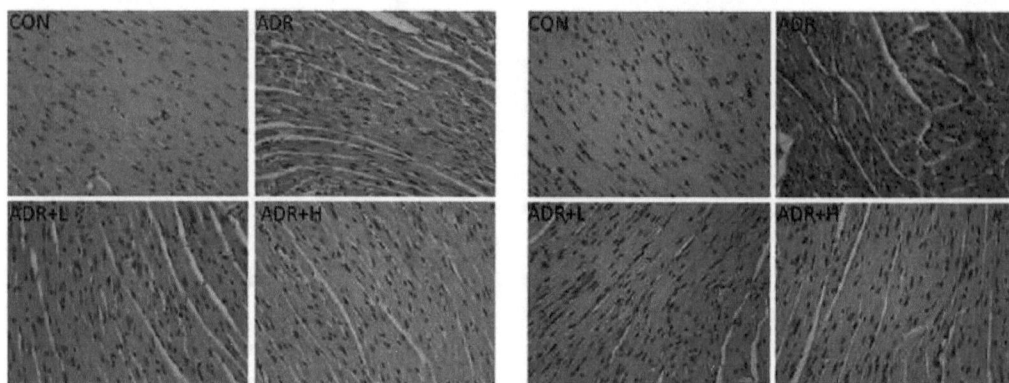

Fig. (2). Fasudil treatment ameliorated adriamycin induced cardiac damage. Representative micrographs of HE (right) and T-COL (left) staining of heart tissue. ADR:adriamycin; L:low dose(3mg/kg) of fasudil; H:high dose (10mg/kg) of fasudil.

Outlook

A large number of studies have confirmed that Rho/Rho kinase signaling pathway is involved in a variety of pathological mechanisms and is closely related to a variety of cardiovascular diseases [87, 88]. Upregulation of Rho kinase expression will promote the occurrence and development of many cardiovascular diseases. At present, many animal experiments have proven that Rho kinase inhibitors can improve and treat cardiovascular diseases, can reduce clinical symptoms, and is superior to some commonly used cardiovascular disease treatment drugs [16, 89]. Therefore, it is necessary to further understand the physiological functions of various subtypes of Rho kinase and the specific inhibitors of various subtypes. Specific and effective pharmacological modulators of Rho kinase signaling pathway are still essential for cardiovascular disease intervention. So far, fasudil is the only Rho kinase inhibitor that has been used in clinical practice. In the future, more Rho kinase inhibitors will be developed and applied in clinic.

RHO KINASE AND ISCHEMIC CEREBROVASCULAR DISEASE

The possible pathogenesis of ROCK in ischemic stroke is to inhibit the expression of myosin light chain phosphorylase and up-regulate the phosphorylation level of myosin light chain, so as to enhance the contraction of vascular smooth muscle and aggravate the ischemia and hypoxia at the cerebral infarction site, thus leading to the enlargement of central necrotic area and the reduction of ischemic penumbra [90]. Rho kinases are also thought [87] to play an important role in hemodynamic abnormalities, inflammatory processes, and the function of many cells, such as the migration of neutrophils and monocytes, and endothelial cell injury caused by the decrease of eNOS.

The Mechanism of Rho Kinase in Cerebral Ischemia

Rho Kinase Mediates Oxidative Stress

Oxidative stress plays an important role in ischemic brain diseases. Reactive oxygen species damage endothelial cell function by promoting lipid oxidation, pro-inflammatory gene expression and oxidative inactivation of endothelial nitric oxide (NO). The activation of RhoA can induce the activation of Rho kinase, promote the production of reactive oxygen species, cause endothelial cell injury, increase the permeability of blood-brain barrier, and induce brain edema [91]. At the same time, reactive oxygen species can also directly damage the nerve cell membrane, resulting in brain cell parenchyma edema. Rac 1, as a small GTP binding protein of Rho kinase family, also plays an important role in the process of ischemic induced oxidative stress in cerebral microvascular endothelial cells [92]. The redox-dependent decrease in Rho activity is required for Rac-induced formation of membrane ruffles and integrin-mediated cell spreading. Nimmual *et al* showed that Rac produced ROS and then resulted in the downregulation of Rho activity, which involves inhibition of the low-molecular-weight protein tyrosine phosphatase (LMW-PTP) and then an increase in the tyrosine phosphorylation and activation of its target, p190Rho-GAP [93]. Hypoxia/reoxygenation can induce the transfer of Rac-1 (NADPH oxidase activator) to cell membrane in porcine brain microvascular endothelial cells. As a weak pleiotropic inhibitor of Rock, Statins have been shown to exert neuronal protection in ischemic stroke. In rat's transient focal ischemia model, atorvastatin could inhibit the activity of Rac-1 and prevent BBB injury induced by ischemia/reperfusion [94]. Rho kinase inhibitor can completely block ROS induced increase endothelial permeability and actin cytoskeleton phosphorylation, reduce BMEC damage and BBB permeability [91]. Fasudil hydrochloride noticeably contributed to the recovery of neurological function, improved the function of blood-brain barrier, inhibited RhoA protein expression, and upregulated growth-associated protein-43 and claudin-5 protein expression following cerebral I/R [95].

Rho Kinase Mediated Cytoskeleton Changes

Rho proteins regulate a diverse spectrum of biological processes including [96] regulation of changes in cytoskeletal organization, superoxide production, gene transcription, cell proliferation and transformation. As an upstream signal molecule of rock, RhoA plays an important role in the regulation of endothelial cell integrity and permeability. Studies using constitutively active and dominant negative forms of Rho GTPases have shown that [97], in some cells, Rho regulate the formation of stress fibers. Rho also plays a positive role in the regulation of cell motility, which was thought to be restricted to the generation of contractile force and focal adhesion turnover needed for tail retraction. Mirvat El-Sibai *et al* demonstrated in carcinoma cells that [98] RhoA activation is kinetically correlated with actin nucleation, and occurs in a broad band that extends throughout the protruding lamellipod and into the lamellar region. Inhibition of Rho or p160ROCK leads to increased protrusion but decreased motility. Inhibition of ROCK leads to a switch in the Rho GTPase that regulates protrusion. Cerebral ischemia can induce the activation of RhoA, then promote the activation of Rho kinase, promote the formation of stress fiber, and then cause the phosphorylation of myosin light chain, and reduce the biological activity of nitric oxide (NO) [99, 100]. NO plays an important role in maintaining the integrity of endothelial cells. ROCK has also been shown to regulate myosin activity by phosphorylating either the regulatory subunit of MLC phosphatase or MLC directly [101, 102]. Therefore, cerebral ischemia can increase cell permeability by activating rock and aggravate the occurrence of ischemic cerebrovascular disease.

Rho Kinase Mediates Inflammatory Response

Ischemic brain damage manifests from a complex series of mechanisms, and neuroinflammation plays critical role of this pathogenesis. Microglial polarization to the anti-inflammatory M2 phenotype is essential in resolving neuroinflammation, making it a promising therapeutic strategy for stroke intervention. Ermei Lu *et al* indicated that [103] profilin 1 mediates microglial polarization induced by ischemia/hypoxia through the RhoA/ ROCK pathway in *in vitro* and *in vivo* models of brain ischemia. ROCK plays an important role in hemodynamic abnormalities and inflammatory response. RhoA, as a cytoskeleton actin regulator, can be activated by some inflammatory substrates such as lipopolysaccharide (LPS), and then induce the activation of rock and promote a series of inflammatory reactions [104]. Inflammatory reaction can promote the migration of neutrophils and monocytes into ischemic injury area. Inhibition of RhoA and its downstream target ROCK, has been proven to promote axon regeneration and function recovery following injury in the central nervous system

[105]. Previous studies have shown that the Rock activity of white blood cells in patients with ischemic stroke were significantly increased [106]. Evidence has shown that [107] sepsis may increase cerebral and cognitive injury through Rho-kinase/ROCK pathway in rats, and ROCK inhibitors may be potentially employed to overcome sepsis-induced deleterious effects in the brain. Additional study also found that ROCK expression and activity increased in the striatum, especially in axons, in the early phase of ischemia [108]. And fasudil reduced this ROCK activity and protected against cerebral infarction by acting directly on neurons. Long non-coding RNAs (lncRNAs) are considered as critical regulators in pathogenesis progression of cerebral ischemia. lncRNA-small nucleolar RNA host gene 14 (SNHG14) was found upregulated in middle cerebral artery occlusion/reperfusion (MCAO/R) treated brain tissues and oxygen-glucose deprivation and reoxygenation (OGD/R) treated PC-12 cells [109]. SNHG14 promoted neurological impairment and inflammatory response through elevating the expression of ROCK1 while decreasing miR-136-5p level in OGD/R induced damage.

Rho Kinase Regulates Phosphatidylinositol Metabolism

RhoA is required to regulate the metabolism of phosphatidylinositol. Related studies have shown that [110, 111] RhoA is involved in the activation of PI3K activated by thrombin receptor (one of G protein coupled receptors) and lysophosphatidic acid receptor (LPA). RhoA indirectly controls cell metabolism, proliferation and survival by regulating PI3K activity. At the same time, RhoA could directly interact with phosphatidylinositol 4,5, which regulates cell survival through glycogen synthase kinase, fructose phosphokinase and a potential survival signal [112].

Rho Kinase Regulates the Expression of eNOS

NO constitutively produced by endothelial NO synthase (eNOS), regulates cerebral blood flow and vascular tone and protects against ischemic stroke by increasing collateral flow to the ischemic area. Indeed, eNOS-deficient (eNOS$^{-/-}$) mice develop larger cerebral infarctions after middle cerebral artery occlusion [113]. Relevant studies have shown that [114] acute cerebral ischemia can induce the activation of Rho kinase, and then down regulate the expression of eNOS, indirectly leading to the impairment of microcirculation function in the surrounding area of cerebral ischemia and expand the scope of ischemic damage. Cerebral ischemia injury can activate Rock in neurons, inhibit the synthesis of phosphatidylinositol-3 kinase, and down regulate the expression of eNOS protein, which further leads to the disintegration of important structures such as phospholipid membrane, cytoskeleton protein and nucleic acid of neurons, eventually leading to neuron damage and apoptosis, aggravating the pathogenesis of cerebral ischemia [115]. Evidence has shown that [116] fasudil could prevent the downregulation of eNOS under hypoxic conditions. In animal model of middle cerebral artery occlusion, fasudil increased eNOS mRNA and protein expression in a concentration-dependent manner [117]. Furthermore, fasudil increased cerebral blood flow to both ischemic and nonischemic brain areas and reduced cerebral infarct size. Therefore, neuroprotective effect of ROCK inhibition is mediated by endothelium-derived NO and suggest that ROCK may be an important therapeutic target for ischemic stroke [117].

Rho Kinase Regulates the Expression of Matrix Metalloproteinase-9

Matrix metalloproteinase 9 (MMP9) is one of extracellular protein degradation enzymes. Activated MMP-9 can induce BBB basement membrane damage and aggravate the occurrence of stroke [118]. A study by liu *et al* has shown that [119] the activation of Rock can induce the increase of MMP9 expression, resulting in the degradation of basement membrane and the increase of BBB permeability, which aggravates the pathogenesis of stroke .

Neuroprotective Effect of Rho Kinase Inhibitor

Rho kinase plays an important role in the pathogenesis of ischemic brain disease. Inhibition of Rho kinase activity can reverse the occurrence of related pathology. Therefore, more and more attention has been paid to the research of Rho kinase inhibitors, which show that Rho kinase inhibitors play an important role in the prevention and treatment of ischemic stroke. Rikitake *et al* [117] and other studies [91] have shown that ROCK inhibitors (fasudil hydrochloride and Y27632) can inhibit the expression of rock in endothelial cells, expand blood vessels, promote local microcirculation, protect the vitality of endothelial cells, and reduce cerebral infarction after stroke.

The enlargement of dead volume promotes the improvement of nerve function. A critical role for Rock in the pathogenesis of cerebral ischemic injury, and the potential utility of the inhibitor as a therapeutic agent in stroke has been demonstrated in animals [117, 120]. Hydroxy fasudil, an active metabolite of an antispastic drug, fasudil, could improve the hemodynamic function and inhibit neutrophil-mediated damage, and contributes to the potency and long duration of the cytoprotective properties of fasudil on ischemic brain damage [121]. Rho kinase inhibitors can also inhibit the infiltration of neutrophils and monocytes to prevent the occurrence of inflammatory reaction, inhibit the overload of Ca^{2+}, reduce the production of oxygen free radicals in neutrophils and cerebral vessels, promote the regeneration of nerve axons and the reconstruction of neural network, and reduce the delayed neuronal damage [122]. The role of ROCK polymorphisms has been investigated in ischemic stroke patients. Zee *et al* demonstrated [123] the potential association of *ROCK1* and *ROCK2* with the risk of ischemic stroke in participants from the Women's Genome Health Study. In this large cohort of 23,294 initially healthy Caucasian women, a significant association of 7 single polymorphisms in *ROCK1* with the risk of ischemic stroke were found, but none of the 15 tested *ROCK2* single nucleotide polymorphisms were associated with ischemic stroke.

Outlook

In conclusion, rock signaling pathway plays an important role in many aspects of ischemic stroke. The research on ROCK signaling pathway will provide a new therapeutic target for clinical treatment of ischemic stroke, nerve injury and other nervous system diseases. Rho kinase inhibitors, which are used in clinic, have significant therapeutic effects on ischemic stroke and other cardiovascular and cerebrovascular diseases, and show a wide range of prospects for clinical prevention and treatment of ischemic stroke. For ischemic cerebrovascular diseases, we should further study Rho kinase signaling pathway, clarify the structure and interaction of various regions of Rho kinase, as well as the activation and regulation mechanism of Rho kinase after brain injury. It is of great significance to develop more effective treatment options for ischemic cerebrovascular diseases.

RHO KINASE AND RESPIRATORY DISEASES

As a key downstream target effector in Rho/Rho kinase signaling pathway, Rho kinase activates downstream response by receiving upstream signal and regulates cell biological behavior. It was found that Rho/Rho kinase signaling pathway plays an important role in the occurrence and development of respiratory diseases, especially in chronic obstructive pulmonary disease (COPD) [124], bronchial asthma [125], idiopathic pulmonary fibrosis [126], and lung cancer [127].

Rho Kinase and COPD

The pathophysiological characteristics of COPD manifests as incomplete reversible airflow limitation. Its essence is chronic small airway inflammation. Repeated injury and repair lead to airway collagen deposition and fibrosis and other structural changes. The main manifestation of COPD patients is inflammatory reaction with neutrophil infiltration in small airway. Rho kinase signaling pathway plays a certain role in the process of neutrophil aggregation in COPD patients [128]. Palani K, *et al.* showed that [129] Rho kinase inhibitor can reduce the level of myeloperoxidase (an indicator of neutrophil content) in sepsis injured lung tissue. In order to slow down the aggregation of neutrophils in lung tissue, F-actin plays an important role in neutrophil infiltration. Rho kinase inhibitor Y-27632 can inhibit the aggregation of F-actin by blocking the synthesis of F-actin in neutrophils [130]. Rho kinase also plays an important role in the airway infiltration of monocytes, neutrophils and T lymphocytes and the release of inflammatory cytokines, which regulates the inflammatory response of COPD [131]. Furthermore, Kondrikov *et al.* found that [132] Rho kinase inhibitor Y-27632 can reduce collagen synthesis and inhibit fibroblast proliferation, suggesting that Rho kinase also participates in airway remodeling of COPD. A series of studies [133] have shown that Rho kinase plays an important role in the occurrence and development of COPD, but the specific mechanism is still not very clear, so further research is needed to fully understand the role of Rho kinase in the pathogenesis of COPD.

Rho Kinase and Asthma

Asthma is a chronic airway inflammatory disease, which is mainly characterized by airway hyperresponsiveness [125] and involved by a combination of different cells (such as eosinophils, mast cells, lymphocytes, neutrophils, *etc.*) and cellular components. Airway inflammation and the increase of airway smooth muscle contractility are the basis of airway hyperresponsiveness. Recent studies have found that [134] Rho kinase plays an important role in regulating airway responsiveness. Plenty of studies have confirmed that [135 - 137] Rho/Rho kinase signaling pathway is involved in airway hyperresponsiveness, increased aggregation of airway inflammatory cells, and secretion and release of inflammatory cytokines. PI3K-dependent activation of ROCK is necessary for agonist-induced human airway smooth muscle cell contraction, and inhibition of PI3K promotes bronchodilation of human small airways [138]. Activation of PI3K mediate inflammation and hyperresponsiveness. Utilizing human precision cut lung slices from non-asthma donors and primary human airway smooth muscle cells from both non-asthma and asthma donors, Koziol-White, C. J. *et al* demonstrated that [137] inhibition of PI3K promotes dilation of human small airways in a Rho kinase-dependent manner. Fasudil, an inhibitor of Rho kinase, can inhibit ovalbumin induced airway hyperresponsiveness in mice [139]. Other studies have confirmed that Rho kinase regulates the contractility of airway smooth muscle and changes airway responsiveness through a series of phosphorylation/dephosphorylation reactions downstream of Rho kinase [140]. In addition, Rho kinase is involved in airway smooth muscle proliferation [141] and plays an important role in airway remodeling in asthmatic patients. With the further study on the mechanism of Rho kinase in asthma, Rho kinase may become a new target for the treatment of asthma [125].

Rho Kinase and IPF

Idiopathic pulmonary fibrosis (IPF) is a kind of interstitial pneumonia characterized by pulmonary fibrosis [142] where, inflammation is the main initiating factor. In the process of inflammatory damage repair, the imbalance between fibrosis and anti-fibrosis leads to abnormal deposition of extracellular matrix and progressive destruction and fibrosis of lung structure, increase of type I collagen in lung interstitium, and decrease of lung compliance. It can induce apoptosis of alveolar epithelial cells. Mair KM *et al.* found that [143] the activation of Rho/Rho kinase signaling pathway promoted the proliferation of lung fibroblasts. Kondrikov *et al.* confirmed that [132] both RhoA activity and collagen synthesis increased in hypoxia induced pulmonary fibrosis model and hypoxia treated lung fibroblasts. Rho kinase inhibitor Y-27632 could reduce collagen synthesis and inhibit fibroblast proliferation [144]. Connective tissue growth factor (CTGF) and its inducible factor transforming growth factor-8 (TGF-8) play a key role in the process of activating fibroblasts and transforming into fibroblasts [145]. Moreover, overexpression of CTGF can lead to abnormal deposition of extracellular matrix and proliferation of fibroblasts [146]. Kono *et al.* found that [147] the plasma CTCF levels were significantly higher in patients with IPF than in those with non-IPF IIPs and healthy volunteers, suggesting that Rho/Rho kinase signaling pathway is involved in the synthesis and activation of CTGF. Watts, *et al.* showed that [148] exotoxin C3, a Rho kinase inhibitor, could inhibit the increase of CTGF synthesis induced by TGF-j3. Therefore, blocking Rho/Rho kinase signaling pathway can inhibit CTGF activity and treat IPF. Rho/Rho kinase signaling pathway may play an important role in the pathogenesis of IPF, and Rho/Rho kinase pathway inhibitors may play a role in the treatment of IPF.

Rho Kinase and Lung Cancer

Lung cancer is a serious threat to human health. In recent years, the incidence of lung cancer is increasing, and the etiology is complex [149] and still unclear. According to the histological classification, lung cancer can be divided into two categories: small cell lung cancer and non-small cell lung cancer (NSCLC). NSCLC accounts for about 75% of cases, including squamous cell carcinoma adenocarcinoma, large cell carcinoma and adenosquamous carcinoma. Cell migration of malignant tumor is the key step of tumor invasion and metastasis. Cell migration mainly depends on actin. Rho/Rho signaling pathway plays an important role in actin contraction and cytoskeleton reorganization by regulating the assembly and retraction of myosin filaments [150], which may be a potential therapeutic target for cancer. It has been found that [151] Rho kinase inhibits migration, invasion, adhesion, and expression of matrix metalloproteinases in tumor cells, and Y-27632 inhibits the motility of NSCLC cells and A549 cells. RhoA protein is located in the process of cell membrane, and its overexpression is positively correlated with the metastasis of tumor cells, and its possible mechanism is to promote the invasion behavior of tumor cells by enhancing the migration of tumor cells [152]. The expression level of RhoA protein in lung cancer cells was much higher than that in normal lung tissues; the expression of RhoA protein and vascular endothelial growth factor were significantly down regulated in lung cancer A549 cells treated with fasudil, a Rho kinase inhibitor [153]. Further studies showed that [154] the migration and invasion activity of NSCIC cells, lung cancer A549 cells and SQ5 cells decreased with Rho dominant negative mutant. The evidence of Rho kinase inhibitors in the treatment of lung cancer is still relatively lacking, and further research is needed [155].

Conclusion and Prospect

Rho kinase participates in the activation and migration of inflammatory cells and the release of mediators, inhibits the contraction and proliferation of airway and pulmonary vascular smooth muscle cells, reduces the proliferation of fibroblasts, and controls the migration and proliferation of lung cancer cells through regulating the phosphorylation of myosin light chain and the occurrence and development of lung cancer. With the deepening of future research and the further elucidation of Rho/Rho kinase signaling pathway in the pathogenesis of these diseases, Rho kinase inhibitors may become a new way to prevent and treat respiratory diseases in the future.

RHO KINASES IN IMMUNE CELLS AND AUTOIMMUNE DISEASES

The guanine nucleotide-binding protein Rho has essential functions in T cell development and is important for the survival and proliferation of T cell progenitors in the thymus. The importance of RhoA in T cell development stems from its ability to mediate proliferative and differentiation signals induced by Src kinase p56Lck and the GTPase Rac-1 in pre-T cells. Thymocyte development is controlled by AgRs, chemokines, and cytokines. The importance of Rho for T cell development has been revealed by studies of transgenic mice that express Clostridium botulinum C3-transferase under the control of T cell-specific promoters in thymocytes [156]. C3-transferase selectively ADP-ribosylates Rho within its effector-binding domain and thereby abolishes its biological function. Transgenic mice that express C3-transferase under the control of the p56Lck promoter have a thymus in which T cell progenitors and subsequent thymocyte subsets are devoid of Rho function. Studies of these mice show that Rho inactivation severely impairs the generation of T cells, resulting in a very small thymus and severely reduced numbers of peripheral T cells. By the way, studies have shown that Rho is also a critical component of survival signaling pathways in T cell progenitors. A complementary strategy to probe Rho function in the thymus has been to examine the effects of a gain of function mutant of RhoA in the thymus [157]. Studies of transgenic mice with T cell-specific expression of an active RhoA mutant, V14RhoA, indicate that [158] activation of RhoA potentiates AgR responses both *in vivo* and *in vitro* . The molecular basis for the role of RhoA in the thymus is not known. However, recent studies revealed that RhoA activation in primary thymocytes is associated with increased (1) integrin mediated cell adhesion [159]. (2) integrin LFA-1 [160]. Integrin-mediated cell adhesion is important for cell migration and evidence indicated that Rho function is necessary for chemokine-induced migration in thymocytes. The directed migration of thymocytes is essential for normal T cell development and any action of RhoA on integrin function could influence the ability of thymocytes to make cell contacts and migrate and could explain why Rho is necessary for thymocyte differentiation.

In the process of inflammation, T cells need to cross the vascular endothelial barrier and enter the tissue to play a role. This process involves the adhesion and polarization of T cells with vascular endothelium, as well as cytokine mediated trans-endothelial migration (TEM). Rho GTPase plays an important role in this process. Mrass *et al.* found that [161] during the migration of T cells from blood to tissue, the front and tail of T cells were polarized, and cell structures such as filiform pseudopodia and plate pseudopodia were extended. RhoA activation was observed in these pseudopods by RhoA biosensor, and RhoA depletion would lead to the disappearance of pseudopodia. The polarity of T cells decreased, and the adhesion and migration of T cells *via* endothelial cells also decreased.

Activation of T cells is the central link in the pathogenesis of many diseases. Some studies have found that under the condition of helper T cell (Th) 17 offset, Rock-2 subtypes in CD[4+] T cells are highly activated. Activated Rock-2 promotes the secretion of inflammatory cytokines such as interleukin (IL) - 17, IL-21 through phosphorylation of interferon regulatory factor 4 (IRF4) [162]. At the same time, Th17 differentiation was impaired in the immature T cells of Rock-2 specific deficient mice, and the expression of transcription factors, retinoid related orphan receptor YT (roryt) and the production of Th17 cytokines such as IL-17 and IL-21 were also decreased. Under the induction of Thl7, through regulating the phosphorylation of signal transducer and activator of transcription 3 (STAT3), ROCK can increase the binding rate of IL-17 and IL-21 promoters, stimulate T cells to secrete IL-10, and play a regulatory role in Thl7/THL signaling pathway.ROCK2-mediated signaling in the cytosol provides a positive feed-forward signal for nuclear ROCK2 to be recruited to the chromatin by STAT3 and potentially regulates TH17/TFH gene transcription [163].

Rho/ROCK signaling pathway also play important role on B lymphocytes. In addition to regulating B-cell skeleton remodeling, RhoA also plays a complex role in the development of B cells. The number of peripheral B cells in CD19 CRE transgenic mice was significantly reduced after RhoA was eliminated [164]. Studies on the dynamics of B cell immune synapse indicate that the internalization of B cell receptor antigen also depends on the activity of ROCK-1 to a great extent. In addition, Azab *et al*. also found that [165] Rocks regulate the adhesion, chemotaxis, migration and other biological activities of B cells.

The process of monocyte migration to inflammatory site and infiltration also involves actin involved cytoskeleton remodeling. By using the rock inhibitor Y27632, it was found that Rocks not only participate in the above process, but also affect the secretion of IL-1β by monocytes [166]. Vemula *et al*. found that [167] selective ROCK-1 ablation can affect the chemotaxis and migration of macrophages *in vivo* and *in vitro* by regulating the phosphorylation and stability of phosphatase and tensihomology (PTEN). In addition [168], in patients with age-related macular degeneration, there is an imbalance of M1/M2. In the classically activated M1 type induced by IL-12 and the selectively activated M2 type induced by IL-10 and transforming growth factor, there is a macrophage polarization mediated by rocks.

Rho/ROCK Signaling Pathway in Systemic Lupus Erythematosus

Systemic lupus erythematosus (SLE) is a chronic autoimmune disease with complex clinical manifestations, which can involve multiple organs at the same time [169]. At present, the pathogenesis of SLE is still not very clear, but in recent years, more and more attention has been paid to the abnormal immune regulation. It was found that [170] in SLE patients, the balance between cells (Th1 cells, Th2 cells, Thl7 cells and regulatory T cells) was lost. Meanwhile, the expression of Thl7 cytokines such as IL-17 and IL-21 was up-regulated in SLE patients and MRL/lpr mice (SLE mouse model) [171]. Therefore, immune disorder plays an important role in the pathogenesis of SLE. In addition, several studies have shown that abnormal activation of Rock-2 has been detected in peripheral blood T cells of SLE patients, and the activity of Rocks decreased after the addition of Rocks inhibitors, and the expression of inflammatory cytokines such as IL-17, IL-21 decreased [170, 172]. The same results were also obtained in animal experiments. After adding Y-27632 into MRL/lpr classic lupus mice model, the production of dsDNA autoantibodies was significantly reduced, and the renal involvement such as proteinuria was also significantly improved [173]. In addition, Apostolidis *et al.* found that [174] protein phosphatase 2A can enhance the activation of rocks, and its catalytic unit is overexpressed in T cells of SLE patients. Based on the regulatory effect of rocks on IL-17, studies have compared the activity of ROCKs in SLE patients with the same gender and age of normal people. Results revealed that [172] the peripheral blood of SLE patients has a significant enhanced rock expression.

The pathological feature of SLE is nonspecific vasculitis. In recent years, some studies have suggested that the pathogenesis of SLE vasculitis is related to ROS [175]. On the one hand, it can directly damage vascular endothelial cells, form indirect damage through protein and lipid peroxidation. In conclusion, ROCKs may be involved in the regulation of SLE through a variety of ways.

Rho/ROCK Signaling Pathway in Rheumatoid Arthritis

Rheumatoid arthritis (RA) is a complex inflammatory autoimmune disease, characterized by synovitis, cartilage degeneration and bone destruction. Recent studies have found that IL-17 plays an important regulatory role in the pathogenesis of RA [176]. IL-17 can promote the secretion of tumor necrosis factor (TNF-a), IL-1 and other inflammatory cytokines in the onset of RA. On the other hand, IL-17 can up regulate the ligand of rank (NF-κB activated receptor factor) and increase the activity of MMPs and promote bone destruction.

The activity of Rocks in peripheral blood mononuclear cells (PBMCs) and synovial cells was significantly higher than that in normal subjects [172]. Stimulation with lipopolysaccharide or TNF-a can promote the activation of Rocks, thus further promoting the production of TNF-a and other inflammatory cytokines by monocytes and fibroblast like synoviocytes by promoting p65 nuclear translocation and activation of NF-κB signaling pathway [177]. In addition, a number of animal experiments have also obtained consistent results [170, 178]. The abnormal increase of Rocks activity was detected in the spleen and synovium of collagen-induced arthritis (CIA) mice mode [178] l, which was similar to SLE animal model experiment [170]. When RA mice were given fasudil, IL-17 and IL-21 were significantly decreased in spleen and joint, and the production of autoantibodies was reduced. Fasudil also inhibits the NF-κB signaling required for binding of NF-κB to specific DNA sequences. Meanwhile, the symptoms of arthritis were relieved [179].

Rho/ROCK Signaling Pathway in Systemic Sclerosis

Systemic sclerosis (SSC) is a chronic fibrosis autoimmune disease [180]. In addition to the skin fibrosis and thickening, the lung, kidney, heart and other organs can also be involved. Its pathogenesis is very complex, including immune dysfunction, microvascular endothelial cell dysfunction and excessive deposition of extracellular matrix (ECM). At present, a number of studies have confirmed that immune imbalance is involved in the pathogenesis of SSC [181]. The immune system is the central stage of SSC. In recent years, an important role for the ROCKs in the regulation of immune responses is also being uncovered [182]. Some evidence showed that ROCK expression is elevated in patients with systemic sclerosis and Rho/ROCK gene polymorphisms have been shown to be associated with this disorder [183]. In hypochlorous acid -treated mice model, fasudil significantly decreased the serum levels of anti-DNA-topoisomerase-1 antibodies, reduced the skin fibrosis and the expression of α-smooth-muscle actin and 3-nitrotyrosine in the fibrotic skin [184]. Other studies have shown that the abnormal activation of Rocks was also observed in another classic fibrotic disease [185]. In addition, the dysfunction of rocks was also observed in the animal models of PAH and Raynaud syndrome [186]. Therefore, it is reasonable to speculate that [184] ROCKs may be related to the formation of vascular complications such as PAH and Raynaud phenomenon in SSC. Consequently, ROCKs inhibitors may become a new therapeutic target for SSC.

CONCLUSION

Rho GTPase/ROCK signaling pathway plays an important role in the activation of immune cells and the secretion of inflammatory cytokines. Its role in the process of inflammation depends on the ability of rocks to regulate cytoskeleton dynamics, cell proliferation and survival, and even gene expression. In recent years, more and more evidence show that this pathway is involved in the pathogenesis of many autoimmune diseases. Therefore, Rocks inhibitors are expected to play a therapeutic role in a variety of autoimmune diseases. However, the molecular mechanism of Rho GTPase/ROCK signaling pathway and the pathogenesis of various diseases are not completely clear, so the therapeutic effect of Rho GTPase/ROCK signaling pathway inhibitors for autoimmune diseases needs to be further improved.

RHO AND CHRONIC KIDNEY DISEASE

Chronic Kidney Disease (CKD) is emerging as a major public health priority worldwide. The main causes of CKD are primary glomerulonephritis, hypertensive renal arteriosclerosis, diabetic nephropathy, secondary glomerulonephritis, renal tubulointerstitial lesions (chronic pyelonephritis, chronic uric acid nephropathy, obstructive nephropathy, drug-induced nephropathy, ischemic nephropathy, hereditary nephropathy (polycystic kidney disease, hereditary nephritis), *etc.* [187]. In developed countries, diabetic nephropathy and hypertensive renal arteriosclerosis have become the main causes of chronic kidney disease [188]. In China, these two diseases still rank after primary glomerulonephritis in various causes, but there is an obvious increase trend in recent years [189]. According to relevant statistics, the prevalence of CKD in American adults (about 200 million) has reached 11.3%. According to some reports in China, the prevalence of CKD is about 10%. The main risk factors of CKD are age (such as old age), family history of CKD (including hereditary and non-hereditary nephropathy), diabetes, hypertension, obesity metabolic syndrome, high protein diet, hyperlipidemia, hyperuricemia, autoimmune diseases, urinary tract infection or systemic infection, hepatitis virus (such as hepatitis B or hepatitis C virus), urinary calculi, urethra obstruction, urinary or systemic tumor, history of nephrotoxic drugs, cardiovascular disease, anemia, smoking, low birth weight, *etc.* Other risk factors include environmental pollution, low economic level, low medical insurance level and low education level. Evidence confirms that [190, 191] Rho kinase system mediates the progress of CKD, and the role of ROCK system in CKD has been paid more and more attention. Many models of different kidney diseases have confirmed that inhibition of Rho/ROCK pathway can improve renal function and reduce renal injury [8, 192]. Surprisingly, *Rock1−/−* mice protected against the development of albuminuria in the model of streptozotocin-induced diabetic kidney disease but are not protected against renal fibrosis in the unilateral ureteral obstruction model [193]. Up to now, the clinical research results of Rho kinase inhibitors in the treatment of kidney diseases are lacking [194].

Rho/ROCK in 5/6 Nephrectomy and Unilateral Ureteral Ligation Model

Kanda *et al.* used 5/6 nephrectomized rats to study the role of Rho/Rho kinase pathway [195]. The results showed that fasudil treatment did not reduce blood pressure, but reduced proteinuria excretion, improved glomerular and tubulointerstitial damage, reduced cell proliferation and renal macrophage infiltration. These results suggest that Rho/Rho kinase pathway is involved in the progression of hypertensive glomerulosclerosis, and inhibition of Rho kinase has non hemodynamic renal protection. Sugano *et al.* confirmed that [196] the use of T-type calcium channel blockers can prevent tubular epithelial cell trans-differentiation and renal interstitial fibrosis in 5/6 nephrectomized animal models, and the mechanism may be down-regulation of Rho kinase activity. Nagatoya k *et al* found that [197] Rho kinase inhibitor Y-27632 alleviated tubulointerstitial fibrosis in rats with unilateral ureteral ligation, but blood pressure did not change significantly, which indicated that Rock was involved in kidney injury of ureteral obstruction animals, and it was probably related to inhibiting the infiltration of inflammatory cells such as macrophages in the early stage and inhibiting the chemotaxis of fibroblasts and neutrophils.

Rho/ROCK in Hypertensive Nephropathy Animal Model

If hypertension is not well controlled for a long time, the structural damage caused by it is difficult to reverse, and renal function damage will gradually appear, even chronic renal failure, and the final serious stage is uremia. Rho/ROCK signaling pathway plays an important role in the pathogenesis of hypertensive nephropathy. Kanda *et al.* found that [195] after 6 weeks of treatment, fasudil could significantly reduce renal Rock activity, reduce proteinuria level, reduce glomerular vascular proliferation and tubulointerstitial inflammatory reaction, down regulate the levels of PCNA and p21 protein in renal glomeruli and tubulointerstitium, and up regulate the level of p27 protein. However, fasudil has no effects on blood pressure. Excessive production of fibrosis is a feature of hypertension-induced renal injury. Activation of Rock axis has been shown in deoxycorticosterone acetate (DOCA)-salt hypertensive rats. Lee TM *et al* found that [198] inhibiting RhoA/Rock axis by selective endothelin receptor blockers can attenuate renal fibrosis in DOCA-salt rats. Moreover, in malignant hypertensive rats, Ishikawa *et al.* found that [199] fasudil treatment for 3 weeks could significantly reduce renal fibrosis, inflammatory cell infiltration and oxygen free radical production, and up regulate the expression of endothelial nitric oxide synthase.

Rho/ROCK in Diabetic Animal Model

RhoA mediates multiple intracellular signaling pathways, and is highly expressed in renal cortex. The ratio of membrane-bound RhoA verses cytosolic RhoA in membrane of renal cortex of STZ diabetic rats was increased by 1.8 times, indicating that actived Rock involved in diabetic renal injury [200]. RhoA/ROCK signaling plays an important role in diabetic nephropathy, and ROCK inhibitor fasudil exerts nephroprotection in experimental diabetic nephropathy but has no effects on blood pressure [201]. Evidence also indicated that [202] fasudil exerts protective actions in STZ-induced diabetic nephropathy by blocking the VEGFR2/Src/caveolin-1 signaling pathway and fibronectin upregulation. Still more, fasudil treatment for 8 weeks could reduce the elevated TNF-α and TGF-β levels and restored the deficit in antioxidant level of the diabetic aorta [203].

Additionally, fasudil markedly improved the endothelial dysfunctionin the diabetic aorta and corrected the dysregulated eNOS expression [203]. Inflammation and fibrosis induced by hyperglycemia are considered to play a critical role in the pathogenesis of diabetic nephropathy. In streptozotocin-induced type 1 diabetic mice model, fasudil significantly decreased urinary protein and serum creatinine, whereas it had no effect on the body weight and blood glucose. Moreover, fasudil increased the number of M2-type macrophages and related anti-inflammatory cytokines, which attenuated renal injury in diabetic mice [204].

Rho/ROCK in Contrast Medium Induced Kidney Injury Model

Contrast medium induced kidney injury is a serious complication of radio-diagnostic procedures [205]. Different strategies have been used [206] for the prevention of nephropathy in different studies. Previously, we found that the mice showed marked increases in the serum Cr, serum BUN and urinary NAG levels following iodixanol administration. However, fasudil treatment attenuated the contrast medium induced increase in the creatinine and urea levels, as well as the structural abnormalities in mouse model. The renal blood flow was detected using color Doppler flow imaging. The administration of iodixanol substantially reduced renal blood flow; the animals displayed increases in renal blood flow and renal vasodilation in response to the high-dose fasudil (10 mg/kg) treatment (Fig. 3). However, low-dose fasudil (3mg/kg) tended to increase renal blood flow non-significantly. Meanwhile, we found that fasudil suppressed renal oxidative stress and inflammation, improved renal antioxidant defense capacity, and modulated the expression of PI-3K/AKT in the kidney, thus inhibiting cellular apoptosis and intracellular vacuolization. These findings support the use of fasudil to combat contrast medium-induced nephrotoxicity [207].

RHO AND PORTAL HYPERTENSION

Portal hypertension (PHT) is an important pathological process during and after the formation of liver cirrhosis [208], which causes many serious complications and seriously affects the quality of life of patients. The pathogenesis of PHT has two theories: forward blood flow and backward blood flow [209]. According to the backward blood flow theory, the increase of intrahepatic vascular resistance is the initial factor of PHT formation, which is the most classic theory of PHT formation. The core of the forward flow theory is that in the later stage of PHT, the visceral hyperdynamic circulation is formed, the vasodilation substances of visceral vessels increase, and the reactivity to vasoconstrictive substances decreases, resulting in vasodilation and increase of portal vein blood flow, thus maintaining portal hypertension. Studies have shown that [210, 211] the abnormal regulation of RhoA/Rho kinase signal pathway in the liver and extrahepatic is involved in the pathogenesis of PHT. The expression of RhoA/Rho kinase signal pathway increased in fibrotic liver tissue and activated hepatic stellate cells (HSC) *in vitro* , which promoted the contraction of HSC and led to the increase of intrahepatic portal venous reflux resistance [212]. However, in extrahepatic tissues, Rho kinase activity decreased, which promoted visceral vasodilation, resulting in PHT worsening. In addition, in PHT animal model, targeting inhibition of Rho kinase activity in liver tissue can significantly reduce portal vein pressure.

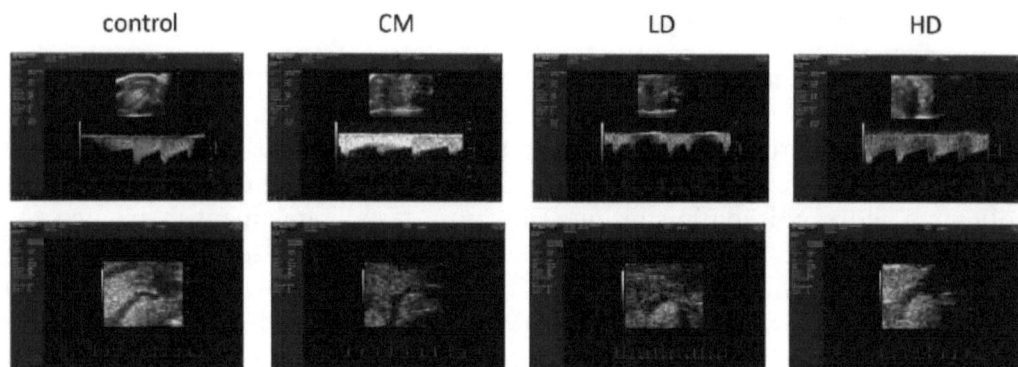

Fig. (3). Fasudil treatment improved the renal blood flow(RBF) in contrast induced renal injury model. Evaluation of RBF was performed with pulse Doppler. The probe was applied to the left flank of each participant and the renal artery was visualized. RBF was automatically calculated from the blood flow velocity and cross-sectional area of the ultrasound echo. CM:contrast medium; LD:low dose(3mg/kg); HD: high dose(10mg/kg).

The increase of intrahepatic vascular resistance during PHT includes two factors: mechanical factors accounted for 70%, functional and changeable factors accounted for 30%. The mechanical factors are mainly manifested as fibroplasia of liver tissue, reconstruction of vascular structure in liver, and increase of portal vein blood reflux resistance. Injury of hepatic sinusoidal endothelial cells and activation of HSC are the key links of PHT. The HSC is located around the endothelial cells of hepatic sinusoids and belongs to another kind of non-parenchymal cells [213]. The HSC around hepatic sinuses experienced morphological and functional changes and became myofibroblast like cells. The activated HSC has the ability to enhance fiber formation, contraction, immune regulation and migration potential. After activation, HSC expressed smooth muscle like protein, which reduced the diameter of hepatic sinusoid, increased the resistance of intrahepatic blood vessels and increased portal pressure; secreted extracellular matrix protein, which led to capillary formation of disc space, and the liver cells and blood could not fully exchange material, which aggravated the damage of liver cells. It has been found that [214] RhoA/Rho kinase signaling pathway in liver tissue has a very important relationship with HSC activation. As early as 1999, Iwamoto H *et al.* found that [215] Rho kinase inhibitor Y-27632 could inhibit the MLC phosphorylation level of cultured HSC *in vitro* , thus weakening the migration and contraction of cultured HSC and reducing the activity of HSC. Zhou *et al.* found that [216] in the PHT model induced by bile duct ligation (BDL), the expression of RhoA and Rho kinase in liver increased at gene and protein levels, and the activity of Rho kinase in liver of cirrhotic rats and patients increased. Systemic and portal hemodynamics in patients with cirrhosis and portal hypertension were measured prior to and 50 min after the initiation of intravenous administration of 30 mg fasudil (n = 15) or placebo (n = 8). After fasudil, significant decreases in mean arterial pressure, systemic vascular resistance, hepatic venous pressure gradient and portal vascular resistance were found [217], whereas the heart rate increased significantly. Intravenous injection of Y-27632 can reduce the sensitivity of isolated perfused liver to vasoconstrictor and reduce portal vein pressure, and the anti-hypertensive effect is dose-dependent [216]. However, the large dose of Y-27632 can reduce the portal vein pressure, and its vasodilation in the visceral circulation also brings about the adverse reactions of reducing the visceral circulation resistance and the mean arterial pressure. Therefore, the key to solve this problem is to develop targeted inhibitors of liver Rho kinase. Kuroda *et al.* combined Y-27632 with the vitamin A (VA)-coupled liposomes carrier for targeted HSCs in steatotic rats [218]. Results have shown that liposomal Y-27632 could inhibit the activation of HSC, inhibit the activity of Rho kinase, reduce intrahepatic vascular resistance, and have no adverse effects on systemic circulation. Xu *et al.* found that [219] salvianolic acid B can also inhibit the activation of RhoA and Rho kinase, weaken the contraction of HSC induced by endothelin-1, and reduce portal pressure. Hennenberg *et al.* found that [220] sorafenib can also inhibit the expression of Rho kinase at protein and messenger RNA levels, reduce the activity of Rho kinase, thus reducing intrahepatic vascular resistance and portal vein pressure. However, sorafenib has no effect on extrahepatic vascular resistance. Therefore, it is speculated that there are other mechanisms regulating the expression of Rho kinase in extrahepatic vessels, which is also one of the problems to be solved in the role of RhoA/Rho kinase signaling pathway in the mechanism of forward flow. In the extrahepatic aspect, RhoA protein expression in the thoracic aorta of BDL rats did not change [216]. However, the expression and activity of Rho kinase decreased in thoracic aorta and mesenteric artery, which was related to the decrease of aortic contractility. Moreover, it is suggested that the signal pathway of RhoA/Rho kinase mainly regulate the contraction of visceral vessels and maintain the resistance of blood circulation. The decrease in Rho kinase expression by Y-27632 can reduce portal vein pressure [221]. In another study, Hennenberg *et al.* found that [222] the expression of MYPT1 and CPI-17, the substrates of Rho kinase in thoracic aorta of BDL rats, decreased the calcium sensitivity of thoracic aorta and promoted the expansion of aorta. According to the current research progress of PHT hyperdynamic circulation, it is not only the thoracic aorta and mesenteric artery dilation, but also the visceral vessels of portal vein in PHT. The changes of RhoA/Rho kinase signaling pathway in visceral blood vessels are unknown. Shi *et al.* treated the patients with portal hypertension caused by liver cirrhosis and complicated by EVB and hypersplenism with phased joint intervention, and measured the expression of Rho, ROCK1 and ROCK2 mRNA and proteins [223]. Results show that phased joint intervention is able to effectively treat EVB and hypersplenism and improve liver function. The efficacy of phased joint intervention may be associated with its role in the regulation of the Rho-ROCK signaling pathway.

OUTLOOK

RhoA/Rho kinase signaling pathway plays an important role in regulating intrahepatic and extrahepatic vascular resistance and increasing portal pressure. Taking this approach as the breakthrough point, the development of drugs for the treatment of PHT will provide a new idea to solve the current dilemma of PHT treatment.

CONCLUSION

In recent years, it has been found that the activation of Rho/ROCK signaling pathway is closely related to the occurrence and development of cardiovascular disease, atherosclerosis, cerebrovascular disease, respiratory diseases, immune cells and autoimmune diseases, and liver disease. As a therapeutic target, Rho/ROCK signaling pathway has attracted more and more attention. Because Rho and rock are widely distributed in the body and involved in complex physiological functions, drugs targeting Rho and Rock have great potential adverse reactions and rarely can be used in clinical practice. At present, there is only fasudil, the ROCK non-specific inhibitors that have been used in the clinic to target Rho/ROCK signaling pathway. However, the systemic inhibition of ROCK affects both the pathological and physiological functions of Rho-kinase, resulting in hypotension, increased heart rate, decreased lymphocyte count, and eventually cardiovascular collapse. In addition, there are many other problems that need to be solved. For example, the physiological functions of the downstream effectors of Rho/ROCK signaling pathway after activation, the interaction between Rho/ROCK signaling pathway and other signaling pathways, the different roles of Rho/ROCK signaling pathway in different tissues and cells, and the different physiological functions caused by different targets of different inhibitors need to be further studied. To further study the physiological function and relationship of

Rho/ROCK signaling pathway with the diseases has important theoretical significance for the development of new target drugs with targeted curative effect, good absorption and less adverse reactions.

ABBREVIATIONS

ROCK	Rho kinase
GTP	Guanosine triphosphate
GEFs	Guanosine nucleoside exchange factors
GAPs	GTPase activating proteins
GDIs	GDP dissociation inhibitors
RBD	Ras binding domain
PHD	Plant homeodomain
CRD	Cysteine rich domain
ADR	Adriamycin
SAH	Subarachnoid hemorrhage
AA	Arachidonic acid
SPC	Sphingosine phosphorylcholine
ROS	Reactive oxygen species
CNS	Central nervus system
VSMC	Vascular smooth muscle cell
PH	Pulmonary hypertension
HPV	Hypoxic pulmonary vasoconstriction
SSc	Systemic sclerosis
AS	Atherosclerosis
MMP	Matrix metalloproteinase
PHT	Portal hypertension
IPF	Idiopathic pulmonary fibrosis
I/R	Ischemia/reperfusion
IRF	Interferon regulatory factor
ERM	Ezrin/Radixin/Moesin
NO	endothelial nitric oxide
NOS	Endothelial nitric oxide synthase
eNOS	Endothelial NO synthase
CAD	Coronary heart disease
CKD	Chronic Kidney Disease
NSCLC	Non-small cell lung cancer

DOCA	Deoxycorticosterone acetate
TNF	Tumor necrosis factor
COPD	Chronic obstructive pulmonary disease
CTGF	Connective tissue growth factor
TGF	Transforming growth factor
MCAO/R	Middle cerebral artery occlusion/reperfusion
OGD/R	Oxygen-glucose deprivation and reoxygenation
SLE	Systemic lupus erythematosus
lncRNAs	Long non-coding RNAs
β-gal	Beta Galactosidase
EF	Left ventricular ejection fraction
HE	Hematoxylin and Eosin
LDH	Lactate dehydrogenase
LV	Left ventricle
MDA	Malondialdehyde
MYPT-1	Myosin light-chain phosphatase
SOD	Superoxide dismutase

CONSENT FOR PUBLICATION

Not applicable.

CONFLICT OF INTEREST

The author declares no conflict of interest, financial or otherwise.

ACKNOWLEDGEMENTS

Declared none.

REFERENCES

[1]   Etienne-Manneville S, Hall A. Rho GTPases in cell biology. Nature 2002; 420(6916): 629-35.
[http://dx.doi.org/10.1038/nature01148] [PMID: 12478284]

[2]   Hall A. Small GTP-binding proteins and the regulation of the actin cytoskeleton. Annu Rev Cell Biol
1994; 10: 31-54.
[http://dx.doi.org/10.1146/annurev.cb.10.110194.000335] [PMID: 7888179]

[3]   Shimizu T, Liao JK. Rho Kinases and Cardiac Remodeling. Circ J 2016; 80(7): 1491-8.
[http://dx.doi.org/10.1253/circj.CJ-16-0433] [PMID: 27251065]

[4]   Zhou J, Yin G, Yu T, *et al.* Rosuvastatin reduces expression of tissue factor through inhibiting
RhoA/ROCK pathway to ameliorate atherosclerosis. Panminerva Med 2019.
[PMID: 31577094]

[5]   Yan Y, Xiang C, Yang Z, Miao D, Zhang D. Rho Kinase Inhibition by Fasudil Attenuates Adriamycin-Induced Chronic Heart Injury. Cardiovasc Toxicol 2020; 20(4): 351-60.
[http://dx.doi.org/10.1007/s12012-019-09561-6] [PMID: 31894538]

[6]   Odagiri K, Watanabe H. Effects of the Rho-kinase inhibitor, fasudil, on pulmonary hypertension. Circ J 2015; 79(6): 1213-4.
[http://dx.doi.org/10.1253/circj.CJ-15-0443] [PMID: 25925979]

[7]   Loirand G, Guérin P, Pacaud P. Rho kinases in cardiovascular physiology and pathophysiology. Circ Res 2006; 98(3): 322-34.
[http://dx.doi.org/10.1161/01.RES.0000201960.04223.3c] [PMID: 16484628]

[8]   Wang Y, Zhang H, Yang Z, Miao D, Zhang D. Rho kinase inhibitor, fasudil, attenuates contrast-induced acute kidney injury. Basic Clin Pharmacol Toxicol 2018; 122(2): 278-87.
[http://dx.doi.org/10.1111/bcpt.12895] [PMID: 28929640]

[9]   Bishop AL, Hall A. Rho GTPases and their effector proteins. Biochem J 2000; 348(Pt 2): 241-55.
[http://dx.doi.org/10.1042/bj3480241] [PMID: 10816416]

[10]   Bustelo XR, Sauzeau V, Berenjeno IM. GTP-binding proteins of the Rho/Rac family: regulation, effectors and functions *in vivo*. BioEssays 2007; 29(4): 356-70.
[http://dx.doi.org/10.1002/bies.20558] [PMID: 17373658]

[11]   Guilluy C, Garcia-Mata R, Burridge K. Rho protein crosstalk: another social network? Trends Cell Biol 2011; 21(12): 718-26.
[http://dx.doi.org/10.1016/j.tcb.2011.08.002] [PMID: 21924908]

[12]   Schofield AV, Bernard O. Rho-associated coiled-coil kinase (ROCK) signaling and disease. Crit Rev Biochem Mol Biol 2013; 48(4): 301-16.
[http://dx.doi.org/10.3109/10409238.2013.786671] [PMID: 23601011]

[13]   Seccia TM, Rigato M, Ravarotto V, Calò LA. ROCK (RhoA/Rho Kinase) in Cardiovascular-Renal Pathophysiology: A Review of New Advancements. J Clin Med 2020; 9(5): E1328.
[http://dx.doi.org/10.3390/jcm9051328] [PMID: 32370294]

[14]   de Sousa GR, Vieira GM, das Chagas PF, Pezuk JA, Brassesco MS. Should we keep rocking? Portraits from targeting Rho kinases in cancer. Pharmacol Res 2020; 160: 105093.
[http://dx.doi.org/10.1016/j.phrs.2020.105093] [PMID: 32726671]

[15]   Sunamura S, Satoh K, Kurosawa R, *et al.* Different roles of myocardial ROCK1 and ROCK2 in cardiac dysfunction and postcapillary pulmonary hypertension in mice. Proc Natl Acad Sci USA 2018; 115(30): E7129-38.
[http://dx.doi.org/10.1073/pnas.1721298115] [PMID: 29987023]

[16]   Hu E, Lee D. Rho kinase as potential therapeutic target for cardiovascular diseases: opportunities and challenges. Expert Opin Ther Targets 2005; 9(4): 715-36.
[http://dx.doi.org/10.1517/14728222.9.4.715] [PMID: 16083339]

[17]   Shi J, Surma M, Yang Y, Wei L. Disruption of both ROCK1 and ROCK2 genes in cardiomyocytes promotes autophagy and reduces cardiac fibrosis during aging. FASEB J 2019; 33(6): 7348-62.
[http://dx.doi.org/10.1096/fj.201802510R] [PMID: 30848941]

[18]   Tawara S, Shimokawa H. Progress of the study of rho-kinase and future perspective of the inhibitor. Yakugaku Zasshi 2007; 127(3): 501-14.
[http://dx.doi.org/10.1248/yakushi.127.501] [PMID: 17329936]

[19]   Bailey KE, MacGowan GA, Tual-Chalot S, *et al.* Disruption of embryonic ROCK signaling reproduces the sarcomeric phenotype of hypertrophic cardiomyopathy. JCI Insight 2020; 5(24): 146654.
[http://dx.doi.org/10.1172/jci.insight.146654] [PMID: 33328387]

[20]   Shimizu Y, Thumkeo D, Keel J, *et al.* ROCK-I regulates closure of the eyelids and ventral body wall

by inducing assembly of actomyosin bundles. J Cell Biol 2005; 168(6): 941-53.
[http://dx.doi.org/10.1083/jcb.200411179] [PMID: 15753128]

[21]   Kher SS, Worthylake RA. Regulation of ROCKII membrane localization through its C-terminus. Exp Cell Res 2011; 317(20): 2845-52.
[http://dx.doi.org/10.1016/j.yexcr.2011.09.009] [PMID: 22001410]

[22]   Okamoto R, Li Y, Noma K, *et al.* FHL2 prevents cardiac hypertrophy in mice with cardiac-specific deletion of ROCK2. FASEB J 2013; 27(4): 1439-49.
[http://dx.doi.org/10.1096/fj.12-217018] [PMID: 23271052]

[23]   Zhang YM, Bo J, Taffet GE, *et al.* Targeted deletion of ROCK1 protects the heart against pressure overload by inhibiting reactive fibrosis. FASEB J 2006; 20(7): 916-25.
[http://dx.doi.org/10.1096/fj.05-5129com] [PMID: 16675849]

[24]   Chitaley K, Weber D, Webb RC. RhoA/Rho-kinase, vascular changes, and hypertension. Curr Hypertens Rep 2001; 3(2): 139-44.
[http://dx.doi.org/10.1007/s11906-001-0028-4] [PMID: 11276396]

[25]   Coleman ML, Sahai EA, Yeo M, Bosch M, Dewar A, Olson MF. Membrane blebbing during apoptosis results from caspase-mediated activation of ROCK I. Nat Cell Biol 2001; 3(4): 339-45.
[http://dx.doi.org/10.1038/35070009] [PMID: 11283606]

[26]   Ark M, Ozdemir A, Polat B. Ouabain-induced apoptosis and Rho kinase: a novel caspase-2 cleavage site and fragment of Rock-2. Apoptosis 2010; 15(12): 1494-506.
[http://dx.doi.org/10.1007/s10495-010-0529-1] [PMID: 20661774]

[27]   Al-Humimat G, Marashdeh I, Daradkeh D, Kooner K. Investigational Rho Kinase Inhibitors for the Treatment of Glaucoma. J Exp Pharmacol 2021; 13: 197-212.
[http://dx.doi.org/10.2147/JEP.S259297] [PMID: 33664600]

[28]   Abbhi V, Piplani P. Rho-kinase (ROCK) Inhibitors - A Neuroprotective Therapeutic Paradigm with a Focus on Ocular Utility. Curr Med Chem 2020; 27(14): 2222-56.
[http://dx.doi.org/10.2174/0929867325666181031102829] [PMID: 30378487]

[29]   Watabe H, Abe S, Yoshitomi T. Effects of Rho-associated protein kinase inhibitors Y-27632 and Y-39983 on isolated rabbit ciliary arteries. Jpn J Ophthalmol 2011; 55(4): 411-7.
[http://dx.doi.org/10.1007/s10384-011-0048-9] [PMID: 21667088]

[30]   Kloner RA, Chaitman B. Angina and Its Management. J Cardiovasc Pharmacol Ther 2017; 22(3): 199-209.
[http://dx.doi.org/10.1177/1074248416679733] [PMID: 28196437]

[31]   Hirooka Y, Shimokawa H. Therapeutic potential of rho-kinase inhibitors in cardiovascular diseases. Am J Cardiovasc Drugs 2005; 5(1): 31-9.
[http://dx.doi.org/10.2165/00129784-200505010-00005] [PMID: 15631536]

[32]   Lai A, Frishman WH. Rho-kinase inhibition in the therapy of cardiovascular disease. Cardiol Rev 2005; 13(6): 285-92.
[http://dx.doi.org/10.1097/01.crd.0000138079.91392.37] [PMID: 16230885]

[33]   Waddingham MT, Edgley AJ, Astolfo A, *et al.* Chronic Rho-kinase inhibition improves left ventricular contractile dysfunction in early type-1 diabetes by increasing myosin cross-bridge extension. Cardiovasc Diabetol 2015; 14: 92.
[http://dx.doi.org/10.1186/s12933-015-0256-6] [PMID: 26194354]

[34]   Zhou H, Li YJ, Wang M, *et al.* Involvement of RhoA/ROCK in myocardial fibrosis in a rat model of type 2 diabetes. Acta Pharmacol Sin 2011; 32(8): 999-1008.
[http://dx.doi.org/10.1038/aps.2011.54] [PMID: 21743486]

[35]   Mihailidou AS. Words Matter: Hypertension and High Normal Blood Pressure Labels. Circ Cardiovasc Qual Outcomes 2021; 14(4): e007751.
[http://dx.doi.org/10.1161/CIRCOUTCOMES.121.007751] [PMID: 33813853]

[36] Kazmi I, Al-Maliki WH, Ali H, Al-Abbasi FA. Biochemical interaction of salt sensitivity: a key player for the development of essential hypertension. Mol Cell Biochem 2020.
[PMID: 33070283]

[37] Xue B, Zhang Y, Johnson AK. Interactions of the Brain Renin-Angiotensin-System (RAS) and Inflammation in the Sensitization of Hypertension. Front Neurosci 2020; 14: 650.
[http://dx.doi.org/10.3389/fnins.2020.00650] [PMID: 32760236]

[38] Gao Q, Zhao X, Ahmad M, Wolin MS. Mitochondrial-derived hydrogen peroxide inhibits relaxation of bovine coronary arterial smooth muscle to hypoxia through stimulation of ERK MAP kinase. Am J Physiol Heart Circ Physiol 2009; 297(6): H2262-9.
[http://dx.doi.org/10.1152/ajpheart.00817.2009] [PMID: 19855056]

[39] Shi J, Zhang YW, Summers LJ, Dorn GW II, Wei L. Disruption of ROCK1 gene attenuates cardiac dilation and improves contractile function in pathological cardiac hypertrophy. J Mol Cell Cardiol 2008; 44(3): 551-60.
[http://dx.doi.org/10.1016/j.yjmcc.2007.11.018] [PMID: 18178218]

[40] Noma K, Oyama N, Liao JK. Physiological role of ROCKs in the cardiovascular system. Am J Physiol Cell Physiol 2006; 290(3): C661-8.
[http://dx.doi.org/10.1152/ajpcell.00459.2005] [PMID: 16469861]

[41] Rikitake Y, Oyama N, Wang CY, *et al.* Decreased perivascular fibrosis but not cardiac hypertrophy in ROCK1+/- haploinsufficient mice. Circulation 2005; 112(19): 2959-65.
[http://dx.doi.org/10.1161/CIRCULATIONAHA.105.584623] [PMID: 16260635]

[42] Yao L, Chandra S, Toque HA, *et al.* Prevention of diabetes-induced arginase activation and vascular dysfunction by Rho kinase (ROCK) knockout. Cardiovasc Res 2013; 97(3): 509-19.
[http://dx.doi.org/10.1093/cvr/cvs371] [PMID: 23250919]

[43] Ito K, Hirooka Y, Sakai K, *et al.* Rho/Rho-kinase pathway in brain stem contributes to blood pressure regulation *via* sympathetic nervous system: possible involvement in neural mechanisms of hypertension. Circ Res 2003; 92(12): 1337-43.
[http://dx.doi.org/10.1161/01.RES.0000079941.59846.D4] [PMID: 12791705]

[44] Awede B, Lemaire MC, Hyvelin JM, Halimi JM, Bonnet P, Eder V. Hemin, a carbon monoxide donor, improves systemic vascular compliance by inhibiting the RhoA-Rhokinase pathway in spontaneous hypertensive rats. Eur J Pharmacol 2010; 626(2-3): 256-61.
[http://dx.doi.org/10.1016/j.ejphar.2009.09.045] [PMID: 19819235]

[45] Ishimaru K, Ueno H, Kagitani S, Takabayashi D, Takata M, Inoue H. Fasudil attenuates myocardial fibrosis in association with inhibition of monocyte/macrophage infiltration in the heart of DOCA/salt hypertensive rats. J Cardiovasc Pharmacol 2007; 50(2): 187-94.
[http://dx.doi.org/10.1097/FJC.0b013e318064f150] [PMID: 17703135]

[46] Calò LA, Ravarotto V, Simioni F, *et al.* Pathophysiology of Post Transplant Hypertension in Kidney Transplant: Focus on Calcineurin Inhibitors Induced Oxidative Stress and Renal Sodium Retention and Implications with RhoA/Rho Kinase Pathway. Kidney Blood Press Res 2017; 42(4): 676-85.
[http://dx.doi.org/10.1159/000483023] [PMID: 29131070]

[47] Yang S, Zhao Y, Tian Y, *et al.* Common variants of ROCKs and the risk of hypertension, and stroke: Two case-control studies and a follow-up study in Chinese Han population. Biochim Biophys Acta Mol Basis Dis 2018; 1864(3): 778-83.
[http://dx.doi.org/10.1016/j.bbadis.2017.12.007] [PMID: 29246448]

[48] Seasholtz TM, Wessel J, Rao F, *et al.* Rho kinase polymorphism influences blood pressure and systemic vascular resistance in human twins: role of heredity. Hypertension 2006; 47(5): 937-47.
[http://dx.doi.org/10.1161/01.HYP.0000217364.45622.f0] [PMID: 16585408]

[49] Rankinen T, Church T, Rice T, Markward N, Blair SN, Bouchard C. A major haplotype block at the rho-associated kinase 2 locus is associated with a lower risk of hypertension in a recessive manner: the

HYPGENE study. Hypertens Res 2008; 31(8): 1651-7.
[http://dx.doi.org/10.1291/hypres.31.1651] [PMID: 18971541]

[50]   Burki TK. Pharmacotherapy for pulmonary arterial hypertension. Lancet Respir Med 2020; 8(11): e81.
[http://dx.doi.org/10.1016/S2213-2600(20)30394-5] [PMID: 32857988]

[51]   Abman SH. Pulmonary hypertension: the hidden danger for newborns. Neonatology 2021; 118(2): 211-7.
[http://dx.doi.org/10.1159/000516107] [PMID: 33951650]

[52]   Turzo M, Spöhr FA, Felix L, Weigand MA, Busch CJ. Kv7 channel inhibition increases hypoxic pulmonary vasoconstriction in endotoxemic mouse lungs. Exp Lung Res 2020; 46(10): 363-75.
[http://dx.doi.org/10.1080/01902148.2020.1818888] [PMID: 32945215]

[53]   Wang XY, Mo D, Tian W, *et al.* Inhibition of RhoA/ROCK signaling pathway ameliorates hypoxic pulmonary hypertension *via* HIF-1α-dependent functional TRPC channels. Toxicol Appl Pharmacol 2019; 369: 60-72.
[http://dx.doi.org/10.1016/j.taap.2019.02.017] [PMID: 30831131]

[54]   Novelli D, Fumagalli F, Staszewsky L, *et al.* Monocrotaline-induced pulmonary arterial hypertension: Time-course of injury and comparative evaluation of macitentan and Y-27632, a Rho kinase inhibitor. Eur J Pharmacol 2019; 865: 172777.
[http://dx.doi.org/10.1016/j.ejphar.2019.172777] [PMID: 31697933]

[55]   Lee AH, Dhaliwal R, Kantores C, *et al.* Rho-kinase inhibitor prevents bleomycin-induced injury in neonatal rats independent of effects on lung inflammation. Am J Respir Cell Mol Biol 2014; 50(1): 61-73.
[PMID: 23947621]

[56]   Oka M, Fagan KA, Jones PL, McMurtry IF. Therapeutic potential of RhoA/Rho kinase inhibitors in pulmonary hypertension. Br J Pharmacol 2008; 155(4): 444-54.
[http://dx.doi.org/10.1038/bjp.2008.239] [PMID: 18536743]

[57]   Fujita H, Fukumoto Y, Saji K, *et al.* Acute vasodilator effects of inhaled fasudil, a specific Rho-kinase inhibitor, in patients with pulmonary arterial hypertension. Heart Vessels 2010; 25(2): 144-9.
[http://dx.doi.org/10.1007/s00380-009-1176-8] [PMID: 20339976]

[58]   Fukumoto Y, Tawara S, Shimokawa H. Recent progress in the treatment of pulmonary arterial hypertension: expectation for rho-kinase inhibitors. Tohoku J Exp Med 2007; 211(4): 309-20.
[http://dx.doi.org/10.1620/tjem.211.309] [PMID: 17409670]

[59]   Abe K, Shimokawa H, Morikawa K, *et al.* Long-term treatment with a Rho-kinase inhibitor improves monocrotaline-induced fatal pulmonary hypertension in rats. Circ Res 2004; 94(3): 385-93.
[http://dx.doi.org/10.1161/01.RES.0000111804.34509.94] [PMID: 14670839]

[60]   Abe K, Tawara S, Oi K, *et al.* Long-term inhibition of Rho-kinase ameliorates hypoxia-induced pulmonary hypertension in mice. J Cardiovasc Pharmacol 2006; 48(6): 280-5.
[http://dx.doi.org/10.1097/01.fjc.0000248244.64430.4a] [PMID: 17204906]

[61]   Zhang Y, Wu S. Effects of fasudil on pulmonary hypertension in clinical practice. Pulm Pharmacol Ther 2017; 46: 54-63.
[http://dx.doi.org/10.1016/j.pupt.2017.08.002] [PMID: 28782712]

[62]   Minelli S, Minelli P, Montinari MR. Reflections on Atherosclerosis: Lesson from the Past and Future Research Directions. J Multidiscip Healthc 2020; 13: 621-33.
[http://dx.doi.org/10.2147/JMDH.S254016] [PMID: 32801729]

[63]   De Flora S, Izzotti A. Mutagenesis and cardiovascular diseases Molecular mechanisms, risk factors, and protective factors. Mutat Res 2007; 621(1-2): 5-17.
[http://dx.doi.org/10.1016/j.mrfmmm.2006.12.008] [PMID: 17383689]

[64]   Wang HW, Liu PY, Oyama N, *et al.* Deficiency of ROCK1 in bone marrow-derived cells protects against atherosclerosis in LDLR-/- mice. FASEB J 2008; 22(10): 3561-70.

[http://dx.doi.org/10.1096/fj.08-108829] [PMID: 18556458]

[65]   Zhou Q, Mei Y, Shoji T, *et al.* Rho-associated coiled-coil-containing kinase 2 deficiency in bone marrow-derived cells leads to increased cholesterol efflux and decreased atherosclerosis. Circulation 2012; 126(18): 2236-47.
[http://dx.doi.org/10.1161/CIRCULATIONAHA.111.086041] [PMID: 23011471]

[66]   Noma K, Rikitake Y, Oyama N, *et al.* ROCK1 mediates leukocyte recruitment and neointima formation following vascular injury. J Clin Invest 2008; 118(5): 1632-44.
[http://dx.doi.org/10.1172/JCI29226] [PMID: 18414683]

[67]   Su Z, Lin R, Chen Y, *et al.* Oxidized Low-Density Lipoprotein-Induced Cyclophilin A Secretion Requires ROCK-Dependent Diphosphorylation of Myosin Light Chain. J Vasc Res 2016; 53(3-4): 206-15.
[http://dx.doi.org/10.1159/000449387] [PMID: 27825172]

[68]   Surma M, Wei L, Shi J. Rho kinase as a therapeutic target in cardiovascular disease. Future Cardiol 2011; 7(5): 657-71.
[http://dx.doi.org/10.2217/fca.11.51] [PMID: 21929346]

[69]   Wu DJ, Xu JZ, Wu YJ, *et al.* Effects of fasudil on early atherosclerotic plaque formation and established lesion progression in apolipoprotein E-knockout mice. Atherosclerosis 2009; 207(1): 68-73.
[http://dx.doi.org/10.1016/j.atherosclerosis.2009.04.025] [PMID: 19473657]

[70]   Dong M, Jiang X, Liao JK, Yan BP. Elevated rho-kinase activity as a marker indicating atherosclerosis and inflammation burden in polyvascular disease patients with concomitant coronary and peripheral arterial disease. Clin Cardiol 2013; 36(6): 347-51.
[http://dx.doi.org/10.1002/clc.22118] [PMID: 23553913]

[71]   Nohria A, Grunert ME, Rikitake Y, *et al.* Rho kinase inhibition improves endothelial function in human subjects with coronary artery disease. Circ Res 2006; 99(12): 1426-32.
[http://dx.doi.org/10.1161/01.RES.0000251668.39526.c7] [PMID: 17095725]

[72]   Förstermann U, Münzel T. Endothelial nitric oxide synthase in vascular disease: from marvel to menace. Circulation 2006; 113(13): 1708-14.
[http://dx.doi.org/10.1161/CIRCULATIONAHA.105.602532] [PMID: 16585403]

[73]   Hamid SA, Bower HS, Baxter GF. Rho kinase activation plays a major role as a mediator of irreversible injury in reperfused myocardium. Am J Physiol Heart Circ Physiol 2007; 292(6): H2598-606.
[http://dx.doi.org/10.1152/ajpheart.01393.2006] [PMID: 17220176]

[74]   Kitano K, Usui S, Ootsuji H, *et al.* Rho-kinase activation in leukocytes plays a pivotal role in myocardial ischemia/reperfusion injury. PLoS One 2014; 9(3): e92242.
[http://dx.doi.org/10.1371/journal.pone.0092242] [PMID: 24638037]

[75]   Zhang YS, Tang LJ, Tu H, *et al.* Fasudil ameliorates the ischemia/reperfusion oxidative injury in rat hearts through suppression of myosin regulatory light chain/NADPH oxidase 2 pathway. Eur J Pharmacol 2018; 822: 1-12.
[http://dx.doi.org/10.1016/j.ejphar.2018.01.007] [PMID: 29337194]

[76]   Gao JY, Yasuda S, Tsuburaya R, *et al.* Long-term treatment with eicosapentaenoic acid ameliorates myocardial ischemia-reperfusion injury in pigs *in vivo*. -Involvement of Rho-kinase pathway inhibition-. Circ J 2011; 75(8): 1843 51.
[http://dx.doi.org/10.1253/circj.CJ-11-0209] [PMID: 21628831]

[77]   Bian H, Zhou Y, Yu B, *et al.* Rho-kinase signaling pathway promotes the expression of PARP to accelerate cardiomyocyte apoptosis in ischemia/reperfusion. Mol Med Rep 2017; 16(2): 2002-8.
[http://dx.doi.org/10.3892/mmr.2017.6826] [PMID: 28656263]

[78]   Cadete VJ, Sawicka J, Polewicz D, Doroszko A, Wozniak M, Sawicki G. Effect of the Rho kinase

inhibitor Y-27632 on the proteome of hearts with ischemia-reperfusion injury. Proteomics 2010; 10(24): 4377-85.
[http://dx.doi.org/10.1002/pmic.201000393] [PMID: 21136592]

[79]   Huang YY, Wu JM, Su T, Zhang SY, Lin XJ. Fasudil, a Rho-Kinase Inhibitor, Exerts Cardioprotective Function in Animal Models of Myocardial Ischemia/Reperfusion Injury: A Meta-Analysis and Review of Preclinical Evidence and Possible Mechanisms. Front Pharmacol 2018; 9: 1083.
[http://dx.doi.org/10.3389/fphar.2018.01083] [PMID: 30327600]

[80]   Li Y, Zhu W, Tao J, *et al.* Fasudil protects the heart against ischemia-reperfusion injury by attenuating endoplasmic reticulum stress and modulating SERCA activity: the differential role for PI3K/Akt and JAK2/STAT3 signaling pathways. PLoS One 2012; 7(10): e48115.
[http://dx.doi.org/10.1371/journal.pone.0048115] [PMID: 23118936]

[81]   Kiss A, Tratsiakovich Y, Gonon AT, *et al.* The role of arginase and rho kinase in cardioprotection from remote ischemic perconditioning in non-diabetic and diabetic rat *in vivo*. PLoS One 2014; 9(8): e104731.
[http://dx.doi.org/10.1371/journal.pone.0104731] [PMID: 25140754]

[82]   Min F, Jia XJ, Gao Q, *et al.* Remote ischemic post-conditioning protects against myocardial ischemia/reperfusion injury by inhibiting the Rho-kinase signaling pathway. Exp Ther Med 2020; 19(1): 99-106.
[PMID: 31853278]

[83]   Li WN, Wu N, Shu WQ, Guan YE, Jia DL. The protective effect of fasudil pretreatment combined with ischemia postconditioning on myocardial ischemia/reperfusion injury in rats. Eur Rev Med Pharmacol Sci 2014; 18(18): 2748-58.
[PMID: 25317813]

[84]   Zhang J, Xu F, Liu XB, Bi SJ, Lu QH. Increased Rho kinase activity in patients with heart ischemia/reperfusion. Perfusion 2019; 34(1): 15-21.
[http://dx.doi.org/10.1177/0267659118787432] [PMID: 30004298]

[85]   Wander DPA, van der Zanden SY, van der Marel GA, Overkleeft HS, Neefjes J, Codée JDC. Doxorubicin and aclarubicin: shuffling anthracycline glycans for improved anticancer agents. J Med Chem 2020; 63(21): 12814-29.
[http://dx.doi.org/10.1021/acs.jmedchem.0c01191] [PMID: 33064004]

[86]   Ma ZG, Kong CY, Wu HM, *et al.* Toll-like receptor 5 deficiency diminishes doxorubicin-induced acute cardiotoxicity in mice. Theranostics 2020; 10(24): 11013-25.
[http://dx.doi.org/10.7150/thno.47516] [PMID: 33042267]

[87]   Amin F, Ahmed A, Feroz A, *et al.* An update on the association of protein kinases with cardiovascular diseases. Curr Pharm Des 2019; 25(2): 174-83.
[http://dx.doi.org/10.2174/1381612825666190312115140] [PMID: 30864507]

[88]   Yu B, Sladojevic N, Blair JE, Liao JK. Targeting Rho-associated coiled-coil forming protein kinase (ROCK) in cardiovascular fibrosis and stiffening. Expert Opin Ther Targets 2020; 24(1): 47-62.
[http://dx.doi.org/10.1080/14728222.2020.1712593] [PMID: 31906742]

[89]   Satoh K, Fukumoto Y, Shimokawa H. Rho-kinase: important new therapeutic target in cardiovascular diseases. Am J Physiol Heart Circ Physiol 2011; 301(2): H287-96.
[http://dx.doi.org/10.1152/ajpheart.00327.2011] [PMID: 21622831]

[90]   Sladojevic N, Yu B, Liao JK. ROCK as a therapeutic target for ischemic stroke. Expert Rev Neurother 2017; 17(12): 1167-77.
[http://dx.doi.org/10.1080/14737175.2017.1395700] [PMID: 29057688]

[91]   Gibson CL, Srivastava K, Sprigg N, Bath PM, Bayraktutan U. Inhibition of Rho-kinase protects cerebral barrier from ischaemia-evoked injury through modulations of endothelial cell oxidative stress and tight junctions. J Neurochem 2014; 129(5): 816-26.
[http://dx.doi.org/10.1111/jnc.12681] [PMID: 24528233]

[92]   Rudrabhatla RS, Selvaraj SK, Prasadarao NV. Role of Rac1 in Escherichia coli K1 invasion of human brain microvascular endothelial cells. Microbes Infect 2006; 8(2): 460-9.
[http://dx.doi.org/10.1016/j.micinf.2005.07.012] [PMID: 16243562]

[93]   Nimnual AS, Taylor LJ, Bar-Sagi D. Redox-dependent downregulation of Rho by Rac. Nat Cell Biol 2003; 5(3): 236-41.
[http://dx.doi.org/10.1038/ncb938] [PMID: 12598902]

[94]   Hong H, Zeng JS, Kreulen DL, Kaufman DI, Chen AF. Atorvastatin protects against cerebral infarction *via* inhibition of NADPH oxidase-derived superoxide in ischemic stroke. Am J Physiol Heart Circ Physiol 2006; 291(5): H2210-5.
[http://dx.doi.org/10.1152/ajpheart.01270.2005] [PMID: 16766636]

[95]   Cui Q, Zhang Y, Chen H, Li J. Rho kinase: A new target for treatment of cerebral ischemia/reperfusion injury. Neural Regen Res 2013; 8(13): 1180-9.
[PMID: 25206412]

[96]   Bouzahzah B, Albanese C, Ahmed F, *et al.* Rho family GTPases regulate mammary epithelium cell growth and metastasis through distinguishable pathways. Mol Med 2001; 7(12): 816-30.
[http://dx.doi.org/10.1007/BF03401974] [PMID: 11844870]

[97]   Nobes CD, Hall A. Rho, rac, and cdc42 GTPases regulate the assembly of multimolecular focal complexes associated with actin stress fibers, lamellipodia, and filopodia. Cell 1995; 81(1): 53-62.
[http://dx.doi.org/10.1016/0092-8674(95)90370-4] [PMID: 7536630]

[98]   El-Sibai M, Pertz O, Pang H, *et al.* RhoA/ROCK-mediated switching between Cdc42- and Rac1-dependent protrusion in MTLn3 carcinoma cells. Exp Cell Res 2008; 314(7): 1540-52.
[http://dx.doi.org/10.1016/j.yexcr.2008.01.016] [PMID: 18316075]

[99]   Liu PY, Liao JK. A method for measuring Rho kinase activity in tissues and cells. Methods Enzymol 2008; 439: 181-9.
[http://dx.doi.org/10.1016/S0076-6879(07)00414-4] [PMID: 18374165]

[100] Sladojevic N, Yu B, Liao JK. Regulator of G-Protein Signaling 5 Maintains Brain Endothelial Cell Function in Focal Cerebral Ischemia. J Am Heart Assoc 2020; 9(18): e017533.
[http://dx.doi.org/10.1161/JAHA.120.017533] [PMID: 32875943]

[101] Satoh S, Kobayashi T, Hitomi A, *et al.* Inhibition of neutrophil migration by a protein kinase inhibitor for the treatment of ischemic brain infarction. Jpn J Pharmacol 1999; 80(1): 41-8.
[http://dx.doi.org/10.1254/jjp.80.41] [PMID: 10446755]

[102] Yano K, Kawasaki K, Hattori T, *et al.* Demonstration of elevation and localization of Rho-kinase activity in the brain of a rat model of cerebral infarction. Eur J Pharmacol 2008; 594(1-3): 77-83.
[http://dx.doi.org/10.1016/j.ejphar.2008.07.045] [PMID: 18703046]

[103] Lu E, Wang Q, Li S, *et al.* Profilin 1 knockdown prevents ischemic brain damage by promoting M2 microglial polarization associated with the RhoA/ROCK pathway. J Neurosci Res 2020; 98(6): 1198-212.
[http://dx.doi.org/10.1002/jnr.24607] [PMID: 32291804]

[104] He P, Guo Y, Wang J, Yan L, Feng A. Protection of ripasudil, a Rho kinase inhibitor, in lipopolysaccharides-induced acute pneumonia in mice. Am J Transl Res 2019; 11(10): 6433-43.
[PMID: 31737195]

[105] Zhang Z, Fauser U, Schluesener HJ. Dexamethasone suppresses infiltration of RhoA+ cells into early lesions of rat traumatic brain injury. Acta Neuropathol 2008; 115(3): 335-43.
[http://dx.doi.org/10.1007/s00401-007-0301-y] [PMID: 17929039]

[106] Silke Dehde, C. v. R.; Stefan Gatzemeier, P. K.; Friedrich Thaiss; Meyer*, T. N., Rho kinase inhibition attenuates LPS-induced renal failure in mice in part by attenuation of NF- B p65 signaling. Am J Physiol Renal Physiol 2009.

[107] Jianjun Z, Baochun Z, Limei M, Lijun L. Exploring the beneficial role of ROCK inhibitors in sepsis-induced cerebral and cognitive injury in rats. Fundam Clin Pharmacol 2021; 35(5): 882-91.
[http://dx.doi.org/10.1111/fcp.12645] [PMID: 33440039]

[108] Yamashita K, Kotani Y, Nakajima Y, *et al.* Fasudil, a Rho kinase (ROCK) inhibitor, protects against ischemic neuronal damage *in vitro* and *in vivo* by acting directly on neurons. Brain Res 2007; 1154: 215-24.
[http://dx.doi.org/10.1016/j.brainres.2007.04.013] [PMID: 17482584]

[109] Zhong Y, Yu C, Qin W. LncRNA SNHG14 promotes inflammatory response induced by cerebral ischemia/reperfusion injury through regulating miR-136-5p /ROCK1. Cancer Gene Ther 2019; 26(7-8): 234-47.
[http://dx.doi.org/10.1038/s41417-018-0067-5] [PMID: 30546117]

[110] Han X, Lan X, Li Q, *et al.* Inhibition of prostaglandin E2 receptor EP3 mitigates thrombin-induced brain injury. J Cereb Blood Flow Metab 2016; 36(6): 1059-74.
[http://dx.doi.org/10.1177/0271678X15606462] [PMID: 26661165]

[111] Yamazaki J, Katoh H, Negishi M. Lysophosphatidic acid and thrombin receptors require both G alpha12 and G alpha13 to regulate axonal morphology in hippocampal neurons. Biol Pharm Bull 2008; 31(12): 2216-22.
[http://dx.doi.org/10.1248/bpb.31.2216] [PMID: 19043202]

[112] Asano S, Ikura Y, Nishimoto M, *et al.* Phospholipase C-related catalytically inactive protein regulates cytokinesis by protecting phosphatidylinositol 4,5-bisphosphate from metabolism in the cleavage furrow. Sci Rep 2019; 9(1): 12729.
[http://dx.doi.org/10.1038/s41598-019-49156-3] [PMID: 31484968]

[113] Huang Z, Huang PL, Ma J, *et al.* Enlarged infarcts in endothelial nitric oxide synthase knockout mice are attenuated by nitro-L-arginine. J Cereb Blood Flow Metab 1996; 16(5): 981-7.
[http://dx.doi.org/10.1097/00004647-199609000-00023] [PMID: 8784243]

[114] Shin HK, Salomone S, Potts EM, *et al.* Rho-kinase inhibition acutely augments blood flow in focal cerebral ischemia *via* endothelial mechanisms. J Cereb Blood Flow Metab 2007; 27(5): 998-1009.
[http://dx.doi.org/10.1038/sj.jcbfm.9600406] [PMID: 17033691]

[115] Yagita Y, Kitagawa K, Oyama N, *et al.* Functional deterioration of endothelial nitric oxide synthase after focal cerebral ischemia. J Cereb Blood Flow Metab 2013; 33(10): 1532-9.
[http://dx.doi.org/10.1038/jcbfm.2013.112] [PMID: 23820645]

[116] Takemoto M, Sun J, Hiroki J, Shimokawa H, Liao JK. Rho-kinase mediates hypoxia-induced downregulation of endothelial nitric oxide synthase. Circulation 2002; 106(1): 57-62.
[http://dx.doi.org/10.1161/01.CIR.0000020682.73694.AB] [PMID: 12093770]

[117] Rikitake Y, Kim HH, Huang Z, *et al.* Inhibition of Rho kinase (ROCK) leads to increased cerebral blood flow and stroke protection. Stroke 2005; 36(10): 2251-7.
[http://dx.doi.org/10.1161/01.STR.0000181077.84981.11] [PMID: 16141422]

[118] Ueno M, Wu B, Nishiyama A, *et al.* The expression of matrix metalloproteinase-13 is increased in vessels with blood-brain barrier impairment in a stroke-prone hypertensive model. Hypertens Res 2009; 32(5): 332-8.
[http://dx.doi.org/10.1038/hr.2009.26] [PMID: 19300451]

[119] Liu K, Li Z, Wu T, Ding S. Role of rho kinase in microvascular damage following cerebral ischemia reperfusion in rats. Int J Mol Sci 2011; 12(2): 1222-31.
[http://dx.doi.org/10.3390/ijms12021222] [PMID: 21541054]

[120] Ishiguro M, Kawasaki K, Suzuki Y, *et al.* A Rho kinase (ROCK) inhibitor, fasudil, prevents matrix metalloproteinase-9-related hemorrhagic transformation in mice treated with tissue plasminogen activator. Neuroscience 2012; 220: 302-12.
[http://dx.doi.org/10.1016/j.neuroscience.2012.06.015] [PMID: 22710066]

[121] Satoh S, Utsunomiya T, Tsurui K, *et al.* Pharmacological profile of hydroxy fasudil as a selective rho kinase inhibitor on ischemic brain damage. Life Sci 2001; 69(12): 1441-53.
[http://dx.doi.org/10.1016/S0024-3205(01)01229-2] [PMID: 11531167]

[122] Song Y, Chen X, Wang LY, Gao W, Zhu MJ. Rho kinase inhibitor fasudil protects against β-amyloi-
-induced hippocampal neurodegeneration in rats. CNS Neurosci Ther 2013; 19(8): 603-10.
[http://dx.doi.org/10.1111/cns.12116] [PMID: 23638992]

[123] Zee RYL, Wang QM, Chasman DI, Ridker PM, Liao JK. Gene variations of ROCKs and risk of ischaemic stroke: the Women's Genome Health Study. Clin Sci (Lond) 2014; 126(12): 829-35.
[http://dx.doi.org/10.1042/CS20130652] [PMID: 24351102]

[124] Cazzola M, Rogliani P, Matera MG. The future of bronchodilation: looking for new classes of bronchodilators. Eur Respir Rev 2019; 28(154): 190095.
[http://dx.doi.org/10.1183/16000617.0095-2019] [PMID: 31871127]

[125] Zhang Y, Saradna A, Ratan R, *et al.* RhoA/Rho-kinases in asthma: from pathogenesis to therapeutic targets. Clin Transl Immunology 2020; 9(5): e01134.
[http://dx.doi.org/10.1002/cti2.1134] [PMID: 32355562]

[126] Zhou Y. Most Good, Least Harm: Isoform-Specific Targeting of ROCK in Pulmonary Fibrosis. Am J Respir Cell Mol Biol 2018; 58(4): 421-2.
[http://dx.doi.org/10.1165/rcmb.2017-0426ED] [PMID: 29717880]

[127] Zhang Z, Nong L, Chen M, *et al.* Baicalein suppresses vasculogenic mimicry through inhibiting RhoA/ROCK expression in lung cancer A549 cell line. Acta Biochim Biophys Sin (Shanghai) 2020; 52(9): 1007-15.
[http://dx.doi.org/10.1093/abbs/gmaa075] [PMID: 32672788]

[128] Bei Y, Duong-Quy S, Hua-Huy T, Dao P, Le-Dong NN, Dinh-Xuan AT. Activation of RhoA/Rho-kinase pathway accounts for pulmonary endothelial dysfunction in patients with chronic obstructive pulmonary disease. Physiol Rep 2013; 1(5): e00105.
[http://dx.doi.org/10.1002/phy2.105] [PMID: 24303177]

[129] Palani K, Rahman M, Hasan Z, *et al.* Rho-kinase regulates adhesive and mechanical mechanisms of pulmonary recruitment of neutrophils in abdominal sepsis. Eur J Pharmacol 2012; 682(1-3): 181-7.
[http://dx.doi.org/10.1016/j.ejphar.2012.02.022] [PMID: 22374257]

[130] Saito H, Minamiya Y, Saito S, Ogawa J. Endothelial Rho and Rho kinase regulate neutrophil migration *via* endothelial myosin light chain phosphorylation. J Leukoc Biol 2002; 72(4): 829-36.
[PMID: 12377953]

[131] Crosby LM, Waters CM. Epithelial repair mechanisms in the lung. Am J Physiol Lung Cell Mol Physiol 2010; 298(6): L715-31.
[http://dx.doi.org/10.1152/ajplung.00361.2009] [PMID: 20363851]

[132] Kondrikov D, Caldwell RB, Dong Z, Su Y. Reactive oxygen species-dependent RhoA activation mediates collagen synthesis in hyperoxic lung fibrosis. Free Radic Biol Med 2011; 50(11): 1689-98.
[http://dx.doi.org/10.1016/j.freeradbiomed.2011.03.020] [PMID: 21439370]

[133] Fernandes LB, Henry PJ, Goldie RG. Rho kinase as a therapeutic target in the treatment of asthma and chronic obstructive pulmonary disease. Ther Adv Respir Dis 2007; 1(1): 25-33.
[http://dx.doi.org/10.1177/1753465807080740] [PMID: 19124345]

[134] Zhang W, Li X, Zhang Y. Rho-kinase inhibitor attenuates airway mucus hypersecretion and inflammation partly by downregulation of IL-13 and the JNK1/2-AP1 signaling pathway. Biochem Biophys Res Commun 2019; 516(2): 571-7.
[http://dx.doi.org/10.1016/j.bbrc.2019.06.072] [PMID: 31235256]

[135] Wang L, Chitano P, Paré PD, Seow CY. Upregulation of smooth muscle Rho-kinase protein expression in human asthma. Eur Respir J 2020; 55(3): 1901785.
[http://dx.doi.org/10.1183/13993003.01785-2019] [PMID: 31727693]

[136] Pazhoohan S, Raoufy MR, Javan M, Hajizadeh S. Effect of Rho-kinase inhibition on complexity of breathing pattern in a guinea pig model of asthma. PLoS One 2017; 12(10): e0187249.
[http://dx.doi.org/10.1371/journal.pone.0187249] [PMID: 29088265]

[137] Koziol-White CJ, Yoo EJ, Cao G, *et al.* Inhibition of PI3K promotes dilation of human small airways in a rho kinase-dependent manner. Br J Pharmacol 2016; 173(18): 2726-38.
[http://dx.doi.org/10.1111/bph.13542] [PMID: 27352269]

[138] Yoo EJ, Cao G, Koziol-White CJ, *et al.* Gα$_{12}$ facilitates shortening in human airway smooth muscle by modulating phosphoinositide 3-kinase-mediated activation in a RhoA-dependent manner. Br J Pharmacol 2017; 174(23): 4383-95.
[http://dx.doi.org/10.1111/bph.14040] [PMID: 28921504]

[139] Xie T, Luo G, Zhang Y, *et al.* Rho-kinase inhibitor fasudil reduces allergic airway inflammation and mucus hypersecretion by regulating STAT6 and NFκB. Clin Exp Allergy 2015; 45(12): 1812-22.
[http://dx.doi.org/10.1111/cea.12606] [PMID: 26245530]

[140] Smith PG, Roy C, Zhang YN, Chauduri S. Mechanical stress increases RhoA activation in airway smooth muscle cells. Am J Respir Cell Mol Biol 2003; 28(4): 436-42.
[http://dx.doi.org/10.1165/rcmb.4754] [PMID: 12654632]

[141] Takeda N, Kondo M, Ito S, Ito Y, Shimokata K, Kume H. Role of RhoA inactivation in reduced cell proliferation of human airway smooth muscle by simvastatin. Am J Respir Cell Mol Biol 2006; 35(6): 722-9.
[http://dx.doi.org/10.1165/rcmb.2006-0034OC] [PMID: 16858009]

[142] Funke-Chambour M. Registries for Idiopathic Pulmonary Fibrosis: When Is It Time to Go Global? Ann Am Thorac Soc 2020; 17(11): 1378-9.
[http://dx.doi.org/10.1513/AnnalsATS.202007-835ED] [PMID: 33124912]

[143] Mair KM, MacLean MR, Morecroft I, Dempsie Y, Palmer TM. Novel interactions between the 5-HT transporter, 5-HT1B receptors and Rho kinase *in vivo* and in pulmonary fibroblasts. Br J Pharmacol 2008; 155(4): 606-16.
[http://dx.doi.org/10.1038/bjp.2008.310] [PMID: 18695640]

[144] Boateng SY, Hartman TJ, Ahluwalia N, Vidula H, Desai TA, Russell B. Inhibition of fibroblast proliferation in cardiac myocyte cultures by surface microtopography. Am J Physiol Cell Physiol 2003; 285(1): C171-82.
[http://dx.doi.org/10.1152/ajpcell.00013.2003] [PMID: 12672651]

[145] Watts KL, Spiteri MA. Connective tissue growth factor expression and induction by transforming growth factor-beta is abrogated by simvastatin *via* a Rho signaling mechanism. Am J Physiol Lung Cell Mol Physiol 2004; 287(6): L1323-32.
[http://dx.doi.org/10.1152/ajplung.00447.2003] [PMID: 15298857]

[146] Shi-wen X, Pennington D, Holmes A, *et al.* Autocrine overexpression of CTGF maintains fibrosis: RDA analysis of fibrosis genes in systemic sclerosis. Exp Cell Res 2000; 259(1): 213-24.
[http://dx.doi.org/10.1006/excr.2000.4972] [PMID: 10942593]

[147] Kono M, Nakamura Y, Suda T, *et al.* Plasma CCN2 (connective tissue growth factor; CTGF) is a potential biomarker in idiopathic pulmonary fibrosis (IPF). Clin Chim Acta 2011; 412(23-24): 2211-5.
[http://dx.doi.org/10.1016/j.cca.2011.08.008] [PMID: 21864521]

[148] Watts KL, Cottrell E, Hoban PR, Spiteri MA. RhoA signaling modulates cyclin D1 expression in human lung fibroblasts; implications for idiopathic pulmonary fibrosis. Respir Res 2006; 7: 88.
[http://dx.doi.org/10.1186/1465-9921-7-88] [PMID: 16776827]

[149] Zhu Z, Li Q, Xu M, Qi Z. Effect of whole-brain and intensity-modulated radiotherapy on serum levels of MIR-21 and prognosis for lung cancer metastatic to the brain. Med Sci Monit 2020; 26: e924640.
[http://dx.doi.org/10.12659/MSM.924640] [PMID: 33125362]

[150] Birukova AA, Adyshev D, Gorshkov B, Bokoch GM, Birukov KG, Verin AD. GEF-H1 is involved in

agonist-induced human pulmonary endothelial barrier dysfunction. Am J Physiol Lung Cell Mol Physiol 2006; 290(3): L540-8.
[http://dx.doi.org/10.1152/ajplung.00259.2005] [PMID: 16257999]

[151]   Hakuma N, Kinoshita I, Shimizu Y, *et al.* E1AF/PEA3 activates the Rho/Rho-associated kinase pathway to increase the malignant potential of non-small-cell lung cancer cells. Cancer Res 2005; 65(23): 10776-82.
[http://dx.doi.org/10.1158/0008-5472.CAN-05-0060] [PMID: 16322223]

[152]   Jeong D, Park S, Kim H, *et al.* RhoA is associated with invasion and poor prognosis in colorectal cancer. Int J Oncol 2016; 48(2): 714-22.
[http://dx.doi.org/10.3892/ijo.2015.3281] [PMID: 26648547]

[153]   Zhu F, Zhang Z, Wu G, *et al.* Rho kinase inhibitor fasudil suppresses migration and invasion though down-regulating the expression of VEGF in lung cancer cell line A549. Med Oncol 2011; 28(2): 565-71.
[http://dx.doi.org/10.1007/s12032-010-9468-5] [PMID: 20300976]

[154]   Shimada T, Nishimura Y, Nishiuma T, Rikitake Y, Hirase T, Yokoyama M. Adenoviral transfer of rho family proteins to lung cancer cells ameliorates cell proliferation and motility and increases apoptotic change. Kobe J Med Sci 2007; 53(3): 125-34.
[PMID: 17684444]

[155]   Zakaria MA, Rajab NF, Chua EW, Selvarajah GT, Masre SF. Roles of Rho-associated kinase in lung cancer (Review). Int J Oncol 2021; 58(2): 185-98. [Review].
[http://dx.doi.org/10.3892/ijo.2020.5164] [PMID: 33491756]

[156]   Tan J, Liu G, Zhu X, *et al.* Lentiviral Vector-Mediated Expression of Exoenzyme C3 Transferase Lowers Intraocular Pressure in Monkeys. Mol Ther 2019; 27(7): 1327-38.
[http://dx.doi.org/10.1016/j.ymthe.2019.04.021] [PMID: 31129118]

[157]   Duke-Cohan JS, Ishikawa Y, Yoshizawa A, *et al.* Regulation of thymocyte trafficking by Tagap, a GAP domain protein linked to human autoimmunity. Sci Signal 2018; 11(534): eaan8799.
[http://dx.doi.org/10.1126/scisignal.aan8799] [PMID: 29895617]

[158]   Wang L, Ellis MJ, Gomez JA, *et al.* Mechanisms of the proteinuria induced by Rho GTPases. Kidney Int 2012; 81(11): 1075-85.
[http://dx.doi.org/10.1038/ki.2011.472] [PMID: 22278020]

[159]   Vielkind S, Gallagher-Gambarelli M, Gomez M, Hinton HJ, Cantrell DA. Integrin regulation by RhoA in thymocytes. J Immunol 2005; 175(1): 350-7.
[http://dx.doi.org/10.4049/jimmunol.175.1.350] [PMID: 15972668]

[160]   Giagulli C, Scarpini E, Ottoboni L, *et al.* RhoA and zeta PKC control distinct modalities of LFA-1 activation by chemokines: critical role of LFA-1 affinity triggering in lymphocyte *in vivo* homing. Immunity 2004; 20(1): 25-35.
[http://dx.doi.org/10.1016/S1074-7613(03)00350-9] [PMID: 14738762]

[161]   Mrass P, Oruganti SR, Fricke GM, *et al.* ROCK regulates the intermittent mode of interstitial T cell migration in inflamed lungs. Nat Commun 2017; 8(1): 1010.
[http://dx.doi.org/10.1038/s41467-017-01032-2] [PMID: 29044117]

[162]   Biswas PS, Gupta S, Chang E, *et al.* Phosphorylation of IRF4 by ROCK2 regulates IL-17 and IL-21 production and the development of autoimmunity in mice. J Clin Invest 2010; 120(9): 3280-95.
[http://dx.doi.org/10.1172/JCI42856] [PMID: 20697158]

[163]   Chen W, Nyuydzefe MS, Weiss JM, Zhang J, Waksal SD, Zanin-Zhorov A. ROCK2, but not ROCK1 interacts with phosphorylated STAT3 and co-occupies TH17/TFH gene promoters in TH17-activated human T cells. Sci Rep 2018; 8(1): 16636.
[http://dx.doi.org/10.1038/s41598-018-35109-9] [PMID: 30413785]

[164]   Zhang S, Zhou X, Lang RA, Guo F. RhoA of the Rho family small GTPases is essential for B

lymphocyte development. PLoS One 2012; 7(3): e33773.
[http://dx.doi.org/10.1371/journal.pone.0033773] [PMID: 22438996]

[165]   Azab AK, Azab F, Blotta S, *et al.* RhoA and Rac1 GTPases play major and differential roles in stromal cell-derived factor-1-induced cell adhesion and chemotaxis in multiple myeloma. Blood 2009; 114(3): 619-29.
[http://dx.doi.org/10.1182/blood-2009-01-199281] [PMID: 19443661]

[166]   Kanno S, Hirano S, Chiba S, *et al.* The role of Rho-kinases in IL-1β release through phagocytosis of fibrous particles in human monocytes. Arch Toxicol 2015; 89(1): 73-85.
[http://dx.doi.org/10.1007/s00204-014-1238-2] [PMID: 24760326]

[167]   Vemula S, Shi J, Hanneman P, Wei L, Kapur R. ROCK1 functions as a suppressor of inflammatory cell migration by regulating PTEN phosphorylation and stability. Blood 2010; 115(9): 1785-96.
[http://dx.doi.org/10.1182/blood-2009-08-237222] [PMID: 20008297]

[168]   Cao X, Shen D, Patel MM, *et al.* Macrophage polarization in the maculae of age-related macular degeneration: a pilot study. Pathol Int 2011; 61(9): 528-35.
[http://dx.doi.org/10.1111/j.1440-1827.2011.02695.x] [PMID: 21884302]

[169]   Rekvig OP. Autoimmunity and SLE: Factual and Semantic Evidence-Based Critical Analyses of Definitions, Etiology, and Pathogenesis. Front Immunol 2020; 11: 569234.
[http://dx.doi.org/10.3389/fimmu.2020.569234] [PMID: 33123142]

[170]   Rozo C, Chinenov Y, Maharaj RK, *et al.* Targeting the RhoA-ROCK pathway to reverse T-cell dysfunction in SLE. Ann Rheum Dis 2017; 76(4): 740-7.
[http://dx.doi.org/10.1136/annrheumdis-2016-209850] [PMID: 28283529]

[171]   Moore E, Huang MW, Jain S, Chalmers SA, Macian F, Putterman C. The T cell receptor repertoire in neuropsychiatric systemic lupus erythematosus. Front Immunol 2020; 11: 1476.
[http://dx.doi.org/10.3389/fimmu.2020.01476] [PMID: 32765512]

[172]   Isgro J, Gupta S, Jacek E, *et al.* Enhanced rho-associated protein kinase activation in patients with systemic lupus erythematosus. Arthritis Rheum 2013; 65(6): 1592-602.
[http://dx.doi.org/10.1002/art.37934] [PMID: 23508371]

[173]   Wang Y, Lu Y, Chai J, *et al.* Y-27632, a Rho-associated protein kinase inhibitor, inhibits systemic lupus erythematosus. Biomed Pharmacother 2017; 88: 359-66.
[http://dx.doi.org/10.1016/j.biopha.2017.01.069] [PMID: 28122300]

[174]   Apostolidis SA, Rauen T, Hedrich CM, Tsokos GC, Crispín JC. Protein phosphatase 2A enables expression of interleukin 17 (IL-17) through chromatin remodeling. J Biol Chem 2013; 288(37): 26775-84.
[http://dx.doi.org/10.1074/jbc.M113.483743] [PMID: 23918926]

[175]   Thieblemont N, Wright HL, Edwards SW, Witko-Sarsat V. Human neutrophils in auto-immunity. Semin Immunol 2016; 28(2): 159-73.
[http://dx.doi.org/10.1016/j.smim.2016.03.004] [PMID: 27036091]

[176]   Doshi G, Thakkar A. Deciphering role of cytokines for therapeutic strategies against rheumatoid arthritis. Curr Drug Targets 2020.
[PMID: 33109042]

[177]   Gong J, Guan L, Tian P, Li C, Zhang Y. Rho Kinase Type 1 (ROCK1) Promotes Lipopolysaccharide-induced Inflammation in Corneal Epithelial Cells by Activating Toll-Like Receptor 4 (TLR4)-Mediated Signaling. Med Sci Monit 2018; 24: 3514-23.
[http://dx.doi.org/10.12659/MSM.907277] [PMID: 29804125]

[178]   Park SY, Lee SW, Lee WS, *et al.* RhoA/ROCK-dependent pathway is required for TLR2-mediated IL-23 production in human synovial macrophages: suppression by cilostazol. Biochem Pharmacol 2013; 86(9): 1320-7.
[http://dx.doi.org/10.1016/j.bcp.2013.08.017] [PMID: 23973526]

[179] He Y, Xu H, Liang L, *et al.* Antiinflammatory effect of Rho kinase blockade *via* inhibition of NF-kappaB activation in rheumatoid arthritis. Arthritis Rheum 2008; 58(11): 3366-76.
[http://dx.doi.org/10.1002/art.23986] [PMID: 18975348]

[180] Utsunomiya A, Oyama N, Hasegawa M. Potential biomarkers in systemic sclerosis: a literature review and update. J Clin Med 2020; 9(11): E3388.
[http://dx.doi.org/10.3390/jcm9113388] [PMID: 33105647]

[181] Yin H, Li R, Lu L, Yan Q. Understanding fibrosis in systemic sclerosis: novel and emerging treatment approaches. Curr Rheumatol Rep 2020; 22(11): 77.
[http://dx.doi.org/10.1007/s11926-020-00953-0] [PMID: 32959073]

[182] Pernis AB, Ricker E, Weng CH, Rozo C, Yi W. Rho kinases in autoimmune diseases. Annu Rev Med 2016; 67: 355-74.
[http://dx.doi.org/10.1146/annurev-med-051914-022120] [PMID: 26768244]

[183] Demiryürek S, Baysalman E, Mammadov A, Demiryürek AT. Contribution of the rho-kinase to systemic sclerosis and Behçet's disease. Curr Pharm Des 2018; 24(29): 3402-9.
[http://dx.doi.org/10.2174/1381612824666180702112137] [PMID: 29962333]

[184] Bei Y, Hua-Huy T, Nicco C, *et al.* RhoA/Rho-kinase activation promotes lung fibrosis in an animal model of systemic sclerosis. Exp Lung Res 2016; 42(1): 44-55.
[http://dx.doi.org/10.3109/01902148.2016.1141263] [PMID: 26873329]

[185] Knipe RS, Tager AM, Liao JK. The Rho kinases: critical mediators of multiple profibrotic processes and rational targets for new therapies for pulmonary fibrosis. Pharmacol Rev 2015; 67(1): 103-17.
[http://dx.doi.org/10.1124/pr.114.009381] [PMID: 25395505]

[186] Fonseca C, Abraham D, Ponticos M. Neuronal regulators and vascular dysfunction in Raynaud's phenomenon and systemic sclerosis. Curr Vasc Pharmacol 2009; 7(1): 34-9.
[http://dx.doi.org/10.2174/157016109787354105] [PMID: 19149638]

[187] Pal R, Rathore V, Galhotra A, Mamidi V. Chronic kidney diseases: A realm for preventive nephrology. J Family Med Prim Care 2020; 9(8): 3810-4.
[http://dx.doi.org/10.4103/jfmpc.jfmpc_1264_19] [PMID: 33110772]

[188] Charles C, Ferris AH. Chronic Kidney Disease. Prim Care 2020; 47(4): 585-95.
[http://dx.doi.org/10.1016/j.pop.2020.08.001] [PMID: 33121630]

[189] Hong T, Su Q, Li X, *et al.* Glucose-lowering pharmacotherapies in Chinese adults with type 2 diabetes and cardiovascular disease or chronic kidney disease. An expert consensus reported by the Chinese Diabetes Society and the Chinese Society of Endocrinology. Diabetes Metab Res Rev 2021; 37(4): e3416.
[http://dx.doi.org/10.1002/dmrr.3416] [PMID: 33120435]

[190] Parrish AR. The cytoskeleton as a novel target for treatment of renal fibrosis. Pharmacol Ther 2016; 166: 1-8.
[http://dx.doi.org/10.1016/j.pharmthera.2016.06.006] [PMID: 27343756]

[191] Dolman ME, Fretz MM, Segers GJ, *et al.* Renal targeting of kinase inhibitors. Int J Pharm 2008; 364(2): 249-57.
[http://dx.doi.org/10.1016/j.ijpharm.2008.04.040] [PMID: 18550305]

[192] Park JW, Park CH, Kim IJ, *et al.* Rho kinase inhibition by fasudil attenuates cyclosporine-induced kidney injury. J Pharmacol Exp Ther 2011; 338(1): 271-9.
[http://dx.doi.org/10.1124/jpet.111.179457] [PMID: 21474569]

[193] Zhou L, Liu F, Huang XR, *et al.* Amelioration of albuminuria in ROCK1 knockout mice with streptozotocin-induced diabetic kidney disease. Am J Nephrol 2011; 34(5): 468-75.
[http://dx.doi.org/10.1159/000332040] [PMID: 21986457]

[194] Hayashi K, Wakino S, Kanda T, Homma K, Sugano N, Saruta T. Molecular mechanisms and

therapeutic strategies of chronic renal injury: role of rho-kinase in the development of renal injury. J Pharmacol Sci 2006; 100(1): 29-33.
[http://dx.doi.org/10.1254/jphs.FMJ05003X6] [PMID: 16397371]

[195] Kanda T, Wakino S, Hayashi K, Homma K, Ozawa Y, Saruta T. Effect of fasudil on Rho-kinase and nephropathy in subtotally nephrectomized spontaneously hypertensive rats. Kidney Int 2003; 64(6): 2009-19.
[http://dx.doi.org/10.1046/j.1523-1755.2003.00300.x] [PMID: 14633123]

[196] Sugano N, Wakino S, Kanda T, *et al.* T-type calcium channel blockade as a therapeutic strategy against renal injury in rats with subtotal nephrectomy. Kidney Int 2008; 73(7): 826-34.
[http://dx.doi.org/10.1038/sj.ki.5002793] [PMID: 18200001]

[197] Nagatoya K, Moriyama T, Kawada N, *et al.* Y-27632 prevents tubulointerstitial fibrosis in mouse kidneys with unilateral ureteral obstruction. Kidney Int 2002; 61(5): 1684-95.
[http://dx.doi.org/10.1046/j.1523-1755.2002.00328.x] [PMID: 11967018]

[198] Lee TM, Chung TH, Lin SZ, Chang NC. Endothelin receptor blockade ameliorates renal injury by inhibition of RhoA/Rho-kinase signalling in deoxycorticosterone acetate-salt hypertensive rats. J Hypertens 2014; 32(4): 795-805.
[http://dx.doi.org/10.1097/HJH.0000000000000092] [PMID: 24463935]

[199] Ishikawa Y, Nishikimi T, Akimoto K, Ishimura K, Ono H, Matsuoka H. Long-term administration of rho-kinase inhibitor ameliorates renal damage in malignant hypertensive rats. Hypertension 2006; 47(6): 1075-83.
[http://dx.doi.org/10.1161/01.HYP.0000221605.94532.71] [PMID: 16636194]

[200] Massey AR, Miao L, Smith BN, *et al.* Increased RhoA translocation in renal cortex of diabetic rats. Life Sci 2003; 72(26): 2943-52.
[http://dx.doi.org/10.1016/S0024-3205(03)00228-5] [PMID: 12706482]

[201] Komers R, Oyama TT, Beard DR, *et al.* Rho kinase inhibition protects kidneys from diabetic nephropathy without reducing blood pressure. Kidney Int 2011; 79(4): 432-42.
[http://dx.doi.org/10.1038/ki.2010.428] [PMID: 20962741]

[202] Jin J, Peng C, Wu SZ, Chen HM, Zhang BF. Blocking VEGF/Caveolin-1 signaling contributes to renal protection of fasudil in streptozotocin-induced diabetic rats. Acta Pharmacol Sin 2015; 36(7): 831-40.
[http://dx.doi.org/10.1038/aps.2015.23] [PMID: 25937636]

[203] Hofni A, Shehata Messiha BA, Mangoura SA. Fasudil ameliorates endothelial dysfunction in streptozotocin-induced diabetic rats: a possible role of Rho kinase. Naunyn Schmiedebergs Arch Pharmacol 2017; 390(8): 801-11.
[http://dx.doi.org/10.1007/s00210-017-1379-y] [PMID: 28493050]

[204] Xie F, Lei J, Ran M, *et al.* Attenuation of diabetic nephropathy in diabetic mice by fasudil through regulation of macrophage polarization. J Diabetes Res 2020; 2020: 4126913.
[http://dx.doi.org/10.1155/2020/4126913] [PMID: 32685556]

[205] Kusirisin P, Chattipakorn SC, Chattipakorn N. Contrast-induced nephropathy and oxidative stress: mechanistic insights for better interventional approaches. J Transl Med 2020; 18(1): 400.
[http://dx.doi.org/10.1186/s12967-020-02574-8] [PMID: 33081797]

[206] Mehran R, Dangas GD, Weisbord SD. Contrast-Associated Acute Kidney Injury. N Engl J Med 2019; 380(22): 2146-55.
[http://dx.doi.org/10.1056/NEJMra1805256] [PMID: 31141635]

[207] Xiang C, Yan Y, Zhang D. Alleviation of the doxorubicin-induced nephrotoxicity by fasudil *in vivo* and *in vitro* . J Pharmacol Sci 2021; 145(1): 6-15.
[http://dx.doi.org/10.1016/j.jphs.2020.10.002] [PMID: 33357780]

[208] Lesmana CRA, Raharjo M, Gani RA. Managing liver cirrhotic complications: Overview of esophageal and gastric varices. Clin Mol Hepatol 2020; 26(4): 444-60.

[http://dx.doi.org/10.3350/cmh.2020.0022] [PMID: 33053928]

[209] Okumura H, Aramaki T, Katsuta Y. Pathophysiology and epidemiology of portal hypertension. Drugs 1989; 37 (Suppl. 2): 2-12.
[http://dx.doi.org/10.2165/00003495-198900372-00003] [PMID: 2680428]

[210] Xu W, Liu P, Mu YP. Research progress on signaling pathways in cirrhotic portal hypertension. World J Clin Cases 2018; 6(10): 335-43.
[http://dx.doi.org/10.12998/wjcc.v6.i10.335] [PMID: 30283796]

[211] Uschner FE, Ranabhat G, Choi SS, *et al.* Statins activate the canonical hedgehog-signaling and aggravate non-cirrhotic portal hypertension, but inhibit the non-canonical hedgehog signaling and cirrhotic portal hypertension. Sci Rep 2015; 5: 14573.
[http://dx.doi.org/10.1038/srep14573] [PMID: 26412302]

[212] Lai SS, Fu X, Cheng Q, *et al.* HSC-specific knockdown of GGPPS alleviated CCl_4-induced chronic liver fibrosis through mediating RhoA/Rock pathway. Am J Transl Res 2019; 11(4): 2382-92.
[PMID: 31105844]

[213] Sato M, Suzuki S, Senoo H. Hepatic stellate cells: unique characteristics in cell biology and phenotype. Cell Struct Funct 2003; 28(2): 105-12.
[http://dx.doi.org/10.1247/csf.28.105] [PMID: 12808230]

[214] Klein S, Van Beuge MM, Granzow M, *et al.* HSC-specific inhibition of Rho-kinase reduces portal pressure in cirrhotic rats without major systemic effects. J Hepatol 2012; 57(6): 1220-7.
[http://dx.doi.org/10.1016/j.jhep.2012.07.033] [PMID: 22878469]

[215] Iwamoto H, Nakamuta M, Tada S, Sugimoto R, Enjoji M, Nawata H. A p160ROCK-specific inhibitor, Y-27632, attenuates rat hepatic stellate cell growth. J Hepatol 2000; 32(5): 762-70.
[http://dx.doi.org/10.1016/S0168-8278(00)80245-7] [PMID: 10845663]

[216] Zhou Q, Hennenberg M, Trebicka J, *et al.* Intrahepatic upregulation of RhoA and Rho-kinase signalling contributes to increased hepatic vascular resistance in rats with secondary biliary cirrhosis. Gut 2006; 55(9): 1296-305.
[http://dx.doi.org/10.1136/gut.2005.081059] [PMID: 16492715]

[217] Fukuda T, Narahara Y, Kanazawa H, *et al.* Effects of fasudil on the portal and systemic hemodynamics of patients with cirrhosis. J Gastroenterol Hepatol 2014; 29(2): 325-9.
[http://dx.doi.org/10.1111/jgh.12360] [PMID: 24033356]

[218] Kuroda S, Tashiro H, Kimura Y, *et al.* Rho-kinase inhibitor targeting the liver prevents ischemia/reperfusion injury in the steatotic liver without major systemic adversity in rats. Liver Transpl 2015; 21(1): 123-31.
[http://dx.doi.org/10.1002/lt.24020] [PMID: 25307969]

[219] Xu H, Zhou Y, Lu C, Ping J, Xu LM. Salvianolic acid B lowers portal pressure in cirrhotic rats and attenuates contraction of rat hepatic stellate cells by inhibiting RhoA signaling pathway. Lab Invest 2012; 92(12): 1738-48.
[http://dx.doi.org/10.1038/labinvest.2012.113] [PMID: 22986787]

[220] Hennenberg M, Trebicka J, Stark C, Kohistani AZ, Heller J, Sauerbruch T. Sorafenib targets dysregulated Rho kinase expression and portal hypertension in rats with secondary biliary cirrhosis. Br J Pharmacol 2009; 157(2): 258-70.
[http://dx.doi.org/10.1111/j.1476-5381.2009.00158.x] [PMID: 19338580]

[221] Kawada N, Seki S, Kuroki T, Kaneda K. ROCK inhibitor Y-27632 attenuates stellate cell contraction and portal pressure increase induced by endothelin-1. Biochem Biophys Res Commun 1999; 266(2): 296-300.
[http://dx.doi.org/10.1006/bbrc.1999.1823] [PMID: 10600496]

[222] Hennenberg M, Trebicka J, Biecker E, Schepke M, Sauerbruch T, Heller J. Vascular dysfunction in human and rat cirrhosis: role of receptor-desensitizing and calcium-sensitizing proteins. Hepatology

2007; 45(2): 495-506.
[http://dx.doi.org/10.1002/hep.21502] [PMID: 17256744]

[223] Shi M, Wei J, Meng WY, Wang N, Wang T, Wang YG. Effects of phased joint intervention on Rho/ROCK expression levels in patients with portal hypertension. Exp Ther Med 2016; 12(3): 1618-24.
[http://dx.doi.org/10.3892/etm.2016.3454] [PMID: 27602079]

CHAPTER 3

Hibernation or Transformation? Challenges in Cardiovascular Drug Development

G. Mercanoglu[1,*] and F. Mercanoglu[2]

[1] *Department of Pharmacology, Hamidiye Faculty of Pharmacy, University of Health Sciences, Istanbul, Turkey*

[2] *Department of Cardiology, Istanbul Medical Faculty, Istanbul University, Istanbul, Turkey*

Abstract: The decline in deaths from cardiovascular diseases in line with scientific developments between 1950-2010 was impressive. Despite these significant advances, cardiovascular (CV) diseases remain the leading cause of death worldwide. According to the World Health Organization (WHO) data, 17.9 million people die due to CV diseases every year, which corresponds to 31% of the total deaths worldwide. Therefore, for many CV diseases, there is still a need for improved treatment, and this is only possible with the development of new drugs.

Although investments in the previous decade have resulted in the development of many innovative drugs in the treatment of CV diseases, today, pharmaceutical companies are less enthusiastic about developing CV drugs, mainly due to financial and regulatory difficulties. Indeed, today, institutes, associations and even organizations such as WHO are taking over the sponsorship role that pharmaceutical industry players have abandoned. In parallel, cardiovascular pipeline activity is shifting from large pharmaceutical companies to small and medium-sized companies and from fast-following drugs to first-in classes. This transformation in CV drug discovery and development reveals significant challenges that require square up to. The aim of this chapter is to discuss the global challenges faced in CV drug discovery and development to find effective solutions.

Keywords: Cardiovascular Drug Development, Cardiovascular Drug Discovery, Challenges in Cardiovascular Drug Development.

INTRODUCTION

It is impossible to disagree with the words of Braunwald, the most well-known cardiologist, during his presentation at the Europen Society of Cardiology (ESC) Congress-2013, that "the pathways of discovery, innovation and therapeutic

---

*Corresponding author G. Mercanoglu:** Department of Pharmacology, Hamidiye Faculty of Pharmacy, University of Health Sciences, Istanbul, Turkey; Tel: +90 (536) 267 38 80; E-mail: guldemiko@gmail.com

M. Iqbal Choudhary (Ed.)

advancement in cardiovascular science and medicine over the past two centuries have been truly remarkable". Especially in the last two centuries, serious progress has been made in the cardiovascular (CV) field, and as a result of the advances in the field, there has been a serious decrease in CV mortality rates. CV mortality rate reported as 450/100,000 in 1950 decreased to 100/100,000 by 2010 [1]. Many clinical developments have contributed to this impressive decline, and these clinical advances are undoubtedly accompanied by new CV agents. Beta-blockers, angiotensin converting enzyme inhibitors (ACE inhibitor), HMGCoA inhibitors (statins) are among the first ones to come to mind (Fig. **1**).

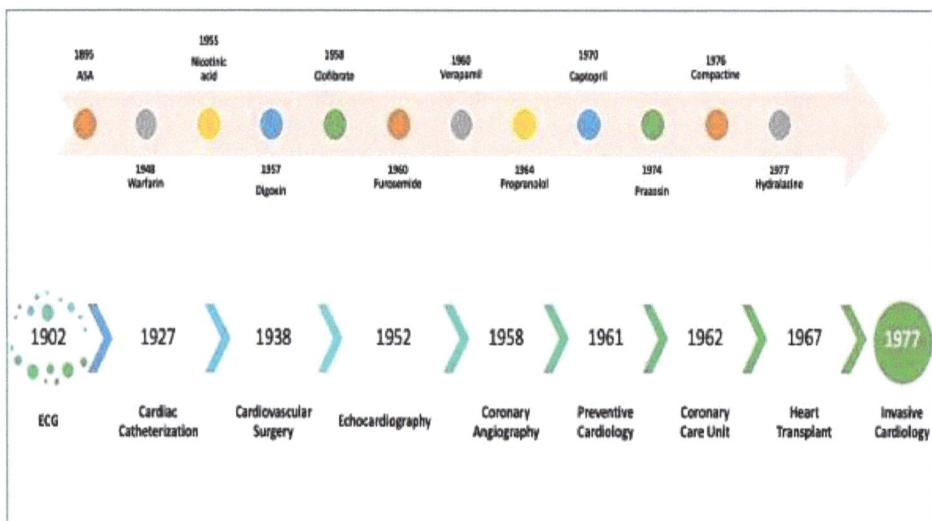

Fig. (1). Milestones in CV therapy and drug development.

Despite these significant advances, CV diseases remain the leading cause of death worldwide. According to the World Health Organization (WHO) data, 17.9 million people die due to CV diseases every year, which corresponds to 31% of the total deaths worldwide [2]. In addition to mortality, the burden of comorbidities accompanying CV diseases, especially diabetes and obesity, and heart failure, which develops following myocardial infarction and has a worse prognosis, continues to be both an important public health problem and an increasing financial problem on a global scale.

New drug development is becoming increasingly difficult and costly for the industry. Introducing a new drug into the market requires 10-12 years of labor and an average investment of 3-5 million$ [3]. Testing each potential new treatment independently of the current treatments used for the related disease requires additional labor and cost [4]. Also, whether the newly developed product will be included in the reimbursement system is another concern [5].

Existing data clearly shows that due to all these concerns, the investment put towards developing new CV drugs is declining day by day. Despite the increasing CV disease load worldwide, CV drug development has come to a standstill, especially within the last two decades. According to the American Food and Drug Administration (FDA) data, only one out of 53 newly approved molecules in 2020 is for CV diseases [6]. Considering the fact that this ratio was 5/22 in 2002, the stagnation in CV drug development becomes clearly visible.

Evaluating the challenges in new drug development specific to the CV field and having a clear picture of the current situation is key to producing effective solutions. Therefore, in this chapter, challenges in developing drugs in the CV field will be evaluated with examples related to the basic steps of developing new drugs. We hope that the analysis of the current situation will be fruitful for all shareholders in terms of bringing effective solutions to the challenges in new CV drug development.

DEVELOPING NEW DRUGS IN THE 21st CENTURY

The process from the identification or creation of a new molecule suitable for a therapeutic goal to its introduction into clinical use is generally referred to as the drug development process. In a broader sense, drug development or drug discovery requires a variety of flows and disciplines in clinical development and pharmaceutical production. Drug discovery is the first major milestone in this labor-intensive marathon that lasted for about a decade. The discovery or synthesis of a promising molecule is followed by the regulatory authority approval phase before the clinical benefit of the related molecule is demonstrated and before it is placed on the market as a drug [7] (Fig. **2**).

The traditional academic research culture that brought us into the twenty-first century, in which chemists, biologists, and other scientists come together under the umbrella of a commercial organization aiming to sell the developed drug globally, has now been replaced by a new operating environment in which new players (internal and external stakeholders) are included. Undoubtedly, the most effective player in this new operating environment is payers (governments or insurance companies) responsible for therapeutic treatments of patients, whose aim is to provide significantly improved treatments with the most affordable drug costs possible. For example, in order for a new medical therapy developed for treating chronic kidney failure to be covered by insurance, the treatment should delay the transition to end-stage renal failure for at least two years. Undoubtedly, the second major player that shapes this operating environment is the investor who aims to get a good financial return from their investments with an annually increasing income, and therefore, waits for quarterly financial reports that greatly affect share prices [8]. So how can the decision to develop a new drug, involving discovery-clinical development and regulatory approval phases, which involve many failures and require a period of 10-12 years, can be taken in line with the objectives of these two big players of the operating environment: "improved therapy"/"quarterly returns"? How do the R&D departments of pharmaceutical companies challenge this paradox? Let us take a look at the challenges that need to be tackled in the basic drug development phases.

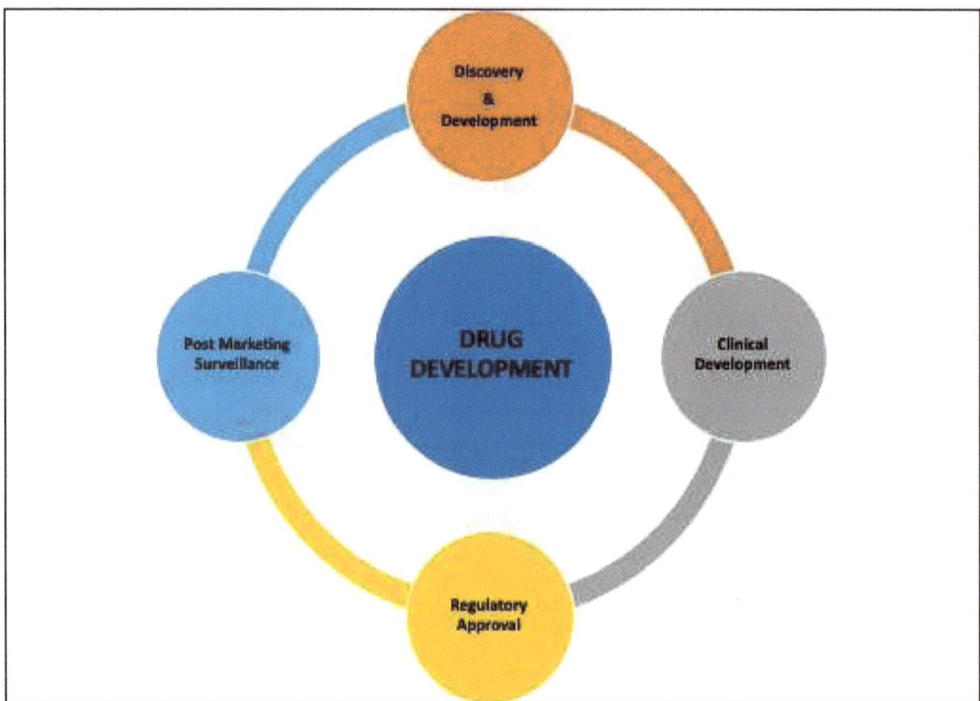

Fig. (2). Drug development stages.

CHALLENGES IN DRUG DEVELOPMENT AND THEIR REFLECTIONS ON THE CARDIOVASCULAR FIELD

DISCOVERY AND DEVELOPMENT

Drug discovery is a multifaceted process aimed at identifying a therapeutically beneficial molecule in the treatment of a disease. Typically, the drug discovery effort aims at a biological target involved in the development of the disease or starts from a molecule with an interesting biological activity. The drug discovery phase includes the identification, synthesis, characterization and analysis of the candidates for their therapeutic effects (Fig. **3**).

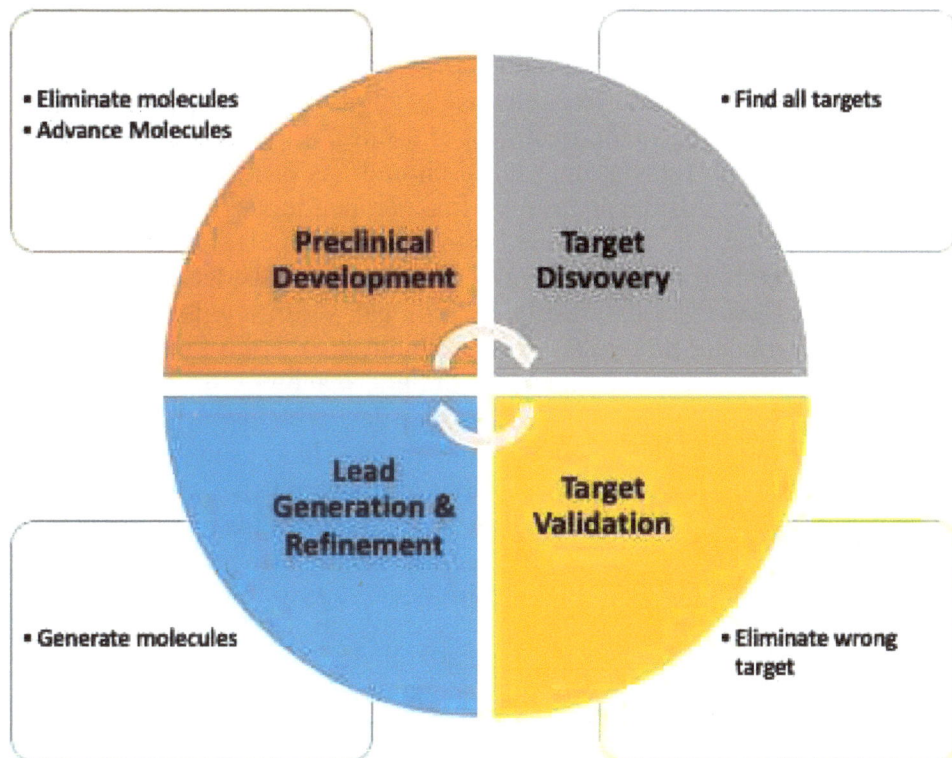

Fig. (3).   Drug discovery and development steps and the main goals. (adopted from https://www.nebiolab.com/drug-discovery-and-development-process/).

The development process of the compound, which is found effective in these tests, begins before clinical trials [9]. Drug discovery and development processes are costly due to the high budgets required for R&D and clinical trials [10]. The average cost for research and development is estimated to be between 900 million and 2 billion dollars per drug. This amount includes the cost of thousands of failures. Because, among the 5.000 – 10.000 compounds scanned, only one can get approval [11]. Success requires serious resources, scientific thinking and logical brains, sophisticated laboratories and technology as well as good project management. Of course, we shouldn't forget about luck [12]. After all, this brings hope and faith to billions of patients in addition to the profit for the manufacturer [13].

Challenges in Strategic Decision Making

In today's drug development environment, which was mentioned in previous sections, the selection and approval of the appropriate research proposal is strategically the biggest challenge. Today, this selection is made in favor of research projects with academic/industry partnership, which is described as translational research. In fact, since the use of digitalis purpurea extract isolated and purified by Withering in the treatment of ascites, the pharmaceutical industry has been familiar with translational research and has used it in drug discovery until the last century. But can a specific therapeutic target with very good preclinical data always be transformed into a safe and potent drug? Today, it is widely accepted that an increase in HDL cholesterol levels decreases the risk of atherosclerosis. However, the results of clinical studies with torceptrapib, a cholesteryl ester transfer protein (CEPT) inhibitor, are the most striking examples of the drug's failure to turn biochemistry and pharmacology into clinical benefit [14]. Another example for failure is omapatrilat, which was developed as a vasopeptidase inhibitor. Although omaprilat has shown very good antihypertensive activity in clinical studies in hypertensive patients, it is not licensed for safety reasons as the incidence of angioedema is higher compared to ACE inhibitors [15]. It seems that the cardiovascular system drugs available in the market have raised the safety bar high up for new drugs to be developed.

So, what are the challenges of this academic/industry partnership from an operational point of view? According to economic research, the main concern in this partnership is that despite academic research being the main source of new scientific concepts, the use of this research in drug discovery means following an unpredictable and tortuous path. In fact, according to the study in which Dusting *et al*. evaluated the strengths and weaknesses of academic/industry collaboration, research institutes often neglect effective cooperation principles and practices [16]. Considering all risks, which direction should the strategic decision take? "Speculative research proposals with unproven therapeutic efficacy? (often referred to as first-in-class)" or "alternatives to the leading molecules of the group with known therapeutic efficacy but with serious disadvantages in clinical practice (usually referred to as fast-following)"? Although the general trend is towards the latter, there are also first-in-class examples that succeeded as a result of the decision to continue despite early failures. The most striking of these examples is the story of the development of the first ACE inhibitor at the Squip Institute for Medical Research. Until the blood pressure lowering effect of teprotidine, the first peptide inhibitor, was shown in 1970, the important role of the renin angiotensin system in the regulation of blood pressure was met with suspicion among clinicians. After this discovery, Squip's pharmacology consultant Prof. Sir John Vane shared with the R&D directors the idea that inhibition of his enzyme could have a therapeutic effect. Although more than two thousand analogs were scanned, no results were obtained, bringing ACE inhibitor studies to a halt [17]. Despite all these problems, the insistence and works of the R&D director Cushman resulted in the discovery of captopril a year later and its subsequent introduction to the market in 1978. This discovery is also deemed one of the best examples of academy/industry cooperation [18]. Another effective project director was Garnet Devis, the research director of the Pharmaceutical Department of the Imperial Chemical Industries, which was the biggest chemistry company of England established in 1926. Under his directorate, the first beta-blocker agents propranolol and tenormin, as well as the first anti-estrogen agent tamoxifen were developed and marketed. We should also not forget the pharmacologist Dr. Paul Janssen, the founder of Johnson & Johnson affiliate Janssen Pharmaceuticals, who invented the first antipsychotic agent, haloperidol, and the narcotic analgesic fentanyl, which we still use today, and who has brought more than 40 products to the market in the last 30 years until 1984 [19].

Challenges in Preclinical Trials

It is essential to show the specificity of the target for the drug candidate molecule and the selectivity of the candidate molecule for this target before moving on to the clinical phase. So, what are the specific targets for new cardiovascular agents? Traditionally, cardiovascular drug development has focused on systemic therapies centered upon large populations such as hypertension and heart failure. However, these conditions result from multiple heterogeneous effects and pathways and have several potential therapeutic biological targets [20]. There are relatively few drug targets that can be completely separated from current targets for cardiovascular disease. Because in the cardiovascular drug groups, there are more than one effective drug (such as statins, antiplatelet drugs, new anticoagulants) that makes differentiation from existing treatments difficult. This is one of the major challenges in developing new agents. Following the well-known targeted treatment strategies for oncology and infectious diseases, today might be the key for overcoming this challenge for cardiovascular diseases as well. If heterogeneous diseases that have been clustered as a result of not examining the rapidly emerging molecular data in the International Classification of Disease (ICD), the basic international classification of the World Health Organization (WHO), coincidental patient characteristics or socio-environmental effects on the disease can be divided into subclasses with an approach that represents the underlying socio-pathophysiology better and is based on biological signatures that allow for a more clear treatment target, understanding the molecular basis of the disease in early drug development steps and developing appropriate biomarkers for therapeutic suitability can be achieved [21]. Identifying appropriate biomarkers for cardiovascular diseases can be used to predict treatment response because these biomarkers allow the disease to be detected in the early stages before the onset of symptoms, which is usually the stage at which the disease can be prevented or most treated [22]. In this context, genomic, proteomic and metabolomic technologies combined with physiological profiling and molecular imaging methods can provide valuable information. Different gene and protein expressions in a disease can provide valuable insight into this process. However, unlike different types of cancer, cardiovascular diseases are not caused by a single gene mutation, but rather reflect the interactions of risk factors with multiple genes, each contributing to a small portion of the risk [23]. Thus, biological targets for cardiovascular disease appear to be somewhat more complex compared to oncology currently. Indeed, the cardiovascular gene therapy agent Mydicar® (AAV1/SERCA2a), originally described as a 'breakthrough', failed to meet the primary and secondary endpoints in Phase IIb CUPID2 trial for systolic heart failure [24].

Studies in regenerative medicine, where rapid advances have been made, especially in the last decade, may also contribute to the development of specific targets for new cardiovascular system agents. Research towards the rate, change, or regeneration mechanisms in cardiac and vascular tissue to restore cardiovascular function following pathology promises much in the identification of new specific targets [25]. In addition to the determination of specific targets, the use of technological approaches such as stem cells, soluble molecules, genetic and tissue engineering and advanced cell therapy alone or in combination also appear as alternative treatment candidates. Stem cell therapies are the most studied of these alternative methods [26]. Although promising results have been reported in preclinical animal and early phase studies on stem cell therapies for ischemic heart muscle regeneration after myocardial infarction and cardiomyopathy, cardiac cells obtained from different sources (embryonic stem cells, fetal and neonatal cardiomyocytes, skeletal myoblasts, bone marrow stem cells) the results of the relatively large clinical trials with cells are contradictory. These contradictory results are thought to be due to differences in stem cell preparation (different strategies for cells obtained from different sources to cardiac muscle cells, *in-vitro* propagation and purification methods of cells, large-scale culture techniques) and transplantation techniques. Although the related studies have produced beneficial results in the early period, especially a decrease in mortality, arrhythmia, which develops as a result of the transplanted cells not being able to integrate structurally and functionally into the host myocardium, is the most serious risk for the related treatments [27]. Therefore, there is still a need for comprehensive clinical studies evaluating the efficacy and safety of stem cell therapies in the long term.

Before the transition to the clinical phase, the safety of the candidate drug molecule must be shown as well as its efficacy. This ensures that the "go/no-go" decision is taken earlier for moving on to clinical trial, avoiding both financial and temporal losses. The rapid identification of drugs that do not meet the safety criteria is a critical element in modern drug discovery strategies. In order to prevent unexpected safety problems in the late stages of the development process, in silico and *in vitro* technological methods, in which in vivo results can be predicted, are alternatives to traditional animal toxicity tests in predicting toxic effects in the early stages of the discovery process. For example, the application of in silico models to cardiac electrophysiology allows the evaluation of drug effects on multiple ion channels. A practical example of this is the demonstration that ranolazine, an antianginal drug, binds prominently to the potassium channels of the cardiac human ether-a-go-go-related gene (hERG), but inhibits Q-T prolongation by acting through other ion channels without causing torsades de pointes [28]. Again, as a classic example, although verapamil, a calcium channel blocker, causes QT prolongation depending on the dose, it does not cause torsades de pointes due to the multiple cardiac ion channel effect [29]. Another type of exciting work in this field is the use of human pluripotent stem cell-derived cardiomyocytes. Such studies conducted on isolated targets alone do not eliminate the need for *in-vivo* studies, since they cannot reflect the *in-vivo* environment as a whole. Again, another disadvantage of these studies is that the related studies cannot reflect the clinical situation in which a new molecule was added to an already existing treatment.

Although new molecules with potential new drug targets and potential cardiovascular applications have been identified as a result of the application of genomic technologies and systems biology approaches, unfortunately, data show that these scientific advances have not been reflected in the development of new cardiovascular drugs. In a study comparing the number of early-stage drugs being developed in two different periods (1990-1999 and 2000-2007), it was reported that an increase of 6.88% in antineoplastic agents was observed between the two periods, whereas a 4.57% decrease in cardiovascular agents was observed [30]. In parallel with these data, the number of antineoplastic drug approvals increased in the related time interval [31]. While oncological drugs ranked first in NDA applications made to the FDA between 2000-2012 with a total of 61 applications, these group of agents also constituted the group that received approval at the first application among all therapeutic groups. In the related period, the number of NDA applications for cardiovascular drugs was 21, and only 7 of these applications were approved at the first application (fist-cycle approval) [32].

Historically, various animal models have been used to determine the etiology, pathogenesis, and pathophysiology of cardiovascular diseases. Animal models are also a valuable tool for drug discovery and the development of new treatment alternatives. As a matter of fact, there are in vivo models used by the pharmaceutical industry for congestive heart failure, cardiac ischemia secondary to atherothrombosis, cardiac dysrhythmia and hypertension. However, experimentally induced pathology in animals is different in terms of cardiovascular and pathophysiological features in humans [33]. Again, the absence of animal models in which genetic, environmental factors and long-term cardiac pathology and accompanying pathology can be reflected does not allow the complex structure of cardiovascular diseases to be demonstrated on a single model. For example, although potential targets for the treatment of congestive heart failure are closely related to the explanation of the tissue anomaly mechanism at the cellular level, there is an unspecific relationship between these targets and the clinical phenotype of congestive heart failure. This is the main reason why many of the agents introduced to the market in recent years are lipoprotein modulators or antithrombotic agents designed to reduce the complications of atherothrombosis. Because such molecular targets are characterized by more robust and predictable mechanistic hypotheses in *in-vivo* animal models [8]. Yet another example is the prevention of ischemia-reperfusion damage and cardiac protection. Targets to be modulated are controversial due to the associated down streaming complexity and complexity of pathophysiological targets. As a matter of fact, many interventions related to the modulation of drug ischemia reperfusion injury (suppression of γδ-T cells; expansion of Treg cells pre and post conditioning, miR-92a inhibition, miR-499 or miR-24, inhibition of apoptosis, activation of autophagy, inhibition of TLR4) are in preclinical or phase II stage [8]. As a result, existing *in-vivo* models cannot fully reflect cardiovascular pathologies and have shortcomings. Therefore, choosing the appropriate animal model in which the results can be translated into humans is a challenging process. Many factors, including research questions, the number of animals, the quality of expected results, and the relevance of results to complications, need to be carefully considered in order to determine the most appropriate animal model. It is also essential to apply the 3R (replacement, reduction, refinement) principle in terms of work ethics [8]. The negative experience of Hofmann-La Roche company is among the best examples of the deficiencies of *in-vivo* animal models. The discovery of endothelin and its receptors in the 1980s made it an exciting target for cardiovascular diseases. As a result of the positive results obtained in *in-vivo* models with bosentan, which was developed as a selective receptor antagonist of the relevant target, phase II evaluation of the molecule in heart failure was started. Unfortunately, clinical trial results were variable and unpredictable [34]. In further studies with the molecule, efficacy could be demonstrated in pulmonary hypertension, but this was not the original target profile. This indication was not found commercially appealing by the company, and the license of the molecule was sold to Actelion, a small biotechnology company, which turned the pulmonary arterial hypertension market into a highly successful project by expanding it beyond its limits [35].

CLINICAL DEVELOPMENT

In its most basic form, clinical research can be defined as a prospective evaluation of the effect and value of intervention against control in humans [36]. Such studies are designed with the aim of either establishing a hypothesis or testing an existing hypothesis. While clinical trials aimed at establishing hypothesis are designed to test new therapies that are established in pre-clinical models or that are biologically feasible but efficacies not yet been determined in humans; testing the hypothesis provides evidence of the efficacy and safety of the existing intervention at a statistical certainty level [37]. Medical treatment development stages start with early Phase I studies in which the safety of the candidate molecule/treatment is evaluated, continues with Phase II studies in which biological efficacy and safety are evaluated and the appropriate dose is determined, ends with Phase III studies required for regulatory authority approval. Phase IV studies are conducted to obtain post-marketing safety data. These studies are also carried out to support and expand the approved indication and sometimes to raise awareness for the new therapy. Depending on the result of the previous one, each gradual progress from Phase I to Phase III maximizes the probability of success while allowing the financially necessary investments to be made sequentially.

The level of evidence required for approval by the regulatory authority or the users in the cardiovascular community depends largely on the disease and the type of treatment. In some cases, as with new antihypertensive agents, lipid-lowering agents, and blood glucose-regulating drugs,the efficacy of new treatments only needs to be demonstrated with a surrogate biomarker for regulatory approval and adoption. However, security concerns, which are almost impossible to identify with low participation efficiency evaluation studies, should be assessed with pre/post approval studies with a sufficient number of volunteers in order to detect safety signals. Phase studies may be less challenging due to the greater number of regulatory approval pathways for relatively rare diseases for which large-scale clinical trials are practically impossible (such as pulmonary hypertension, hypertrophic cardiomyopathy and amyloid heart disease) and for diseases where few effective treatments are available [38]. For example, in May 2019, tafamidis, transthyretin was approved by the FDA as an orphan drug for the treatment of cardiac amyloidosis. Accelerated approval was given due to the ATTR-ACT (Transthyretin Amyloidosis Cardiomyopathy Clinical Trial) study, in which the effectiveness of the drug was evaluated over 30 months in 441 patients *versus* placebo [39]. Priced as 225.000 $/year it became the most expensive CV drug. According to a cost-effectiveness analysis based on the ATRR-ACT study, the cost of the drug was calculated as 880.000 $ per quality-adjusted life-years [40]. Another CV agent approved as an orphan drug is evolocumab, which is a PCSK9 (proprotein convertase subtilisin/kexin type 9) inhibitor. The drug received FDA approval for the treatment of homozygous familial hypercholesterolemia in June 2016 with the TESLA (Trial Evaluating PCSK9 Antibody in Subjects with LDL Receptor Abnormality) study [41], conducted on 49 patients. The drug was priced at more than 14,000 $ per patient per year, but as a result of the payer's refusal to accept this price, the price of the drug was reduced by 60% [42].

Challenges in Clinical Trials

BIO, the world's largest association representing biotech companies, academic institutions, state biotech centers and related organizations in the United States and more than 30 countries, scanned 7455 clinical drug development programs registered in FDA carried out by 1103 companies registered in the Biomed tracker database between 2006-2015 and analyzed the phase transition success rates [43]. In the mentioned analysis, phase transition was defined as the transition to the next stage of drug development or suspension by the sponsor, while the phase transition success rate was calculated for four phases as the ratio of the number of programs moving on to the next stage, the total progress and suspended programs: Phase I (preclinical phase) Phase II (early clinical phase), Phase III (late clinical phase) and preparation of the application files for the regulatory authority. Accordingly, Phase II transition success rates were the lowest among all other phases. Phase I and Phase III rates were significantly higher than that of Phase II and Phase I rate is relatively higher compared to that of Phase III. The highest success rate is the preparation of regulatory authority application (NDA, INDA) files, which is the last step of the development phase. In the relevant analysis, the Phase I transition success rate was stated as 63.2%, and this success rate is due to the fact that the safety tests of the drug candidate molecule were conducted in the relevant phase and the transition to the advanced phase was independent from the efficacy results. The Phase II transition success rate, which reaches this stage as a concept and is the first stage in which this concept is tested in humans, is the lowest among the four phases with 30.7%. This phase is also the turning point in which the go/no-go decision is made in the drug development program for many reasons, including Phase III studies, which is the most expensive phase, and commercial applicability. Phase III transition success rate was 58.1% (Table **1**) [43].

Table 1. Phase transition success.

	Phase I to Phase II		Phase II to Phase III		Phase III to NDA		NDA to approval	
	N	Success (%)	N	Success (%)	N	Success (%)	N	Success (%)
Cardiovascular	209	58.9	237	24.1	110	55.5	76	84.2
All indications	3582	63.2	3862	30.7	1491	58.1	1050	85.3
n:total number of transitions (advanced or suspended)								

According to the analysis, the probable success rate for the transition from Phase I to FDA approval (Likelihood of approval, LOA) was only 9.6% (Table 2) [43].

Table 2. LOA of CV Drugs.

	Phase I to Phase II		Phase II to Phase III		Phase III to NDA		NDA to approval	
	n*	LOA (%)	N	LOA (%)	n	LOA (%)	N	LOA (%)
Cardiovascular	632	6.6	423	11.2	186	46.7	76	84.2
All indications	9985	9.6	6403	15.3	2541	49.6	1050	85.3
n: total number of transitions (advanced or suspended); LOA: probability of FDA approval for drugs from this phase of development								

In the subgroup analysis of the relevant data for 21 diseases and 558 indications, Hematology ranked first with an LOA of 26.1%, followed by infectious diseases with 19.1% and ophthalmology with 17.1%. CV is third from the last with 6.6% LOA (Table 2). On the other hand, NDA application success rate for cardiovascular drug candidate molecules is 85%, and it ranks 4th among all diseases (Table 3) [43].

Table 3. Time to FDA approval and percent approved by FDA.

	% Approved on 1st review	% Approved by 2nd review	% Approved
Cardiovascular	69	83	85
All diseases	61	80	86

Clinical trials are time-consuming, expensive, and often inconvenient for patients. Failure in these studies may occur due to many reasons (*e.g.* , inadequate efficacy, problems regarding safety, insufficient financial resources to complete the study, *etc.*). Therefore, it is very important to make the decision to continue the study by producing accurate and sufficient results at every stage of clinical studies. Let's take a brief look at the main causes of failure in clinical trials in general:

Efficacy and Safety: The main reason for failure in clinical trials is the inability to demonstrate efficacy. Hwang *et al.* found that 54% of 640 Phase III clinical trials with potential candidate molecules failed and 57% of these failed trials were due to insufficient efficacy [44]. Similarly, Li *et al.*, with their analysis, determined that there were 12 new CV drug candidates terminated during the phase study between 2016-2018, 6 of them were terminated due to efficiency and safety reasons, and the others were terminated due to strategic or unspecified reasons [45]. Researchers reported that 3 of the total 12 candidate molecules were terminated in Phase I, 6 in Phase II and 3 in Phase III. Safety should be evaluated in all drug development phases. However, the safety data of the candidate molecule can only be evaluated with large-scale controlled studies. Nesiritide was approved by the FDA in 2001 for the treatment of acute decompensated heart failure. Following approval, the drug was shown to be associated with mortality and deterioration of renal function in two meta-analyzes, including small, randomized trials. Thereupon, although the safety of the drug was shown in the ASCEND-HF (Acute Study of Clinical Effectiveness of Nestiritide in Decompensated Heart Failure) study conducted on 7141 patients in 331 centers, its superiority to placebo could not be demonstrated in terms of efficacy [46]. The number of CV candidate molecules terminated for reasons of efficiency and safety by years is summarized in Fig. (**4**).

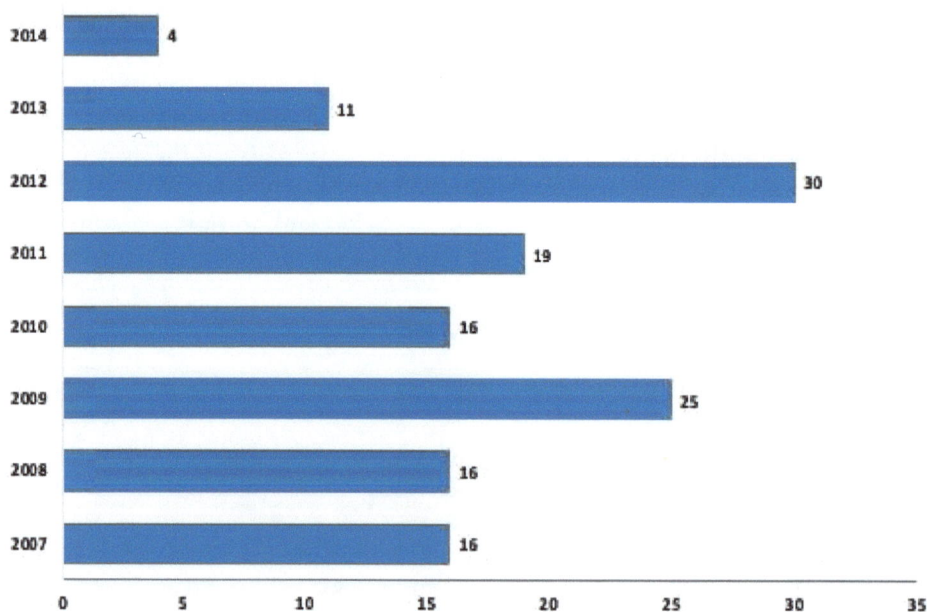

Fig. (4). Numbers of CV drug developments terminated due to efficacy and safety reasons.

Financial Reasons: The main reason for the search for innovative clinical trials by drug development parties, especially industry, is undoubtedly the rapidly increasing drug development costs. The cost of developing a new drug has increased approximately 13-fold in the last thirty years. The estimated amount of the stages from the discovery of an active substance to it being placed on the market may exceed 2.5 billion $. The cost per patient of Phase II and Phase III trials for new diabetes drugs and factor Xa inhibitors is estimated at approximately 35,000 and 47,000 $ respectively, and the total cost of Phase III is half a billion dollars. Despite these high costs, Hwang *et al* point out that 22% of the phase III trials that fail are due to insufficient financial resources [44]. Most studies do not get the chance to produce a positive result due to insufficient resources as a result of high financial burdens. This has led some pharmaceutical companies, who perceive relatively greater potential returns from investments in non-CV areas, to move away from the CV arena.

Eligibility/Inclusion Criteria: Ideally, a suitable patient population and a number of patients who can provide statistically meaningful data should be reached. This undoubtedly means that adverse effects are seen more in cases where comorbidities are high. This situation also brings along the risk of volunteers not being able to continue with the study at a higher rate. The choice of inclusion and exclusion criteria profoundly impacts the duration and cost of clinical trials, and the preservation of the participant required to reach adequate participation rates and to reach a statistical conclusion throughout the study. The eligibility criteria selected without a meticulous planning leads to an inadequate number of participants in studies, a prolonged participant selection process and, consequently, changes in study protocols. Getz *et al* state that 16% of the changes made in the study protocols are changes in the eligibility criteria [47]. Many CV clinical trials can be shown as an example for being successful due to appropriate selection of inclusion criteria. For example, in the COMPANION (Comparison of Medical Therapy, Pacing, and Defibrillation in Heart Failure) study, with the addition of "QRS interval equal to or higher than 12 ms" in the inclusion criteria, a 20% reduction in all-cause deaths or hospitalizations was shown with chronic resynchronization therapy. The researchers acknowledge that the study outcome would be negative if this treatment was applied to the entire heart failure population [48]. With the addition of the inflammatory marker, high C-reactive protein, into the inclusion criteria, a decrease in major CV events with Rosuvastatin was shown in JUPITER (Justification for the Use of Statins in Prevention: An Intervention Trial Evaluating Rosuvastatin) trial [49]. Although TOPCAT (Treatment of Preserved Cardiac Function Heart Failure with an Aldosterone Antagonist) study with spironolactone gave negative results in patients with preserved ejection fraction, specific patient population with high brain natriuretic peptide (BNP) value may benefit from the treatment [50].

Another challenge is to include various populations in terms of gender, race, and ethnicity in studies. Gender is the most important parameter affecting the pharmacokinetic and pharmacodynamic properties of drugs. Women's participation in CV studies has tended to increase in recent years. While only one-third of CV clinical study participants were women between 2011-2015, more than half of the approved drug study populations in 2018 consisted of women. However, a review of clinical studies between 2005 and 2015 shows that women were significantly underrepresented in studies of heart failure, coronary artery disease, and acute coronary syndrome compared with the overall disease incidence. In two of the 10 CV studies approved by the FDA in 2015, no gender-related activity statement was reported, while the female population ratio was below 50% in eight studies [37].

Patient Participation and Continuity, Concerns of the Patients: Patients often tend to participate in studies where they may find the opportunity to receive better treatment or studies, they think will benefit others. Feller reported that 25% of the cancer studies did not reach a sufficient number of patients, and 18% of the studies were concluded with less than half of the targeted number of participants in 3 years or longer [51]. Similarly, patient participation in cardiovascular clinical studies is also low. According to the study conducted by Udel *et al.*, it was shown that the participation of patients with acute myocardial infarction decreased from 5.2% in 2008 to 3.29% in 2011 [51]. In another analysis, it was reported that this rate decreased to 0.8% in 2014. Participation in clinical trials is limited for high-risk groups, such as the elderly and patients living in rural areas, who face more logistical barriers than other groups. Concerns by patients may be listed as possible adverse effects of the treatment, additional tests they may have to go through, financial concerns (disruption of work life) and the uncertainty of whether the treatment will be successful or not. Again, the concerns of the patients about being assigned to the control group rather than taking the active drug negatively affects the study participation and continuation rates. The extra financial burden and time investment that studies can bring also significantly affects participation and continuation. Based on this, it can be said that the selection of the centers where the studies will be carried out is one of the most important factors affecting the success of the studies [52]. Low number of patient participation in clinical studies may result in the failure to demonstrate the efficacy of the candidate molecule in the study due to the insufficient sample size in the related studies. For example, in ALECARDIO, which is a phase III study conducted in a total of 720 centers in 26 different countries, the planned number of patients could be reached in only 18.2% of the study centers (no patients were registered in 10% of the centers). The study was terminated early because sufficient population could not be reached to demonstrate the targeted efficacy. If carried out properly, large, simple studies may be successful despite the treatments recommended by the guidelines that are known to improve results when used extensively. The best example of this is the PARADIGM-HF (Prospective Comparison of ARNI [Angiotensin Receptor–Neprilysin Inhibitor] with ACEI [Angiotensin-Converting–Enzyme Inhibitor] to Determine Impact on Global Mortality and Morbidity in Heart Failure Trial) study comparing the neprilysin inhibitor LCZ696 (sacubitril + valsartan), which is a new agent in heart failure with low ejection fraction, with enapril. The study, with 8442 participants, has the largest sample size ever made in this group of patients, and was terminated early due to its effectiveness in the LCZ696 arm, and received marketing authorization by the FDA within a year [53].

In today's conjuncture, clinical trials are designed/conducted to answer the questions of manufacturers, clinicians, decision-makers and regulators who are involved in drug development. Patients are less involved in clinical trials. However, patients have significant perspectives and experiences in the design and/or development of clinical trials to improve the significance of clinical trial results. Therefore, by planning patient-centered clinical studies, eliminating the patient concerns mentioned above will increase clinical study efficiency by increasing patient admission and patient continuity to clinical studies, and at the same time, reducing the cost of the study by reducing the patient intake, which is the costliest step in clinical studies [37].

Today, high-quality large, randomized, controlled clinical trials that produce scientifically sound evidence of efficacy and safety remain the standard pathway for drug approval. The contribution of randomized controlled studies, which effectively change daily treatment practices, to the field of medicine cannot be denied. However, according to Reith *et al.*, clinical trials have become an industry, in many ways an inflated and inefficient system that prevents effective cardiovascular drug development and practically does not benefit patients [54]. Many scientific organizations, notably the European Society of Cardiology, are also concerned about the declining interest in developing innovative treatments for cardiovascular diseases. As a matter of fact, the pharmaceutical industry data are the basic evidence that this concern is legitimate. While the rates of CV drug candidate molecules in the total Phase II and Phase III studies between 1990-1995 were 16% and 21%, respectively, this rate was reported as 0.5% and 7%, respectively, between 2005-2012. In parallel with industry data, regulatory authorities around the world, especially the FDA, also express a significant decline in new CV drug approvals. Only one of four CV studies entering Phase I can reach the FDA approval stage [55].

The production of cardiovascular evidence is more difficult than in other specialties for various reasons (Fig. **5**) [55]. First, with a few exceptions in general, the chronic nature of cardiovascular diseases makes long-term treatment necessary to effectively treat CV system diseases. Potential products should therefore be evaluated over a longer period of time to adequately measure the intended effect. Second, most cardiovascular enhancement programs include event-focused studies where the annual incidence of events is low while the population at risk is high. For example, the prevention of stroke in atrial fibrillation, where the subjects participating in the study will not experience the event, whether in the new treatment arm or not. Despite the difficulty in execution and the need for a large number of participants, such studies produce clear results from which reliable predictions of efficacy and safety can be made. Third, CV drug development is more focused on heart failure and hypertension. However, these conditions result from many factors and pathways and have a variety of potential therapeutic biological targets. Fourth, due to a large number of effective agents in existing treatment groups such as statins, anti-platelet agents, new anticoagulants, there are relatively few new drug targets that can be completely separated from the potential overlap with existing targets. Still, recent scientific advances, including those in the field of molecular biology and genetics, promise to provide many new drug targets through multiple pathways related to CV diseases such as thrombosis, lipid metabolism and atherosclerosis. Fifth, as a result of past effective innovations, it is not enough to demonstrate the effectiveness and safety of the newly developed treatments, but also the superiority to the current standard treatment must be clearly demonstrated. On the one hand, this means that the efficacy and safety of the candidate molecule in the clinical study to be conducted will be compared with the treatment alternatives available in more than one arm, on the other hand, it means the inclusion of a large number of diverse participant populations through which statistical significance can be achieved. All these result in the formation of a large and complex infrastructure for newly designed clinical studies. Sixth, CV studies in the past have been conducted in large, unselected patient groups (*e.g.* heart failure, atrial fibrillation, *etc.*). Various disease mechanisms that are not affected by the tested molecule may be active in these groups. Finally, surrogate endpoints are biomarkers used to determine whether a particular treatment has an assumed positive effect and can be used as an indicator of clinical trial success. Lowering blood pressure and LDL, increasing plasma HDL, decreasing NT-proBNP have been used as surrogate markers in CV diseases. Undoubtedly, it has been questioned how accurate intermediates these are on the path between disease and outcome. However, the relationship between them is not that simple. For example, while 120 mmHg systolic blood pressure is associated with the event rate, there is not sufficient evidence that lowering the blood pressure below 140 mmHg with medical treatment in hypertensive patients will decrease the event rate. Moreover, in some studies, similar decrease rates in blood pressure had different outcomes on key endpoints such as mortality and stroke. Currently, the number of surrogates accepted for evaluation of new treatments and their use in predicting response to treatment is relatively limited. Because many promising surrogate endpoints have failed to accurately predict clinical outcomes. For example, although high plasma HDL cholesterol levels have been shown to be beneficial in epidemiological studies, and torcetrapib and long-acting niacin have been shown to significantly increase plasma HDL cholesterol, many large clinical studies have not shown cardiovascular benefit with the related agents; on the contrary, significant cardiovascular harm has been shown due to their off-target effects. Again, although favorable results have been shown with surrogate endpoints, death has been reported in other clinical studies with the use of class IC antiarrhythmic agents in myocardial infarction, despite successful suppression of premature ventricular contractions. Similarly, although improvement in hemodynamic parameters was observed, the use of inotropic agents in cardiogenic shock has been associated with mortality. In light of these failures with surrogate endpoints, there is a consensus in the cardiovascular community for the use of proven clinical trial results [56, 57].

Main Challenges in CV Clinical Trials	
1	The chronic nature of cardiovascular diseases requires long-term treatment for effective treatment of CV system diseases.
2	Most cardiovascular enhancement programs include event-focused studies where the annual incidence of events is low while the population under risk is high.
3	A wide variety of mechanisms are involved in the pathogenesis of CV diseases, and this increases the variety of potential therapeutic biological targets.
4	Due to the large number of effective agents in existing treatment groups, there are relatively few new drug targets that can be completely separated from potential overlap with existing targets.
5	Demonstrating incremental risk reduction often requires extremely large sample sizes.
6	Successful drug developments in the past have set the bar very high for new studies to come.
7	There is a need for validated surrogate endpoints to evaluate treatment efficacy.
8	Cardiovascular disease involves a wide variety of mechanisms unaffected by the agent being studied, making it difficult to identify patients likely to benefit.
9	CV studies require a more complex infrastructure compared to other fields.

Fig. (5). Challenges in CV clinical trials.

Considered together, these factors create an environment where new candidate molecules need to undergo extensive trials with large amounts of data collected over a long period. Indeed, the analysis of significant clinical research evidence required for FDA approval between 2005 and 2012 is striking: CV diseases, diabetes mellitus, and hyperlipidemia trials were conducted in a larger (median 651 and 266 patients for CV and others, respectively), longer-term (median 24 and 18.5 weeks in CV and cancer trials, respectively), randomized (93.2% of CV trials and 27.3% of cancer trials) and double-blind (93.2% of CV trials and 27.3% of cancer trials) manner than those in other therapeutic areas, and a placebo or active control (97.2% of CV trials and 47.3% of cancer trials) was used almost identically in the comparison arm [58]. It is an inevitable fact that the costs of these extensive and comprehensive studies are higher than their equivalents. The average CV clinical trial cost is estimated to be around 157 million $, according to a recent study. This is 3 times more than its cancer counterpart and 6 times more than most other disease areas.

Identifying those likely to benefit from the new therapy benefits not only drug developers but also patients. Even a moderately beneficial (15-25% risk reduction) treatment will help avoid thousands of events each year in cardiovascular conditions such as myocardial infarction, heart failure. However, this approach requires the treatment of many patients who would not benefit from it, including those who would not develop an event without treatment. Therefore, the need for a better refined classification of cardiovascular diseases and determination of specific patient characteristics is now voiced more loudly by all stakeholders, especially academia and drug developers. Developing sensitive treatments for specific patient groups is only possible with the development of "personalized medicine". New developments in scientific methods such as imaging, genomics and proteogenomics that contribute to the formation of Big Data are among the most important steps taken in this direction. For example, in a genome-based study, thirteen new sensitivity loci (points) were defined for coronary artery disease, all of them were found to be more important than PCK9, while only three of them were associated with traditional, established risk factors [58]. This analysis shows that there are many potential unconventional targets associated with the pathogenesis of coronary artery disease. Again, a strong relationship was found between the titin protein and dilated cardiomyopathy with next generation sequencing [60]. For this, new preclinical disease models may be needed to characterize disease mechanisms and to identify patients in whom such disease mechanisms are active. Again, the complex interaction between genetic susceptibility, integration of environmental stressors, and multiple pathways common to CV diseases may be clinically necessary to strengthen 'mechanism-based' research. Identification and validation of specific patient groups can be achieved with increasingly earlier use of large genetic biobanks linked to phenotypes of interest, using approaches such as Mendelian randomization to assess possible causation. Thus, better disease classification, phenotyping and biomarker development in CV diseases may be possible.

REGULATORY APPROVAL

Thousands of compounds are analyzed and those with therapeutic value are sought. During six to seven years of preclinical testing, the synthesis and purification of the drug is completed, and *in-vitro* and *in-vivo* tests are performed on a limited number of animals. Only five of the more than five thousand compounds tested show promising results for the New Drug Application for Research Purposes (IND). If the IND application is approved by the regulatory authority (Institutional Review Board in FDA), the manufacturer can start the first stage of development [61].

IND stage consists of three stages. In Phase I, clinical trials are conducted in a small number of healthy individuals to determine the basic properties of the drug and its safety profile in humans. Typically, this stage lasts 1 to 2 years. In Phase II, the drug is administered to the volunteers of a small number of target population and efficacy trials begin. At the end of this phase, the manufacturer meets with regulatory authority officials to discuss the regulatory development process, ongoing human testing, and Phase III protocols (this step may differ depending on how the regulatory authority functions). In the IND phase, the producer can receive the accelerated review. When Phase III is complete, the manufacturer prepares a new Drug Application (NDA) file. In the NDA stage, the drug's effectiveness, safety, efficacy and label information (labeling, SPC and PIL) are analyzed. The drug that receives a marketing authorization can be put on the market with the label approved by the authority. It takes, on average, 1 to 2 years for the related application to be examined by the authority. The total drug development and approval (IND and NDA phases) takes about nine years. Extensive efficacy and safety data (adverse events) related to the drug, which has the opportunity to be used on a wide range of people after being put on the market, are collected by the regulatory authority. In the light of this information, the regulatory authority requests changes in label information and informs healthcare personnel and the public about newly emerging contraindications. If the regulatory authority considers the safety concerns about the drug serious as a result of the reported adverse events, it ensures that the drug is withdrawn from the market [55].

Regulatory authority regulations and requirements for drug approval have increased over time. In the 1980s, thirty clinical trials involving approximately 1,500 patients were sufficient for drug approval, while in the mid-1990s, this number increased up to about sixty clinical trials in which approximately 5,000 patients were included [55]. The process of placing a drug on the market, from the first test to the final regulatory approval, is summarized in Fig. (**6**) .

Duration, Target Population, Goal and Success Rates of Drug Discovery and Development Stages					
Preclinical Development	Clinical Development			Regulatory Review	Post Approval
	Phase I	Phase II	Phase III		
6,5 years	1,5 years	2,0 years	3,5 years	1,5 years	During marketing
In-vitro animals	20-100 healthy volunteers	100-500 patient volunteers	1.000-5.000 patient volunteers	Review and approval	Post approval surveillance
Assess safety, biological activity and formulation	Determine safety and dosage	Evaluate effectiveness and side effects	Confirm effectiveness, monitor adverse reactions		
1/5.000 compounds	5 enter trial			1 approved	

IND SUBMISSION — NDA SUBMISSION — APPROVAL

Fig. (6). Drug discovery, development and approval process. (Adopted from Pharmaceutical Research and Manufacturers of America, www.pharma.org)

Regulatory Uncertainty

It is evident that many drug samples, which were found to be harmful for the patient in post-marketing studies following regulatory approval, created intense public pressure on the regulatory approval process [62]. This is the root cause of perceived complexity and legal uncertainty in managing drug approval processes. It is a fact that the pharmaceutical industry has always played a dominant role in financing for drug development. In fact, according to published studies, 40-80% of randomized clinical trials published in high-level journals are financed by the pharmaceutical industry [63, 64]. In economic analysis, legal uncertainty is defined as the most important unpredictable variable in the return on business investments [65]. The regulatory authority is the most important external environment component in capital investment and market entry decision. While some drugs are approved in a shorter time following the known regulatory pathway, the regulatory pathway for other drugs is not fully defined or has been influenced by prior decisions for therapies in a similar class. This causes the approval period of the drugs to be prolonged or unpredictable. In addition, the lack of experience with new therapies and indications makes the evaluation of innovative drugs difficult by regulatory authorities, making the approval process of the related agents even more uncertain. In addition to all these uncertainties, regulatory complexity, perceived bureaucratic and expensive regulatory environment, especially in the European Medicines Agency (EMA), caused CV clinical studies to shift out of western countries. As it is known, EMA is still a more decentralized organization, and each country has its own regulatory authority and regulation [66]. Again, in the Brexit process that started with the departure of the UK from the European Union, in March 2019, it moved its headquarters from London to Amsterdam and initiated the necessary changes in legal regulations. Although drug approval by the FDA is faster compared to EMA and Canada [67], according to a published study, the number of studies organized by the FDA outside the USA has increased by 15% in the last decade, while studies from USA have decreased by 5.5% annually within the same period [68]. This globalization in clinical studies brings up geographical differences in patient selection, which is the most important parameter affecting study results [69, 70]. As a matter of fact, the distinctly different data obtained from the volunteers from Russia and Georgia in the TOPCAT (Treatment of Preserved Cardiac Function Heart Failure with Aldosterone Antagonist) study, which is one of the clinical studies conducted over the years, seriously changed the results of the study [71]. In the PLATO (Study of Platelet Inhibition and Patient Outcomes) study conducted with ticagrelor, which is also an antiplatelet agent, low participation from USA caused confusing results by causing incompatible treatment results with other geographical regions in USA [72]. Thus, the globalization of CV clinical studies contributes to regulatory uncertainty on the one hand, and complicates the regulatory review process of clinical trial results on the other.

Requirements for regulatory approval differ between countries and regulatory authorities interpret the same data-sets differently. This is the main challenge for global drug development programs. The process, which becomes complex with different license trials in different regions in line with different regulatory requirements, is a problem especially for new drugs that aim to improve existing therapy approaches. Increased use of common scientific advice by regulatory authorities appears to be the primary means of overcoming this challenge. Stakeholders from academia, industry and government gathered in Washington in July 2014 to reach a consensus on improving the CV drug development environment. At the meeting, the high costs of drug development were expressed in a way to include perceived complexities and barriers in managing the regulatory drug approval process. At the meeting, drug representatives highlighted "regulatory uncertainty", rather than a common concern shared by the industry, as an important factor in the decision to develop innovative CV drugs as a result of the high costs caused by regulatory failures in drug development [73, 74]. This suggests that although the critical role of the FDA and other regulatory authority in balancing the public's need for protection from harmful drugs with the timely approval of effective treatments has been voiced and supported by all stakeholders, "regulatory uncertainty" is a deep-seated and serious concern in the pharmaceutical industry. At the meeting, in response to these voiced concerns, the FDA expressed its strong desire and intention to engage with industry representatives early on to discuss drug development plans to provide guidance and feedback on potential regulatory pathways for promising treatments, prior to the launch of key approval trials. As a matter of fact, this intention was put into practice with the publication of the guide named "Interacting with the FDA on complex innovative trial designs for drugs and biological products" in 2020 in order to assist the sponsors and executives in the complex innovative study design of the FDA. Undoubtedly, the ways mentioned in the guide are limited to new and potential applications, and it takes more than a guide to bring the regulator, industry and payers together by changing the existing practice. Similarly, as of February 2021, a virtual training module has been created at the EMA under the Clinical Trials Information System (CTIS) to support the academy, non-commercial sponsors, micro, small and medium sized SMEs. (more information can be found at:https://www.ema.europa.eu/en/human-regulatory/researc--development/clinical-trials/clinical-trial-regulation/clinical-trials-infor-ation-system-ctis-training-programme#overview-section). These practices should be considered as important steps taken in this way.

Optimal CV drug development is possible through partnerships of academicians, physicians, regulatory authorities, industry representatives, scientists, clinical researchers, each representing the needs of patients with CV disease. Inclusion of academic clinical researchers in the study team, who are experts in CV disease status, clinical research operations, and who have a command of relations with regulatory authorities, is important in the design and execution of preliminary CV approval studies [75]. Academic researchers can specifically assist the pharmaceutical industry in identifying unmet clinical needs and transforming action mechanisms of drugs into clinical scenarios where benefits can outweigh risks. Again, academic researchers with their expertise in clinical practice can facilitate discussions between regulatory agencies and the pharmaceutical industry with medical treatment and patient-centered care expertise perspectives.

Health-related Economic Challenges

In addition to the effectiveness and safety of newly developed drugs, potential costs must also be determined. Because the end use of these agents depends on whether they are covered by various public and private paying agencies. Data that would allow economic evaluations (*e.g.* benefit on quality of life) are often not available from studies conducted within a clinical development program. Therefore, many times, there is a need for additional studies, which means increased time and cost for the drug development program [55]. This is a major problem in the evaluation of new CV agents, which are planned to be used as chronic treatment in common CV diseases, based on local data. Although health technology assessment analyses are based on systematically collected post-approval "real world" data sets, it may be beneficial to include basic economic measures in studies within the clinical development program so that these evaluations can be initiated in a timely manner. In fact, these basic economic measures can be requested by the legal authority within the scope of the studies carried out within the clinical development program. The FDA's Center for Devices and Radiological Health (CDRH) established the "Payor Communication Task Force" to facilitate communication between device manufacturers and payers to potentially shorten the time between FDA approval and coverage decision (more information can be found at: https://www.fda.gov/about-fda/cdr- -innovation/payor-communication-task-force'de). Similar structures can be created for drugs within the regulatory authority.

FINANCIAL CHALLENGES

Return Potential of Investment

The cost of launching a new agent is estimated at 1.5 billion $ (approximately 1.2 billion Euros). When the failures in the development phase are added, these figures reach 4-5 billion $ [76]. In fact, costs of up to 12 billion $ have been reported as a result of failure in late-phase clinical trials [77]. The main problem is that despite increasing R&D expenses, the number of new drugs approved per expense is decreasing [78]. The low return on investment associated with significant development costs is the main reason why CV drug pipelines are weak. The reimbursement scope of CV drugs is more limited compared to other groups. For example, while all cancer drugs are covered by reimbursement, this coverage is limited for CV drugs. Again, low-cost generic drugs limit the reimbursement scope of more costly drug alternatives [79]. CV drugs that have been recently put on the market have low net prices and sales figures compared to treatments for other ailments [80].

Patent Cliff

Patent protection ensures that original drugs are unique in the market in the time required to compensate for development costs. As a matter of fact, the patent expiration of many blockbuster products that generate high revenue for companies has seriously affected the CV pharmaceutical market in the last decade. This process started in 2011 with the abolition of the patent protection of Lipitor (atorvastatin), Pfizer's cholesterol drug that broke sales records. From 1996 when it was launched in the USA to the end of 2010, Lipitor was the most profitable drug, with a cumulative sale of 118 billion $. This was followed by Caduet (amlodipine/atorvastatin), whose patent expired that same year, and the best-selling anticoagulant drug Plavix in 2012. Total losses for 2011 and 2012 were reported as 12 and 30 million $, respectively, which corresponds to 20% of the turnover of the pharmaceutical industry in 2013 [81 - 83]. Again, almost all of the widely used angiotensin-II receptor antagonists (ACE inhibitors), including losartan (Cozaar/Hyzaar), irbesartan (Avapro), candesartan (Atacand), and valsartan (Diovan), have lost their patent protection (Table 4) [84].

Table 4. Important CV patent cliffs.

Drug	Active Substance	Patent Expiration Date	US Sales in Year Before Patent Expiration ($ Billions)
Lipitor	Atorvastatin	2011	10,7
Plavix	Clopidogrel	2012	6,9
Avapro	Irbesartan	2012	281
Diovan	Valsartan	2012	2,3
Atacand	Candersartan	2012	110
Integrilin	Eptifibatid	2014	288
Benicar	Olmesartan	2016	2,4
Caduet	Amlodipine/Atorvastatin	2018	339

Despite the revenue losses, big demand for new drugs, and heart disease and stroke being predicted as the leading cause of death [85], the number of CV drugs in development is about one-fifth of oncologic drugs [86]. As a matter of fact, these rates are also reflected in the regulatory authority NDAs. While the ratio of CV drugs that received NDA approval by the FDA in 2002 to all NDA approvals was 5/22, this rate was reported as 1/23 for 2010 and 1/53 for 2020 (Fig. 7).

The slowness of processes in clinical trials conducted in large patient populations (*e.g.* patient recruitment, study approval, *etc.*) are among the most important factors slowing down market approval and patient access for new therapies. These types of delays leave the industry a short period of time to compensate for development and post-approval costs before the patent expires [87].

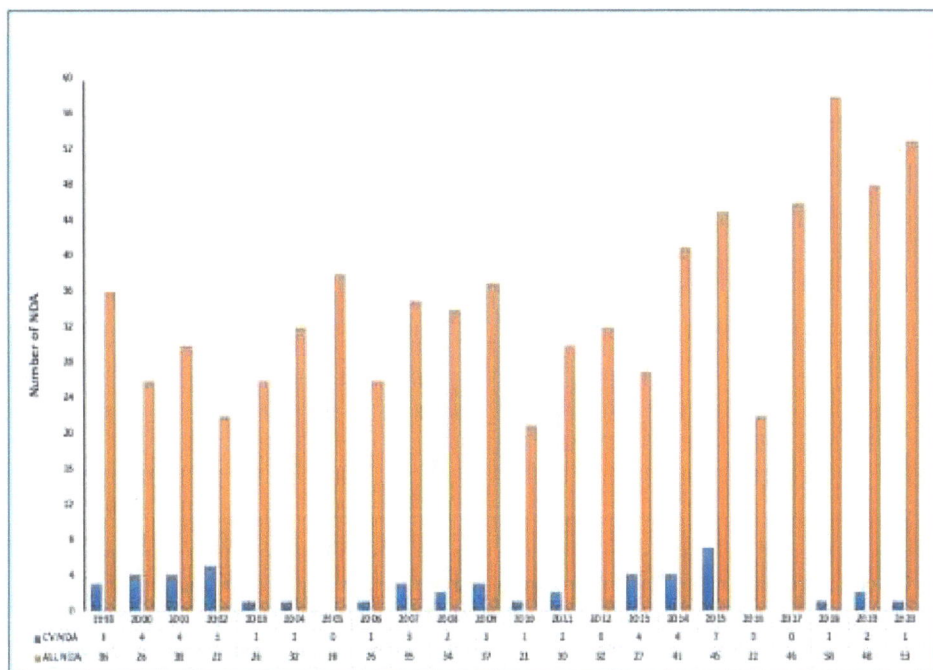

Fig. (7). New CV drug approvals by the FDA.(NDA: New Drug Approval, CV NDA: NDAs specified under the title of heart, lung and circulatory system diseases in the annual drug approval reports published by the FDA)

Insufficient Incentives (Funding)

CV drug development suffers from few incentives compared to other fields, particularly oncology. "Push" financing policies aim to stimulate the pharmaceutical industry by lowering costs in the R&D phase, while "pull" mechanisms create incentives for the pharmaceutical industry by creating market demand for new treatments addressing unmet clinical needs [88]. Push mechanisms can partially offset R&D by securing some of the costs, while pull mechanisms reward positive trial results for new treatments [55]. For example, in the financing pillar, studies conducted in cooperation with academia-industry, where new candidate molecules that may have commercialization potential can be marketed, are supported by the National Institutes of Health (NIH) in the United States. The National Cancer Institute (NCI), which is under this general umbrella, is the institution with the highest grants allocated since 1980. The budget of NIH for 2021 has been approved as 42.9 million $ [89], and 5.56 million $ of this budget has been transferred to NCI. On the other hand, the budget of the National Heart, Lung and Blood Institute (NHBI) is 3.29 million $ for the relevant period

[90]. A special program is also underway within the FDA to accelerate the approval of newly developed drugs for medical drugs not covered. A detailed analysis of the related program shows that the largest percentage of application for all subgroups is for oncological treatments. Comparison of CV drug applications with oncology on the basis of subgroups in the related analysis was stated as: orphans (9% *vs* 38%), priority review (4% *vs* 53%), accelerated approval (8% *vs* 32%) and fast follow-up (% 1 *vs* 56%) [91]. Oncology is also dominant in donation campaigns, which have an important place among the push mechanisms. While 911 million $ was collected in the campaign carried out by Movember with the Prostate Cancer Foundation [92], only 1.3 million $ was collected in the Jump Rope for Health and Hoops for Heart campaigns initiated by the American Heart Association (AHA) [93]. Oncology is also dominant in crowdfunding, which are initiatives that collect small amounts of money, especially over the internet. For example, according to a study of 97 crowdfunding campaigns focusing on cancer research, an average of 45,629 $ was collected from donations, which were 186 $ on average [94]. In response, AHA first used crowdfunding for its Power to End Stroke (later renamed Together the End Stroke) campaign in 2003. Again, in its 2014 session, AHA announced that it started a new funding application to finance early-stage products [95]. Given that cancer diagnosis brings out a much greater emotional response than CV diseases, the scope and success of fundraising campaigns for cancer and CV diseases clearly demonstrates the society's view of the "unmet need" despite the global CV disease burden.

Insufficient Investment

Although the biotechnology sector continues to show interest in drug development, trends towards venture capital financing priorities show a shift away from cardiovascular disease. Especially between 2005-2012, purchases and mergers in companies with products related to oncology and infectious diseases were 4 times more than the CV arena [55]. As a matter of fact, at the meeting held in Washington in 2014, where industry representatives, academics, payers and regulators gathered, the consensus expressed was; despite the venture capital investor's interest in biotechnology, the risk appetite was lower compared to historical trends and accordingly, investment companies' interest in CV drug development programs was lower considering the uncertain ROI. At the same meeting, it was also stated that companies are ready to accept lower ROI in return for a lower drug development risk compared to blockbuster treatments previously developed by biotech companies.

However, it is useful to highlight the change in the CV field as of 2015. New healthcare trends in particular have reshaped the CV market: 1) the shift from volume-based pay-per-service models, particularly in the US, to models focusing on quality and patient outcomes; 2) Increasing use of innovative therapy technologies such as transcatheter aortic valve replacement (TAVR) and 3D printers; 3) adoption of digital solutions such as smart phone and watch apps 4) evolving provider and care service [96]. These trends caught the attention of Technology (MedTec) companies and over time made them players of the CV market. For example, in 2015, AHA collaborated with Verily, a Google Life Science company, to support new strategies for the treatment of coronary heart disease for 50 million $. The goal of this five-year commitment, the largest one-time research investment in AHA's history, was to understand, prevent and reverse coronary heart disease. This partnership between a non-profit organization and a non-traditional MedTec company was also quite contrary to traditional clinical research models. Another example is the collaboration of Qualcomm Inc. and Northern Arizona Healthcare (NAH) companies in 2011 to create advanced wireless care technologies to provide remote healthcare services to patients by seamlessly transferring the biometric information of post-operative CV patients to the physician [97]. During this period, in addition to the non-traditional MedTech companies, established MedTech companies also chose to consolidate with CV companies. The most important example of this is the acquisition of St. Jude Medical, the fourth largest player in the market, by Abbott, the second largest company in the CV market, in 2015 (Table **5**) [98].

Table 5. Important CV consolidations.

Consolidation	Value (B $)	Date
Abbott-St. Jude Medical	25,0	Jan 2017
Medtronic-HeartWare	2,7	Aug 2016
St Jude-Thoratec Corp	3,3	Oct 2015
Cardinal Health-Cordis	1,9	Oct 2015
Cyberonics-Sorin	2,7	Feb 2015
(adopted from https://www2.deloitte.com/)		

Although medical technology companies have brought a significant movement to the CV market, 2019 market data is in favor of oncology. The global oncology market size, which has increased at a compound annual growth rate (CAGR) of 9.8% since 2015, reached a value of approximately 167.9 billion $ in 2019. The market volume for CV for the same year was reported as 92.5 billion $ [99]. These data clearly show that although a recovery in the CV industry has been observed, investment firms are typically more interested in oncology treatments with a clear regulatory pathway.

Late-stage Failures

Reluctance to bear the risk of costly failure contributes to the reduction of the pharmaceutical industry's investment in CV drug development. Despite promising Phase I and Phase II results, there are many CV studies with disappointing results in Phase III studies. For example, PROTECT-1 study evaluating the use of adenosine A1 receptor antagonist Rolofylline in patients with acute heart failure [100], OVERTURE study comparing ACE and neutral endopeptidase (NEP) inhibitor omaprilat with enalapril in chronic heart failure (ILLIMINATE study evaluating the combination of a cholesteryl ester transfer protein (CETP) inhibitor torcetrapib with atorvastatin in patients with high risk of coronary events [14], SOLID-TIMI 52 study evaluating the effect of lipoprotein-associated phospholipase A2 (Lp-PLA2) inhibitor darapladib on plaque stabilization in patients with myocardial infarction [101], HPS2-THRIVE study evaluating the effect of prostaglandin D2 antagonist laropiprant and extended release niacin combination on the incidence of vascular events in high-risk patients [102]. As discussed in the previous chapters, although broad indication targets have been successful in drug development in large patient groups in the past, targeting the population that will gain the maximum benefit from the relevant treatment, producing solid scientific evidence, may be a more accurate and efficient approach for reducing resource and time-based failure costs. Another approach is to use Phase II experiments as leverage to inform Phase III trials. While there is a need to design Phase III trials for regulatory approval and use Phase II research data to predict Phase III results, it is equally important to use the collected data to understand the impact of a new therapy on biology and disease pathways in planning further development steps. In fact, biomarkers can be appropriately used in Phase II trials to screen promising new therapies through the evaluation of biological activity [103]. Therefore, phase II studies should focus on evaluating and improving important variables such as dosing, pharmacokinetic modeling, side effects, as well as the effect of new therapy on biomarkers. Again, the adaptive design model is another strategy [104]. This approach allows for the review of collected information that might suggest changing research characteristics during research, thus removing uncertainty about choices made during planning. Thus, in light of the information gathered, it allows updating predetermined parameters such as maximum sample size, study duration, treatment group allocation, dose, number of treatment arms, or study endpoint. These sponsors can reduce risks, but the main problem here is the difficulty in examining this wide range of changes in ongoing work by the regulatory authority. In fact, the FDA has been wary of accepting all applicable design trials for approval due to a similar difficulty [105].

In previous chapters, we addressed the main reasons for failure in clinical trials, the inability to demonstrate the effectiveness of the candidate molecule, and the importance of safety concerns. According to Dimasi, commercial reasons are more prominent than efficiency and safety reasons among CV drug development failures (over %40) [106]. However, in the analysis of Hwang *et al.* including 63 clinical studies, this rate was reported as 17% (11 out of 63 studies) [107]. Commercial failure can generally be caused by two main reasons: 1) an increase in projected costs for further steps; 2) reduction in expected revenues due to increased competition or the need to narrow the target profile in light of the results of the study. Therefore, the strategic decision in drug development should be able to analyze the existing and possible future economic situations.

CONCLUSION AND FUTURE PERSPECTIVE

CV diseases rank first among the causes of death in the world. According to WHO data, ischemic heart disease, which is responsible for 16% of all deaths, ranks first among the causes of death in the world. Deaths due to ischemic heart disease, which was reported as 2 million in 2000, reached 8.9 million as of 2019 [108]. In addition to the increasing prevalence of CV diseases, the increase in comorbidities such as diabetes, arrhythmia, and dyslipidemia is also very important [109]. Given the expected increase in CV diseases, comorbidities and associated diagnosis and treatment, the financial burden of CV diseases also increases. The direct cost of CV diseases, which was 320 billion $ in 2011 in the USA, doubled in 2015 to 649 billion $ [110]. Therefore, scientific studies for the effective treatment of CV diseases, which are the main public health problem for the whole world, continue at an increasing pace. Indeed, today, institutes, associations and even organizations such as WHO are taking over the sponsorship role that pharmaceutical industry players have abandoned. In parallel, cardiovascular CV pipeline activity is shifting from large pharmaceutical companies to small and medium-sized companies and from fast-following drugs to first-in classes. Therefore, it would be appropriate to evaluate this situation we witnessed in CV drug development as a process of transformation rather than hibernation. As a matter of fact, both the advances in basic sciences, especially molecular biology and genetics, and the rapid developments in the field of medical devices and medical technology after 2015 find response in the CV field is a proof of this. Undoubtedly, this transformation will reshape the CV drug market, as well. As a matter of fact, both strategic partnerships (for example, the launch of Anthos Therapeutics in 2019 by Novartis AG and Blackstone Life Sciences to develop a new generation of antithrombotic agents, the partnership of Pfizer and Bristol Mayers Squib in the development of a new oral anticoagulant, apixaban) and acquisitions (acquisition of The Medicines Company, the developer of PCSK9 inhibitor Inclisiran by Novartis in 2019; BMS buying Celgene and MyoKardia, CV drugs at development stage, with 1 year interval) are the footsteps of this transformation in the rapidly changing CV market player profile.

Taking the current picture with situation analysis is the key to taking the right steps forward. Therefore, in the light of the challenges mentioned in this section, we think that the starting point for effective CV drug development is the determination and development of potential therapeutic goals through pre-clinical and early phase development programs to be carried out in cooperation with academia using public programs. New CV agents can be developed to meet the unmet clinical needs by seeking answers with clinical trials, in which new operational approaches to be carried out on the target population are applied to scientific questions refined with early phase developments. This undoubtedly requires a coordinated effort between academia, regulators, industry and payers.

CONSENT FOR PUBLICATION

Not Applicable.

CONFLICT OF INTEREST

The author declares no conflict of interest, financial or otherwise.

ACKNOWLEDGMENTS

Declared none.

REFERENCES

[1] Nabel EG, Braunwald E. A tale of coronary artery disease and myocardial infarction. N Engl J Med 2012; 366(1): 54-63.
[http://dx.doi.org/10.1056/NEJMra1112570] [PMID: 22216842]

[2] Cardiovascular Diseases WHO https://www.who.int/health-topics/cardiovascular-diseases

[3] Hwang TJ, Lauffenburger JC, Franklin JM, Kesselheim AS. Temporal trends and factors associated with cardiovascular drug development, 1990 to 2012. JACC Basic Transl Sci 2016; 1(5): 301-8.
[http://dx.doi.org/10.1016/j.jacbts.2016.03.012] [PMID: 30167520]

[4] Fordyce CB, Roe MT, Ahmad T, *et al.* Cardiovascular drug development: is it dead or just hibernating? J Am Coll Cardiol 2015; 65(15): 1567-82.
[http://dx.doi.org/10.1016/j.jacc.2015.03.016] [PMID: 25881939]

[5] DiMasi JA, Feldman L, Seckler A, Wilson A. Trends in risks associated with new drug development: success rates for investigational drugs. Clin Pharmacol Ther 2010; 87(3): 272-7.
[http://dx.doi.org/10.1038/clpt.2009.295] [PMID: 20130567]

[6] Advancing Health Through Innovation: New drug theraphy approvals 20220. FDA 2021. www.fda.gov

[7] The Drug Development Process at. https://www.fda.gov/patients/learn-about-drug-and-de-ice-approvals/drug-development-process

[8] Gromo G, Mann J, Fitzgerald JD. Cardiovascular drug discovery: a perspective from a research-based pharmaceutical company. Cold Spring Harb Perspect Med 2014; 4(6): 014092.
[http://dx.doi.org/10.1101/cshperspect.a014092] [PMID: 24890831]

[9] Prakash N, Devangi P. Drug Discovery. JAA 2010; 2: 63-8.

[10] Deore AB, Dhumane JR. The stages of drug discovery and development process. AJPRH 2019; 7: 62-7.

[11] Moffat JG, Vincent F, Lee JA, Eder J, Prunotto M. Opportunities and challenges in phenotypic drug discovery: an industry perspective. Nat Rev Drug Discov 2017; 16(8): 531-43.
[http://dx.doi.org/10.1038/nrd.2017.111] [PMID: 28685762]

[12] DiMasi JA, Hansen RW, Grabowski HG. The price of innovation: new estimates of drug development costs. J Health Econ 2003; 22(2): 151-85.
[http://dx.doi.org/10.1016/S0167-6296(02)00126-1] [PMID: 12606142]

[13] Gashaw I, Ellinghaus P, Sommer A, Asadullah K. What makes a good drug target? Drug Discov Today 2012; 17 (Suppl.): S24-30.
[http://dx.doi.org/10.1016/j.drudis.2011.12.008] [PMID: 22155646]

[14] Barter PJ, Caulfield M, Eriksson M, *et al.* ILLUMINATE Investigators. Effects of torcetrapib in patients at high risk for coronary events. N Engl J Med 2007; 357(21): 2109-22.
[http://dx.doi.org/10.1056/NEJMoa0706628] [PMID: 17984165]

[15] Packer M, Califf RM, Konstam MA, *et al.* Comparison of omapatrilat and enalapril in patients with chronic heart failure: the Omapatrilat *Versus* Enalapril Randomized Trial of Utility in Reducing Events (OVERTURE). Circulation 2002; 106(8): 920-6.
[http://dx.doi.org/10.1161/01.CIR.0000029801.86489.50] [PMID: 12186794]

[16] Chin-Dusting J, Mizrahi J, Jennings G, Fitzgerald D. Outlook: finding improved medicines: the role of academic-industrial collaboration. Nat Rev Drug Discov 2005; 4(11): 891-7.
[http://dx.doi.org/10.1038/nrd1879] [PMID: 16247439]

[17] Cushman DW, Ondetti MA. Design of angiotensin converting enzyme inhibitors. Nat Med 1999; 5(10): 1110-3.
[http://dx.doi.org/10.1038/13423] [PMID: 10502801]

[18] Fitzgerald JD. Trails of discovery: A close call: The discovery of the ACE inhibitors. Dialogues Cardiovasc Med 2001; 6: 38-42.

[19] Ivany Oransky. Paul Janssen. Lancet 2004; 363: 251.
[http://dx.doi.org/10.1016/S0140-6736(03)15357-3]

[20] Prashant AP. Global Challenges in Cardiovascular Drug Discovery and Clinical Trials. Mol Biol 2017; 6: 193.

[21] Committee on a Framework for Development a New Taxonomy of Disease; National Research Council Toward Precision Medicine: Building a Knowledge Network for Biomedical Research and a New Taxonomy of Disease. Washington, DC: National Academies Press 2011.

[22] Ahmad T, Fiuzat M, Pencina MJ, *et al.* Charting a roadmap for heart failure biomarker studies. JACC Heart Fail 2014; 2(5): 477-88.
[http://dx.doi.org/10.1016/j.jchf.2014.02.005] [PMID: 24929535]

[23] Kathiresan S, Srivastava D. Genetics of human cardiovascular disease. Cell 2012; 148(6). 1242-57.
[http://dx.doi.org/10.1016/j.cell.2012.03.001] [PMID: 22424232]

[24] Greenberg B, Butler J, Felker GM, *et al.* Calcium upregulation by percutaneous administration of gene therapy in patients with cardiac disease (CUPID 2): a randomised, multinational, double-blind, placebo-controlled, phase 2b trial. Lancet 2016; 387(10024): 1178-86.
[http://dx.doi.org/10.1016/S0140-6736(16)00082-9] [PMID: 26803443]

[25] Ohlstein EH. The grand challenges in cardiovascular drug discovery and development. Front Pharmacol 2010; 1: 125.
[http://dx.doi.org/10.3389/fphar.2010.00125] [PMID: 21811459]

[26] Földes G, Mioulane M, Wright JS, *et al*. Modulation of human embryonic stem cell-derived cardiomyocyte growth: a testbed for studying human cardiac hypertrophy? J Mol Cell Cardiol 2011; 50(2): 367-76.
[http://dx.doi.org/10.1016/j.yjmcc.2010.10.029] [PMID: 21047517]

[27] Rosenstrauch D, Poglajen G, Zidar N, Gregoric ID. Stem celltherapy for ischemic heart failure. Tex Heart Inst J 2005; 32(3): 339-47.
[PMID: 16392214]

[28] Noble D, Noble PJ. Late sodium current in the path- ophysiology of cardiovascular disease: Consequences of sodium-calcium overload. Heart 2006; 92: 1-5.
[http://dx.doi.org/10.1136/hrt.2005.078782]

[29] Fletcher K, Shah RR, Thomas A, *et al*. Novel approaches to assessing cardiac safety-proceedings of a workshop: regulators, industry and academia discuss the future of *in silico* cardiac modelling to predict the proarrhythmic safety of drugs. Drug Saf 2011; 34(5): 439-43.
[http://dx.doi.org/10.2165/11591950-000000000-00000] [PMID: 21513366]

[30] Pammolli F, Magazzini L, Riccaboni M. The productivity crisis in pharmaceutical R&D. Nat Rev Drug Discov 2011; 10(6): 428-38.
[http://dx.doi.org/10.1038/nrd3405] [PMID: 21629293]

[31] Kaitin KI, DiMasi JA. Pharmaceutical innovation in the 21st century: new drug approvals in the first decade, 2000-2009. Clin Pharmacol Ther 2011; 89(2): 183-8.
[http://dx.doi.org/10.1038/clpt.2010.286] [PMID: 21191382]

[32] Sacks LV, Shamsuddin HH, Yasinskaya YI, Bouri K, Lanthier ML, Sherman RE. Scientific and regulatory reasons for delay and denial of FDA approval of initial applications for new drugs, 2000-2012. JAMA 2014; 311(4): 378-84.
[http://dx.doi.org/10.1001/jama.2013.282542] [PMID: 24449316]

[33] Eltzschig HK, Eckle T. Ischemia and reperfusion from mechanism to translation. Nat Med 2011; 17(11): 1391-401.
[http://dx.doi.org/10.1038/nm.2507] [PMID: 22064429]

[34] Teerlink JR. Recent heart failure trials of neurohormonal modulation (OVERTURE and ENABLE): approaching the asymptote of efficacy? J Card Fail 2002; 8(3): 124-7.
[http://dx.doi.org/10.1054/jcaf.2002.126486] [PMID: 12140803]

[35] Clozel JP, Ertel EA, Ertel SI. Discovery and main pharmacological properties of mibefradil (Ro 40-5967), the first selective T-type calcium channel blocker. J Hypertens Suppl 1997; 15(5): S17-25.
[http://dx.doi.org/10.1097/00004872-199715055-00004] [PMID: 9481612]

[36] Friedman LM, Furberg CD, DeMets DL, Eds. Fundamental of Clinical Trials. 4th ed., New York: Springer 2010.
[http://dx.doi.org/10.1007/978-1-4419-1586-3]

[37] Solomon SD, Pfeffer MA. Future of clinical trials in cardiovascular medicine. Circulation 2016; 133(25): 2662-70.
[http://dx.doi.org/10.1161/CIRCULATIONAHA.115.020723] [PMID: 27324361]

[38] Guha M. First-in-class guanylate cyclase stimulator approved for PAH. Nat Biotechnol 2013; 31(12): 1064.
[http://dx.doi.org/10.1038/nbt1213-1064b] [PMID: 24316627]

[39] Maurer MS, Schwartz JH, Gundapaneni B, *et al*. ATTR-ACT Study Investigators. Tafamidis treatment for patients with transthyretin amyloid cardiomyopathy. N Engl J Med 2018; 379(11): 1007-16.
[http://dx.doi.org/10.1056/NEJMoa1805689] [PMID: 30145929]

[40]   Gurtwitz J, Maurer MS. Initial monthly cost of tafamidis-price for patients-reply. JAMA Cardiol 2020; 5: 848.
[http://dx.doi.org/10.1001/jamacardio.2020.0866]

[41]   Raal FJ, Honarpour N, Blom DJ, *et al.* TESLA Investigators. Inhibition of PCSK9 with evolocumab in homozygous familial hypercholesterolaemia (TESLA Part B): a randomised, double-blind, placebo-controlled trial. Lancet 2015; 385(9965): 341-50.
[http://dx.doi.org/10.1016/S0140-6736(14)61374-X] [PMID: 25282520]

[42]   Khan MS, Vaduganathan M, Butler J. Orphan drug development in cardiovascular medicine. Circ Cardiovasc Qual Outcomes 2020; 13(7): e006509.
[http://dx.doi.org/10.1161/CIRCOUTCOMES.119.006509] [PMID: 32552063]

[43]   BIO Indusrty Analysis Clinical Development Success Rate 2016.

[44]   Hwang TJ, Carpenter D, Lauffenburger JC, Wang B, Franklin JM, Kesselheim AS. Failure of Investigational Drugs in Late-Stage Clinical Development and Publication of Trial Results. JAMA Intern Med 2016; 176(12): 1826-33.
[http://dx.doi.org/10.1001/jamainternmed.2016.6008] [PMID: 27723879]

[45]   Li T, Jiang S, Ni B, Cui Q, Liu Q, Zhao H. Discontinued Drugs for the Treatment of Cardiovascular Disease from 2016 to 2018. Int J Mol Sci 2019; 20(18): 4513.
[http://dx.doi.org/10.3390/ijms20184513] [PMID: 31547243]

[46]   O'Connor CM, Starling RC, Hernandez AF, *et al.* Effect of nesiritide in patients with acute decompensated heart failure. N Engl J Med 2011; 365(1): 32-43.
[http://dx.doi.org/10.1056/NEJMoa1100171] [PMID: 21732835]

[47]   Getz K. Improving protocol design feasibility to drive drug development economics and performance. Int J Environ Res Public Health 2014; 11(5): 5069-80.
[http://dx.doi.org/10.3390/ijerph110505069] [PMID: 24823665]

[48]   Bristow MR, Saxon LA, Boehmer J, *et al.* Comparison of Medical Therapy, Pacing, and Defibrillation in Heart Failure (COMPANION) Investigators. Cardiac-resynchronization therapy with or without an implantable defibrillator in advanced chronic heart failure. N Engl J Med 2004; 350(21): 2140-50.
[http://dx.doi.org/10.1056/NEJMoa032423] [PMID: 15152059]

[49]   Ridker PM, Danielson E, Fonseca FA, *et al.* JUPITER Study Group. Rosuvastatin to prevent vascular events in men and women with elevated C-reactive protein. N Engl J Med 2008; 359(21): 2195-207.
[http://dx.doi.org/10.1056/NEJMoa0807646] [PMID: 18997196]

[50]   Pitt B, Pfeffer MA, Assmann SF, *et al.* TOPCAT Investigators. Spironolactone for heart failure with preserved ejection fraction. N Engl J Med 2014; 370(15): 1383-92.
[http://dx.doi.org/10.1056/NEJMoa1313731] [PMID: 24716680]

[51]   Feller S. 2015.One in Four Cancer Trials Fails to Enroll Enough Participants https://www.upi.com/Health_News/2015/12/30/One-in-four-cancer-trials-fails-to-enroll-enough-participants/2611451485504/

[52]   Liu Z, Delavan B, Roberts R, Tong W. Lessons learned from two decades of anticancer drugs. Trends Pharmacol Sci 2017; 38(10): 852-72.
[http://dx.doi.org/10.1016/j.tips.2017.06.005] [PMID: 28709554]

[53]   McMurray JJ, Packer M, Desai AS, *et al.* PARADIGM-HF Investigators and Committees. Angiotensin-neprilysin inhibition *versus* enalapril in heart failure. N Engl J Med 2014; 371(11): 993 1004.
[http://dx.doi.org/10.1056/NEJMoa1409077] [PMID: 25176015]

[54]   Reith C, Landray M, Devereaux PJ, *et al.* Randomized clinical trials-removing unnecessary obstacles. N Engl J Med 2013; 369(11): 1061-5.
[http://dx.doi.org/10.1056/NEJMsb1300760] [PMID: 24024845]

[55]   Fordyce CB, Roe MTR, Ahmad T, *et al.* Cardiovascular drug development: is it dead or just hibernating? J Am Coll Cardiol 2015; 65(15): 1567-82.
[http://dx.doi.org/10.1016/j.jacc.2015.03.016] [PMID: 25881939]

[56]   Echt DS, Liebson PR, Mitchell LB, *et al.* Mortality and morbidity in patients receiving encainide, flecainide, or placebo. The Cardiac Arrhythmia Suppression Trial. N Engl J Med 1991; 324(12): 781-8.
[http://dx.doi.org/10.1056/NEJM199103213241201] [PMID: 1900101]

[57]   Felker GM, Benza RL, Chandler AB, *et al.* OPTIME-CHF Investigators. Heart failure etiology and response to milrinone in decompensated heart failure: results from the OPTIME-CHF study. J Am Coll Cardiol 2003; 41(6): 997-1003.
[http://dx.doi.org/10.1016/S0735-1097(02)02968-6] [PMID: 12651048]

[58]   Downing NS, Aminawung JA, Shah ND, Krumholz HM, Ross JS. Clinical trial evidence supporting FDA approval of novel therapeutic agents, 2005-2012. JAMA 2014; 311(4): 368-77.
[http://dx.doi.org/10.1001/jama.2013.282034] [PMID: 24449315]

[59]   Schunkert H, König IR, Kathiresan S, *et al.* CARDIoGRAM Consortium; Cardiogenics. Large-scale association analysis identifies 13 new susceptibility loci for coronary artery disease. Nat Genet 2011; 43(4): 333-8.
[http://dx.doi.org/10.1038/ng.784] [PMID: 21378990]

[60]   Herman DS, Lam L, Taylor MR, *et al.* Truncations of titin causing dilated cardiomyopathy. N Engl J Med 2012; 366(7): 619-28.
[http://dx.doi.org/10.1056/NEJMoa1110186] [PMID: 22335739]

[61]   Drug Development and Approval Process. FDA Review Org https://www.fdareview.org/issues/the-drug-development-and-approval-process/

[62]   Eichler HG, Pignatti F, Flamion B, Leufkens H, Breckenridge A. Balancing early market access to new drugs with the need for benefit/risk data: a mounting dilemma. Nat Rev Drug Discov 2008; 7(10): 818-26.
[http://dx.doi.org/10.1038/nrd2664] [PMID: 18787530]

[63]   Lundh A, Krogsbøll LT, Gøtzsche PC. Sponsors' participation in conduct and reporting of industry trials: a descriptive study. Trials 2012; 13: 146.
[http://dx.doi.org/10.1186/1745-6215-13-146] [PMID: 22920226]

[64]   Lundh A, Barbateskovic M, Hróbjartsson A, Gøtzsche PC. Conflicts of interest at medical journals: the influence of industry-supported randomised trials on journal impact factors and revenue - cohort study. PLoS Med 2010; 7(10): e1000354.
[http://dx.doi.org/10.1371/journal.pmed.1000354] [PMID: 21048986]

[65]   Morgan DP. Rating banks: risk and uncertainty in an opaque industry. Am Econ Rev 2002; 92: 874-88.
[http://dx.doi.org/10.1257/00028280260344506]

[66]   Glickman SW, McHutchison JG, Peterson ED, *et al.* Ethical and scientific implications of the globalization of clinical research. N Engl J Med 2009; 360(8): 816-23.
[http://dx.doi.org/10.1056/NEJMsb0803929] [PMID: 19228627]

[67]   Downing NS, Aminawung JA, Shah ND, Braunstein JB, Krumholz HM, Ross JS. Regulatory review of novel therapeutics-comparison of three regulatory agencies. N Engl J Med 2012; 366(24): 2284-93.
[http://dx.doi.org/10.1056/NEJMsa1200223] [PMID: 22591257]

[68]   Getz KA. Global clinical trials activity in the details: individual countries hold the key to finding hot spots in growth regions like Central and Eastern Europe 2009. http://www.appliedclinical trialsonline.com/appliedclinicaltrials/article/articleDetail.jsp?id1

[69]   Mentz RJ, Kaski JC, Dan GA, *et al.* Implications of geographical variation on clinical outcomes of cardiovascular trials. Am Heart J 2012; 164(3): 303-12.

[http://dx.doi.org/10.1016/j.ahj.2012.06.006] [PMID: 22980295]

[70] Fiuzat M, Califf RM. Conduct of clinical trials in acute heart failure: regional differences in heart failure clinical trials. Heart Fail Clin 2011; 7(4): 539-44.
[http://dx.doi.org/10.1016/j.hfc.2011.06.004] [PMID: 21925437]

[71] Pfeffer MA, Claggett B, Assmann SF, *et al.* Regional variation in patients and outcomes in the treatment of preserved cardiac function heart failure with an aldosterone antagonist (TOPCAT) trial. Circulation 2015; 131(1): 34-42.
[http://dx.doi.org/10.1161/CIRCULATIONAHA.114.013255] [PMID: 25406305]

[72] Wallentin L, Becker RC, Budaj A, *et al.* PLATO Investigators. Ticagrelor versus clopidogrel in patients with acute coronary syndromes. N Engl J Med 2009; 361(11): 1045-57.
[http://dx.doi.org/10.1056/NEJMoa0904327] [PMID: 19717846]

[73] Whitford AB. The reduction of regulatory uncertainty: evidence from transfer pricing policy. St Louis Univ Law J 2010; 55: 269-306.

[74] Hoffmann VH, Trautmann T, Schneider M. A taxonomy for regulatory uncertainty—application to the European Emission Trading Scheme. Environ Sci Policy 2008; 11: 712-22.
[http://dx.doi.org/10.1016/j.envsci.2008.07.001]

[75] Brass EP, Hiatt WR. Improving the FDA's advisory committee process. J Clin Pharmacol 2012; 52(8): 1277-83.
[http://dx.doi.org/10.1177/0091270011412962] [PMID: 21908879]

[76] Ferrandiz J Mestre-, J Sussex, A Towse. The R&D cost of a new medicine. Office of Health Economics 2012.

[77] Hersher R. The price of failure: new estimate puts drug R&D in the billions per agent http://blogs.nature.com/spoonful/2012/02/the-price-of-failure-   new-estimate-puts-drug-rd--n-the-billions-per-agent.html/

[78] Scannell JW, Blanckley A, Boldon H, Warrington B. Diagnosing the decline in pharmaceutical R&D efficiency. Nat Rev Drug Discov 2012; 11(3): 191-200.
[http://dx.doi.org/10.1038/nrd3681] [PMID: 22378269]

[79] Warraich HJ, Xu H, DeVore AD, *et al.* Trends in hospice dis- charge and relative outcomes among Medicare patients in the Get with The Guidelines–Heart Failure Registry. JAMA Cardiol 2018; 3(10): 917-26.
[http://dx.doi.org/10.1001/jamacardio.2018.2678] [PMID: 30167645]

[80] Packer M. The imminent demise of cardiovascular drug development. JAMA Cardiol 2017; 2(12): 1293-4.
[http://dx.doi.org/10.1001/jamacardio.2017.3753] [PMID: 29117286]

[81] Harrison C. Patent watch: the patent cliff steepens. Nat Rev Drug Discov 2011; 10(1): 12-3.
[http://dx.doi.org/10.1038/nrd3356] [PMID: 21193859]

[82] Garber AM. An uncertain future for cardiovascular drug development? N Engl J Med 2009; 360(12): 1169-71.
[http://dx.doi.org/10.1056/NEJMp0808414] [PMID: 19297568]

[83] Darrow JJ, Kesselheim AS. Drug development and FDA approval, 1938-2013. N Engl J Med 2014; 370(26): e39.
[http://dx.doi.org/10.1056/NEJMp1402114] [PMID. 24963591]

[84] Stern CS, Lebowitz J. Latest drug developments in the field of cardiovascular disease. Int J Angiol 2010; 19(3): e100-5.
[http://dx.doi.org/10.1055/s-0031-1278379] [PMID: 22477616]

[85] World Health Organization. Cardiovascular Diseases (CVDs). Geneva, Switzerland: WHO 2012.

[86] Access Communications. Cardiovascular Product and Disease Land- scape Analysis Playbook:

Prepared for the American College of Cardiology. San Francisco, CA: Access Communications 2012.

[87]   Komajda M, Coats A, Cowie MR, Jackson N, Svensson A, Vardas P. Cardiovascular Round Table. Championing cardiovascular health innovation in Europe. Eur Heart J 2013; 34(33): 2630-5.
[http://dx.doi.org/10.1093/eurheartj/eht211] [PMID: 23832552]

[88]   Grace C, Kyle M. Comparative advantages of push and pull incentives for technology development: lessons for neglected disease technology development.

[89]   Budget Updates from 2021.https://www.niaid.nih.gov/grants-contracts/budget-updates-january-2021

[90]   2021.https://officeofbudget.od.nih.gov/insti_center_subs.html

[91]   Milne CP. Prospects for rapid advances in the development of new medicines for special medical needs. Clin Pharmacol Ther 2014; 95(1): 98-109.
[http://dx.doi.org/10.1038/clpt.2013.155] [PMID: 23917473]

[92]   Prostate Cancer Fpundation https://www.pcf.org/take-action/movember-pcf/

[93]   American Heart Association At https://www.heart.org/idc/groups/heart-public/

[94]   Dragojlovic N, Lynd LD. Crowdfunding drug development: the state of play in oncology and rare diseases. Drug Discov Today 2014; 19(11): 1775-80.
[http://dx.doi.org/10.1016/j.drudis.2014.06.019] [PMID: 24973645]

[95]   AHA Scientific Statemant. Use of Mobile Devices, Social Media, and Crowdsourcing as Digital Strategies to Improve Emergency Cardiovascular Care. Circulation 2016; 134: e87-e108.

[96]   The American Heart Association and Google Life Sciences Announce Collaboration to Change Trajectory of Heart Disease. 2015.http:// newsroom.heart.org/news/the-american-heart-associat-on-and-google-life-sciences-announce-collaboration-to-change-trajectory-of

[97]   Qualcomm and Northern Arizona Healthcare Expand Home Health Monitoring Program to Enhance the Care of Cardiac, Pulmonary and Post-operative Patients, Qualcomm news room> 2015.http://www. healthitoutcomes.com/doc/qualcomm-enhance-cardiac-pulmonary-post-

[98]   Getting to the heart of the cardiovascular market | New realities and expectations for CVD MedTech companies. Deloitte Development LLC 2017.

[99]   Oncology Drugs Market - Opportunities And Strategies - Global Forecast To 2030. The Business Research Company https://www.thebusinessresearchcompany.com/

[100]   Massie BM, O'Connor CM, Metra M, *et al.* PROTECT Investigators and Committees. Rolofylline, an adenosine A1-receptor antagonist, in acute heart failure. N Engl J Med 2010; 363(15): 1419-28.
[http://dx.doi.org/10.1056/NEJMoa0912613] [PMID: 20925544]

[101]   O'Donoghue ML, Braunwald E, White HD, *et al.* SOLID-TIMI 52 Investigators. Effect of darapladib on major coronary events after an acute coronary syndrome: the SOLID-TIMI 52 randomized clinical trial. JAMA 2014; 312(10): 1006-15.
[http://dx.doi.org/10.1001/jama.2014.11061] [PMID: 25173516]

[102]   Landray MJ, Haynes R, Hopewell JC, *et al.* HPS2-THRIVE Collaborative Group. Effects of extended-release niacin with laropiprant in high-risk patients. N Engl J Med 2014; 371(3): 203-12.
[http://dx.doi.org/10.1056/NEJMoa1300955] [PMID: 25014686]

[103]   Fleming TR, DeMets DL. Surrogate end points in clinical trials: are we being misled? Ann Intern Med 1996; 125(7): 605-13.
[http://dx.doi.org/10.7326/0003-4819-125-7-199610010-00011] [PMID: 8815760]

[104]   Kairalla JA, Coffey CS, Thomann MA, Muller KE. Adaptive trial designs: a review of barriers and opportunities. Trials 2012; 13: 145.
[http://dx.doi.org/10.1186/1745-6215-13-145] [PMID: 22917111]

[105]   U.S. Department of Health and Human Services, Food and Drug Administration, Center for Drug Evaluation and Research, Center for Biologics Eval- uation and Research. Guidance for Industry:

Adaptive Design Clinical Trials for Drugs and Biologics 2010. Rockville, MD: U.S. Department of Health and Human Services.

[106] DiMasi JA. Causes of clinical failures vary widely by therapeutic class, phase of study. Tufts CSDD Impact Report 2013; 15: 1-4.

[107] Hwang TJ, Lauffenburger JC, Franklin JM, Kesselheim AS. Temporal trends and factors associated with cardiovascular drug development, 1990 to 2012. JACC Basic Transl Sci 2016; 1(5): 301-8.
[http://dx.doi.org/10.1016/j.jacbts.2016.03.012] [PMID: 30167520]

[108] WHO. The top 10 causes of death 2010.https://www.who.int/news-room/fact-sheets/detail/the-to--10-causes-of-death

[109] Managing Comorbidities in Patients With Chronic Heart Failure. Am J Cardiovasc Drugs 2015; 15: 171-84.
[http://dx.doi.org/10.1007/s40256-015-0115-6] [PMID: 25837622]

[110] Heidenreich PA, Trogdon JG, Khavjou OA, *et al.* American Heart Association Advocacy Coordinating Committee; Stroke Council; Council on Cardiovascular Radiology and Intervention; Council on Clinical Cardiology; Council on Epidemiology and Prevention; Council on Arteriosclerosis; Thrombosis and Vascular Biology; Council on Cardiopulmonary; Critical Care; Perioperative and Resuscitation; Council on Cardiovascular Nursing; Council on the Kidney in Cardiovascular Disease; Council on Cardiovascular Surgery and Anesthesia, and Interdisciplinary Council on Quality of Care and Outcomes Research. Forecasting the future of cardiovascular disease in the United States: a policy statement from the American Heart Association. Circulation 2011; 123(8): 933-44.
[http://dx.doi.org/10.1161/CIR.0b013e31820a55f5] [PMID: 21262990]

CHAPTER 4

New Approaches in P2Y$_{12}$ Receptor Blocker Drugs Use

Dolunay Merve Fakioğlu[1] and **Sevgi Akaydin**[1,*]

[1] *Department of Biochemistry, Faculty of Pharmacy, Gazi University, Ankara, Turkey*

Abstract: Thienopyridine-derived clopidogrel, prasugrel, cyclopentyltriazole pyrimidine-derived ticagrelor, and non-thienopyridine-derived ATP analogue cangrelor block the P2Y$_{12}$ component of ADP receptors on the platelet surface. This prevents activation of the GPIIb/IIIa receptor complex, thereby reduces platelet aggregation. The platelet activation pathway caused by ADP is blocked by P2Y$_{12}$, and therefore, these drugs have a crucial role in preventing ischemic complications in patients undergoing acute coronary syndrome, including unstable angina, myocardial infarction, and percutaneous coronary intervention. In addition, the use of P2Y$_{12}$ inhibitors for secondary prevention has also been focused on in clinical studies. The results of recent studies show a lot of variances in terms of duration of use, dosage, and individualized treatment management.

The main concern in the clinical use of P2Y$_{12}$ is dual antiplatelet therapy (with aspirin and a P2Y$_{12}$ receptor blocker) following intracoronary stenting to prevent stent thrombosis. However, there are also other multifactorial variables in terms of P2Y$_{12}$ inhibitor use. In this chapter, current and precise medicines regarding P2Y$_{12}$ inhibitor use are evaluated, from gene testing to escalation and de-escalation strategies. Taking all these into account, providing appropriate drugs selection considering treatment time, onset time, duration of use, side effect profile, treatment limitations, and evaluating and interpreting differences in clinical use based on randomized trials will shed light on coronary heart disease treatment choice.

Keywords: Acute coronary syndromes, Clopidogrel resistance, CYP2C19 gene testing, De-escalation, Dual antiplatelet treatment, Escalation, Gene polymorphisms, Ischemic stroke, P2Y$_{12}$ inhibitors, Precision medicine, Triple antithrombotic therapy, Vascular heart disease.

PRIMARY AND SECONDARY HEMOSTASIS

Under normal conditions, platelets circulate freely in the blood system. With the

* **Corresponding author Sevgi Akaydın:** Department of Biochemistry, Faculty of Pharmacy, Gazi University, Ankara, Turkey; Tel: +90(535) 277 11 06; E-mail: sevgiy@gazi.edu.tr

M. Iqbal Choudhary (Ed.)

occurrence of any vascular damage, a series of events are triggered, and platelet-rich clot formation occurs. Platelets are the main components in blood clot formation. This process, called primary hemostasis, results in the formation of thrombosis. This cellular formation process is examined under four general categories: adhesion, activation, secretion, and aggregation [1]. A platelet adheres immediately to the dysfunctional and damaged vascular endothelium. Through adhesive proteins that are exposed in the damaged area and recognized by platelet membrane glycoproteins, the adhesion event of the platelets materialize as required, and the first phase of primary hemostasis begins. When there is vascular damage, the A1 region of the von Willebrand factor binds to GPIbα, the essential elements of the GPIb-IX-V complex, on the platelet surface, to enable the platelet adhesion. Also, GPVI helps adhesion in the interaction between sub-endothelial matrix collagen and platelet through GPa2b1 (GPIA-IIA) and Talin-1 [2]. Platelets change shape quickly from disk to sphere with adhesion to the damaged wall endothelium [3]; thus, they also increase the adhesive surface area. Platelet activation can be triggered by a number of biochemical and mechanical stimuli in addition to platelet adhesion. Most of these biochemical agonists are produced or released by the platelets after adhesion to the vascular wall, and the response to each stimulus continues increasingly. Collagen, Adenosine Diphosphate (ADP), Thromboxane A_2 (TxA$_2$), thrombin are the most soluble platelet agonists, and fluid shear stress also mediates platelet activation. TxA$_2$, together with thrombin and ADPs, binds to specific receptors in the platelet membrane and activates these receptors [4]. The strongest element of platelet activation is undoubtedly the thrombin. The first activation of platelets is induced by binding of thrombins to specific receptors on the surface of the platelets, thereby initiating a signal transduction cascade.

Platelets contain at least three different types of granules; α-granules, dense granules, and lysosomes [5]. Dense granules store and secrete a series of small molecules that are not protein-shaped and are released during activation such as ADP, ATP, GDP, 5-HT, pyrophosphate, magnesium and calcium, α-granules secrete fibrinogen and VWF (Von Willebrand factor), which support platelet-platelet and platelet-endothelial cell interactions. In addition, the fibrinogen receptor αIIβ3 (GPIIb-IIIa), collagen receptor GPVI, and VWF receptor complex GPIb-IX-V components in α-granules are expressed on the platelet surface and then promote platelet adhesion. Thus, all these processes are a series of reactions that stimulate each other [6].

In order to activate other platelets in the plasma, secretion of stored secondary substances, such as ADP, ATP and TxA2 synthesis from arachidonic acid is stimulated, thereby stimulating greater platelet activation and spreading across the wall [7].

Platelet aggregation is the center of ADP-centered thrombus formation. ADP stimulates two G protein-bound P2Y receptors on the platelet surface: Gq-mediated P2Y1 and Gi-mediated P2Y12. The fibrinogen binding GP IIb-IIIa receptor is revealed by stimulation of the P2Y1 and P2Y12 receptor [8]. Inactivated GP IIb-IIIa receptors in platelets have low affinity for ligands. First ADP; TxA2, GPIb-IX-V and GPVI components contribute to the activation of the GPIIb / IIIa complex *via* the inside-out signaling pathway [9]. The GPIIb / IIIa complex is a multifunctional receptor and binds at least four sticky proteins on the activated platelet: fibrinogen, von Willebrand factor, and fibronectin. Following the platelet activation, with the conformational change in GP IIb-IIIa (inside-out signaling), it binds fibrinogen and aggregation begins [10]. Binding of the ligand to aIIbb3 induces integrin aggregation and activation so that an out-in signaling pathway is formed, finally platelet aggregates become more stable and platelet plugins are formed (Fig. **1**).

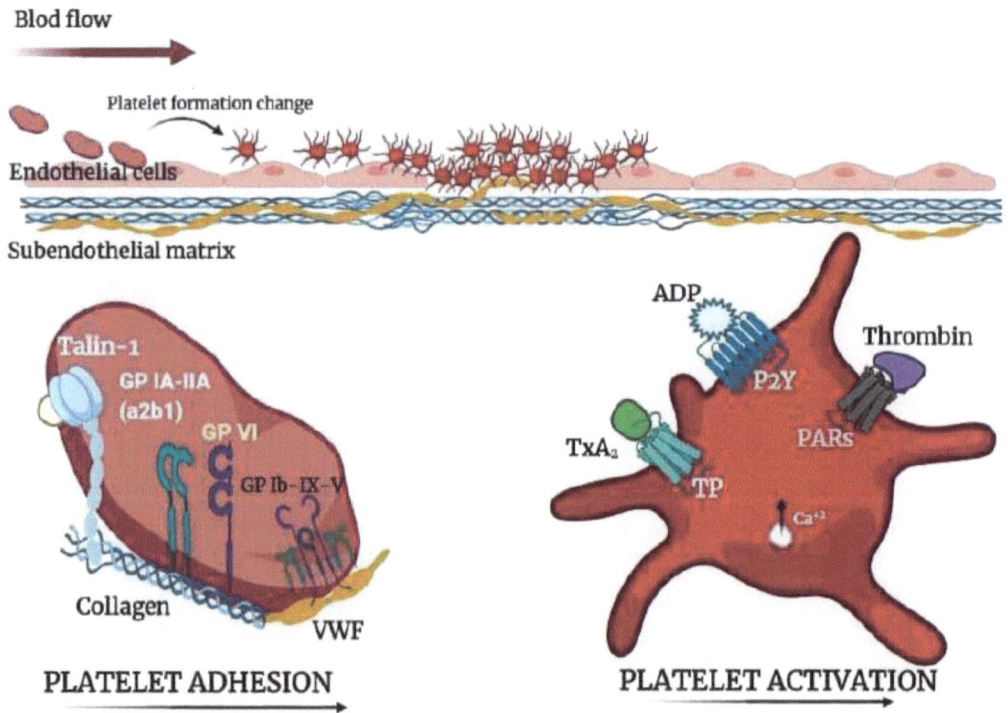

PLATELET ADHESION　　　　PLATELET ACTIVATION

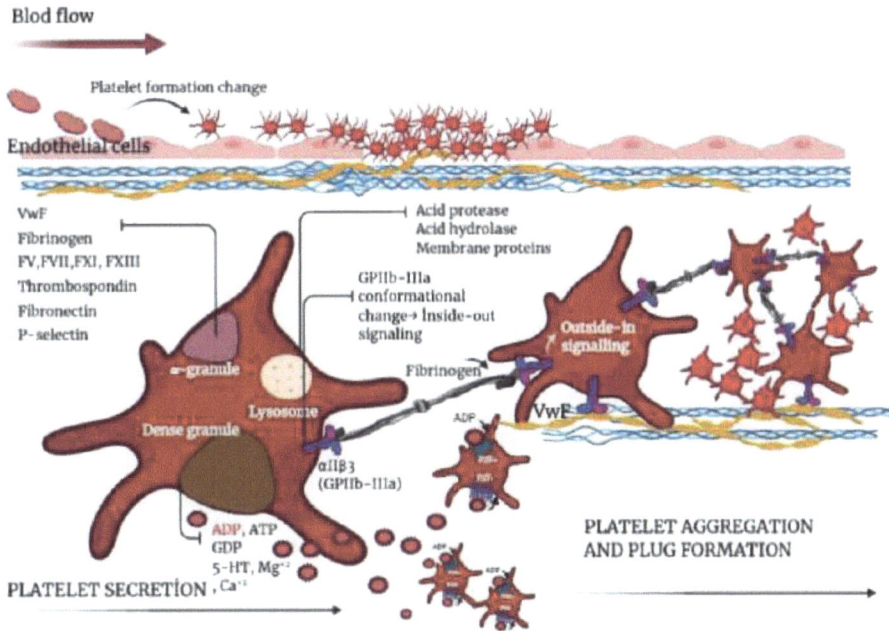

Fig. (1). Platelet Adhesion, Activation, Secretion and Plug formation.

The platelet plug formed after these processes are still delicate, and the coagulation phase or secondary hemostasis phase begins (hemostatic plug formation). This phenomenon is the transformation of the delicate platelet plug into a stable clot (cross-linked fibrin) by binding to the fibrin fibers. Thrombin (Factor 2a) mediated fibrin polymerization occurs, and cross-linked fibrin polymers are comprised [11].

P2Y$_1$ AND P2Y$_{12}$ (ADP RECEPTORS)

P2Y receptors are receptors activated by nucleoside derivatives such as ATP (adenosine triphosphate), UDP (uridine diphosphate), UTP (uridine 5'-triphosphate) or uridine 5'-diphosphoglucose. P1 receptors are activated by adenosine and are available in four subtypes A$_1$, A$_{2A}$, A$_{2B}$, and A$_3$ [12]. P2 receptors are ligand-gated P2X$_1$, G protein-bound P2Y$_1$ and P2Y$_{12}$ [13]and an anti-inflammatory role P2Y$_{14}$ [14]. There are three different purigenic receptors proven to play a role in hemostasis on platelets; these are the G protein-bound P2Y$_1$ and P2Y$_{12}$ and the Ligand-Gated Ion Channels receptor P2X$_1$ [15].

P2Y$_1$, the first identified purinergic receptor, is commonly found in many tissues and has about 150 P2Y$_1$ binding sites on platelets [16]. P2Y$_1$ receptor is Gα / q protein-coupled. Stimulation of the P2Y$_1$ receptor with ADP causes phospholipase C activation-mediated inositol 1,4,5-trisphosphate (IP3) to form calcium release, thereby stimulating the change in platelets and initiating reversible platelet aggregation [17]. In addition, P2Y$_1$ receptors regulate hemostasis in protein expression adjustment. While upregulation increases the risk of platelet aggregation followed by arterial thrombosis [18], downregulation of P2Y$_1$ receptors inhibits platelet aggregation by causing A2B-mediated cAMP (adenosine 3 ', 5'-cyclic monophosphate) levels [19]. Therefore, although P2Y$_1$ receptors appear to have weak and temporary effects on the platelet aggregation pathway, they are in the center of regulating hemostasis.

The P2Y$_{12}$ receptors have approximately 400 binding sites on each platelet [20]. The tissue distribution of this receptor has long been thought to be limited to platelets and sub-regions of the brain. Subsequent studies revealed its expression and functions in microglial cells, vascular smooth muscle cells (VSMCs), dendritic cells (DCs), macrophages, and leukocytes that have not yet been identified [21]. P2Y$_{12}$ receptors located in the center of hemostasis are responsible for irreversible completion of aggregation initiated by P2Y$_1$ receptors. Activation of P2Y$_{12}$ receptors by ADP following platelet activation also stimulates platelet secretion, and stabilizes thrombus formation by enhancing pro-coagulant activity and aggregation [22]. Phosphoinositide 3-kinase (PI3-K) is activated following P2Y$_{12}$ receptor-mediated activation of G protein Gα / i$_2$ G protein subtype [23]. GP IIb-IIIa is activated and maintained by serine-threonine protein kinase B / Akt (PKB / Akt), and by small GTPaseRAP1 [24] in the PI3K downstream pathway and RAP1 regulators such as RASA 3 [25].

Unlike P2Y$_{12}$, the ligand-gated cation receptor, P2X$_1$, is activated by ATP. Following P2X$_1$ activation, intracellular Ca^{++} levels rise very quickly and contribute to platelet deformation and aggregate formation [22].

P2Y$_{12}$ RECEPTOR INHIBITORS AND POTENTIAL CLINICAL USE

The structures of purigenic receptors and subsequent elucidation of the structure-activity studies have resulted in the discovery of a large number of agonist and antagonist drugs acting on these receptors. In particular, P2 receptors have been extensively involved in molecular modeling studies in drug discovery.

According to its mechanisms; direct-acting reversible agents and prodrug irreversible agents represent two essential classes of P2Y$_{12}$receptor inhibitors [26]. Thienopyridines (first approved Ticagrelor $\rightarrow$ Clopidogrel $\rightarrow$ Prasugrel), representing the prodrug group, are the first marketed class of P2Y$_{12}$ receptor inhibitors (Fig. **2**). Ticagrelor and cangrelor are members of the direct-acting reversible group, so they do not require metabolic activation [27]. While clopidogrel, prasugrel, and ticagrelor are the agents that are used orally and for a certain period to provide adequate $P2Y_{12}$ inhibition, cangrelor is preferred intravenously for a shorter period, as an intermediate step to avoid platelet inhibition gap in elective emergency interventions [28].

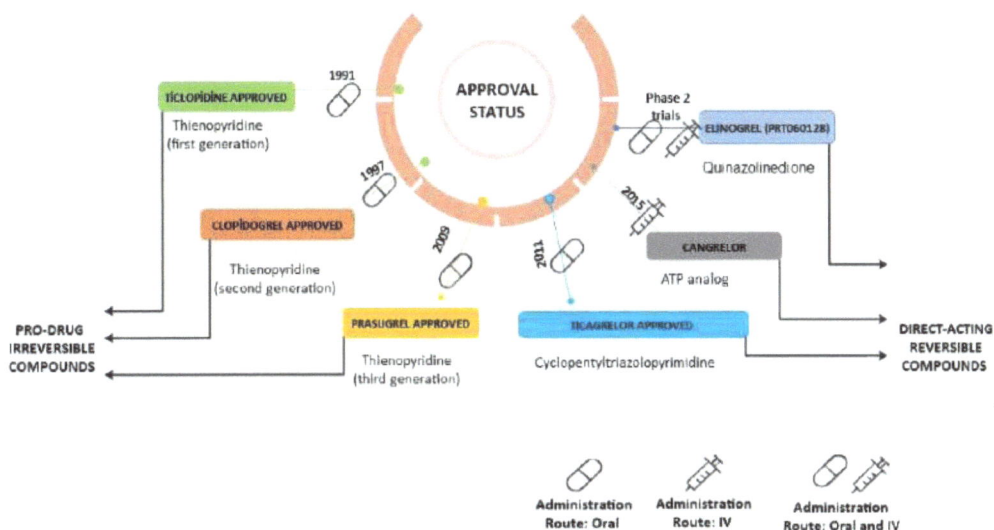

Fig. (2). Features of P2Y12 receptor antagonists.

Ticlopidine is not preferred today, due to severe hematological side effects caused by it. Clopidogrel is the $P2Y_{12}$ inhibitor, which is included in clinical researches the most. Approximately 85% of the absorbed drug turns inactive, and the remaining 15% pro-drug portion is required for oxidation steps managed by hepatic enzymes to be active [29]. The prasugrel is the last generation thienopyridine; shortly after ingestion, the intermediate metabolite is hydrolyzed, and this product turns into an active metabolite in the liver in one step; thus, platelet inhibition begins [29]. Prasugrel onset time is shorter than clopidogrel, thus providing a faster platelet inhibition. In terms of drug metabolism, it is different from clopidogrel. A small amount of clopidogrel, as little as 15%, turns into an active drug after the first hydrolysis, while a large amount of prasugrel turns into an active drug; besides, prasugrel's hepatic activation is provided in one step, whereas the hepatic activation of clopidogrel takes place in two different steps [30]. Like the clopidogrel and prasugrel, orally active ticagrelor binds to a different region from the ADP binding site, unlike thienopyridines, providing platelet inhibition by direct effect [31]. The differences and critical features between $P2Y_{12}$ inhibitors are summarized in Fig. (**3**).

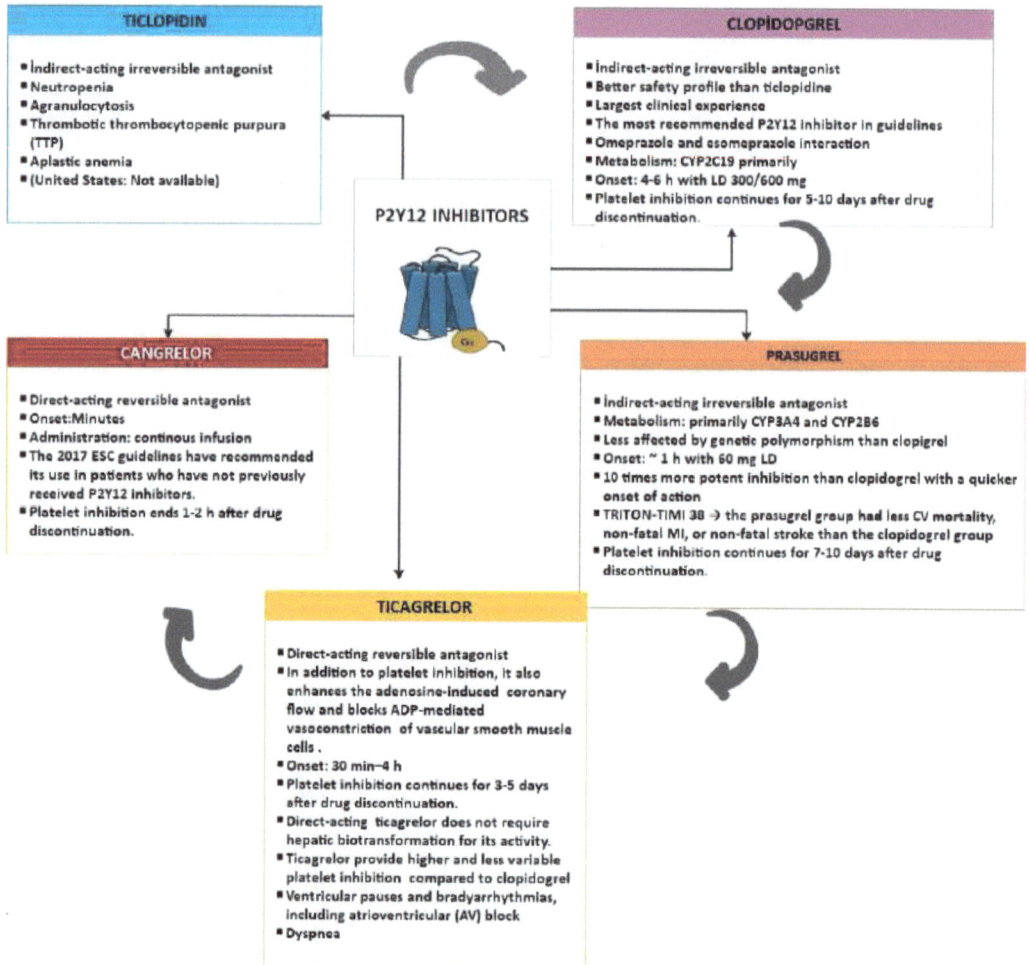

Fig. (3). The main differences of P2Y$_{12}$ inhibitors.

P2Y$_{12}$ inhibitory agents have a wide range of applications in acute coronary syndromes that undergo percutaneous coronary intervention, secondary prevention of atherosclerotic vascular diseases (including stroke, stable coronary artery disease, peripheral artery disease).

Stable Ischemic Heart Disease

Stable ischemic heart disease (SIHD) is myocardial ischemia, which is a result of decreased myocardial oxygen supply and increased myocardial oxygen demand due to one or more stenosis in epicardial coronary arteries. Anginal symptoms are a clinical manifestation of ischemia. Coronary artery disease (CAD) is the leading etiology of ischemic heart disease and is typically characterized by atherosclerotic plaque in the epicardial vessels. Guideline directed medical therapy (GDMT), also called optimal treatment in SIHD management, is the first way to improve disease symptoms and survival [32]. This optimal treatment is composed of lipid management, blood pressure management, antiplatelet therapy, as well as changes in lifestyle such as diet, exercise, and weight control [33].

The basis of antiplatelet therapy in SIHD is provided by aspirin through COX-1 inhibition. In patients who cannot take aspirin due to allergies and intolerance, clopidogrel is used alone. In the CAPRIE study, in which more than 19,000 atherosclerotic vascular patients (previous MI, stroke, or peripheral arterial disease) have been included and followed for three years, it has been shown that long-term use of clopidogrel reduced the risk of developing cardiac events such as myocardial infarction stroke. Still, this study has not provided sufficient data for the use of clopidogrel alone for subgroup analysis, such as SIHD [34]. In a meta-analysis, it has been revealed that the use of clopidogrel alone in SIHD was not more beneficial than aspirin, in terms of mortality, cardiac death, stroke, MI, *etc* [35]. The effectiveness of dual antiplatelet therapy (DAPT), defined as the use of a $P2Y_{12}$ receptor inhibitor (clopidogrel, ticagrelor or prasugrel) and aspirin, is not adequately available in randomized and controlled studies evaluated within the optimal treatment approach in SIHD. In the CHARISMA study, it has been shown that the combination of clopidogrel and low dose aspirin did not considerably reduce the risk of subsequent death, stroke, MI for cardiovascular causes compared to aspirin alone [36].

Revascularization treatment to correct the blood flow to tissues plays a significant and growing role in SIHD. Revascularization options usually consist of coronary artery bypass grafting (CABG) surgery or percutaneous coronary interventions (PCI) with or without a stent. The primary goal with revascularization is to prolong lifetime, whereas the secondary goal is to eliminate or to reduce the symptoms. The revascularization method is particularly useful in stage II SIHD to provide myocardial oxygen support and patients with coronary artery stenosis, despite optimal medical therapy ($\geq$70% diameter). PCI or CABG can be preferred depending on CAD stages and disease symptoms [37].

The term PCI covers the use of stent placement and balloon angioplasty, as well as other lesser-used intracoronary procedures such as rotational atherectomy and aspiration thrombectomy. Owing to the rupture of the atherosclerotic plaque by the balloon during PCI, it requires antithrombotic therapy to prevent acute thrombosis and sudden vessel closure in preoperative procedures [38]. Physical damage to the atherosclerotic plaque during PCI with stent placement stimulates platelet uptake and activation, leading to the potential for thrombus formation.

Therefore, antithrombotic and anticoagulant therapy are required before and after the procedure to achieve a successful outcome [38]. Before elective PCI, clopidogrel and aspirin at the loading dose treatment is recommended [39]. The guidelines recommend the dual antiplatelet therapy (DAPT) approach with clopidogrel+aspirin to be used for a minimum of one month and a maximum of one year, depending on the type of stent used in patients in stage I and stage II after PCIs [40].

CABG is a bypass surgery of the vessels required to provide the necessary myocardial oxygen to the heart muscles. As with PCI, the choice and duration of perioperative and postoperative antiplatelet therapy are determined by the degree of CAD. It is recommended to discontinue P2Y$_{12}$ antagonists five days before the surgery [32].

Acute Coronary Syndromes

Ischemic heart disease appears in a broad clinical spectrum ranging from silent ischemia to sudden death. Acute coronary syndromes (ACSs) are acute atherothrombotic events of atheroma plaques, expressing several conditions compatible with acute myocardial ischemia and / or infarction due to a sudden decrease in coronary blood flow. ACS, characterized by acute change of ischemic symptoms, is pathophysiologically different from SIHD, plaque rupture and subsequent formation of clot formation on the ruptured plaque, and its induction, activation and aggregation of platelet through compounds such as collagen, tissue factors TXA2, ADP. Thrombin-mediated fibrin formation (fibrin clot) stabilizes the clot and traps red blood cells, giving the clot a red appearance. Therefore, the clot consists of cross-linked platelets and fibrin threads [41, 42].

According to ECG changes; ACS, which can be classified as Sn T elevation myocardial infarction (STEMI), a non-ST elevation myocardial infarction (NSTEMI) or unstable angina (UA), is the most common cause of cardiovascular deaths. Acute coronary syndrome includes all clinical syndromes compatible with acute MI, resulting from an imbalance between myocardial oxygen demand and supply [43, 44].

Treatment approach in STEMI and NSTE-ACS (acute coronary syndromes without ST elevation) consists of hospitalization, oxygen supplementation (saturation <90%), pain relief in case of IV nitroglycerin ST elevation, revascularization therapy and subsequently antiplatelet and anticoagulant therapy. Secondary pharmacological treatment is composed of high-density statin, ACE (angiotensin-converting enzyme) inhibitors, and Angiotensin receptor blockers (ARB), blow-blockers and aldosterone antagonists [45, 46]. In STEMI, the preference for revascularization is primarily the PCI. In STEMI patients unsuitable for PCIs, fibrinolytic therapy is preferred. In NSTE-ACS, the first choice according to the TIMI (The Thrombolysis in Myocardial Infarction) score is the medical management of ischemia. However, early invasive procedures (PCI or CABG) may be preferred for those with a high TIMI score. It has not yet been established whether an early invasive strategy reduces the risk of CV or total mortality [47]. In both cases, antiplatelet and anticoagulant therapy are the cornerstones of treatment.

Secondary Prevention of Ischemic Stroke

The stroke is classified into two groups: hemorrhagic (subarachnoid hemorrhage and spontaneous intracerebral hemorrhage) and ischemic stroke (IS), with the highest etiology (87%) [48]. While IS is manifested as a neurological dysfunction that occurs with more than one day of focal cerebral, spinal or retinal infarction, transient ischemic attack (TIA) is manifested by transient symptoms without acute infarction [49]. TIA symptoms vary from minutes to hours, while IS symptoms persist for more than 24 hours.

There are basically two approaches, primary and secondary, in the treatment of IS [50]. Primary prevention is based on lifestyle modifications according to individual risk factors (age, gender, atrial fibrillation, diabetes, smoking, *etc.*), and the antiplatelet approach is not recommended for primary prevention of IS [51]. However, a stroke may predict different cerebrovascular accident (CVA), especially in the first three months after the acute period. Although anticoagulants are used in cardio-embolic strokes, antiplatelet therapy is the treatment of non-cardio embolic strokes, but the optimal approach is controversial [52].

In the MATCH study, which was the first study to evaluate the efficacy of DAPT in IS patients, DAPT treatment did not provide any additional benefit in ischemic stroke, and these findings were attributed to the lacunar stroke population in the study [53], and the results were also supported by further studies [54]. In the subgroup analysis of the CHARISMA study, it was thought that the maximum benefit after acute IS could be seen within the first 30 days [46]. Stroke is a highly heterogeneous disease, unlike CAD, and therefore the heterogeneity of randomized controlled trials may not be sufficient to analyze which population will benefit most from DAPT treatment. In the CHANGE study involving a more specific population, minor IS and high-risk TIA populations were included [55]. According to the results of this study, it was shown that the application of clopidogrel and aspirin administered within the first 24 hours after the onset of minor and high-risk TIA symptoms reduced the recurrence of 3-month stroke without increasing the bleeding rate. In addition, the one-year follow-up reports also reduced the one-year stroke recurrence with clopidogrel monotherapy applied for 90 days, following the aspirin + clopidogrel regimen for 21 days [56]. In the POINT study, the effects of 600 mg clopidogrel loading dose and concomitant aspirin use after acute minor IS and high-risk TIA were evaluated according to aspirin alone, and it was concluded that 90 DAPT times increased the risk of bleeding [57].

In the SOCRATES study conducted in acute minor IS or high-risk TIA patients, it was shown that the ticagrelor regimen alone was not superior to the aspirin regimen [58]. In the PRINCE study conducted in the same population, 90-day DAPT with ticagrelor and aspirin increased platelet reactivity, particularly in patients with P450 2C19 polymorphism, but also increased minor bleeding events [59]. DAPT and monotherapy in acute minor IS, or high-risk TIA patients are shown in Fig. (**4**).

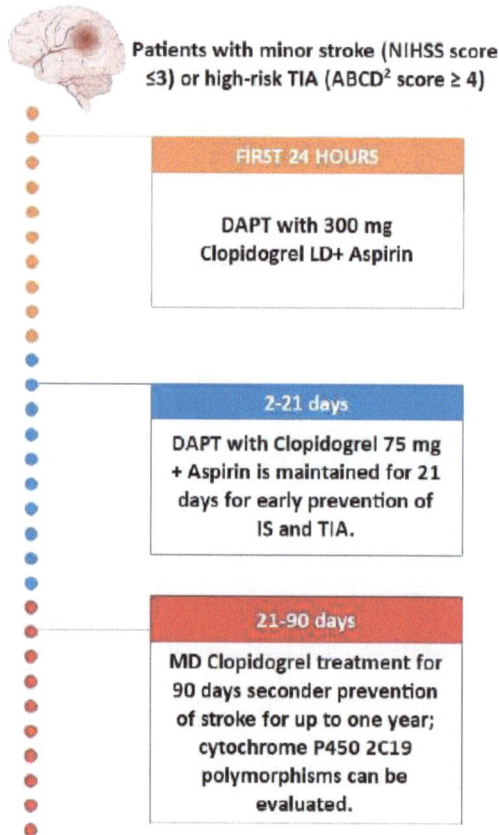

Patients with minor stroke (NIHSS score ≤3) or high-risk TIA (ABCD^2 score ≥ 4)

FIRST 24 HOURS

DAPT with 300 mg Clopidogrel LD+ Aspirin

2-21 days

DAPT with Clopidogrel 75 mg + Aspirin is maintained for 21 days for early prevention of IS and TIA.

21-90 days

MD Clopidogrel treatment for 90 days seconder prevention of stroke for up to one year; cytochrome P450 2C19 polymorphisms can be evaluated.

Fig. (4). Antiplatelet treatment for patients with minor stroke or high-risk transient ischemic attack (TIA), DAPT: Dual antiplatelet therapy, LD: Loading dose, MD: Maintenance dose, IS: Ischemic stroke, NIHSS: National Institutes of Health Stroke Scale, ABCD^2: Score for TIA.

Prosthetic Heart Valves Triple Treatment

Valvular heart diseases have an important place among cardiovascular diseases with frequent prevalence and high valve replacement rates [60]. Mechanical, bioprosthetic, and transcatheter biological valves are the most common types [61]. Mechanical valves are highly thrombogenic, often preferred in young adults due to their durable nature, and require the use of lifelong vitamin K antagonists (warfarin) with INR in the target range [62]. Bioprosthetic valve patients are treated with systemic anticoagulation for a shorter period (preferably six months) following implantation [63].

Today, the DAPT regimen, which is continued with clopidogrel and aspirin in patients using mechanical valves, has been evaluated as an inadequate strategy due to the high risk of embolic events. Although bioprosthetic valves have less anticoagulation requirement, they are more easily degenerated than mechanical valves later on [64]. Therefore, Trans-catheter aortic valve replacement (TAVR) biologicals are preferred, especially in patients with severe aortic stenosis [61]. The ACC / AHA Valve guideline recommends a six-month DAPT regimen at the C evidence level maintained with 75 mg clopidogrel + 75-100 mg aspirin in patients using TAVR [65].

PRECISION MEDICINE IN DUAL ANTIPLATELET REGIMES STRATEGIES (DE-ESCALATION, ESCALATION, CHANGE STRATEGIES FOR DUAL ANTIPLATELET THERAPY)

Individualized therapy in dual antiplatelet therapy is a complete form of many strategies, such as antiplatelet escalation, dose reduction, use of different $P2Y_{12}$ inhibitors, and reduction of $P2Y_{12}$ treatment duration, or continuing treatment with a single agent. De-escalation for DAPT states all definitions from treatment intensity (transition to monotherapy, duration reduction, use of an agent that makes less platelet inhibition) to dose reduction. Both escalation and de-escalation are integral parts of the individualized treatment. When and how to apply these strategies are essential for individualized treatment [66].

De-Escalation *via* a Duration of Dual Antiplatelet Treatment

DAPT is strongly recommended to reduce the risk of stent thrombosis after PCI. However, optimal DAPT duration and selection of an appropriate $P2Y_{12}$ inhibitor agent are still unknown. In 2001, the CURE study demonstrated the superiority of DAPT in monotherapy aspirin use in terms of preventing ischemic coronary events [67], led to the paradigm shift to the duration of DAPT. The optimal DAPT (clopidogrel + aspirin) duration is nine months (3-12 months) in the CURE study, and current guidelines after the CURE study suggest that DAPT therapy should be continued for 6-12 months in the case of ACS [40, 68]. However, prolonged DAPT duration decreases the risk of ischemic adverse events while increasing the risk of bleeding [69]. In addition, the latest technological advances in drug-eluting stents (DES) could allow DAPT duration to be shortened [70]. Clarification of this sharp line between the ischemic event and the bleeding risk with open algorithms will inform clinicians on where to stand.

To date, short and long DAPTs have been evaluated in various meta-analyses, and although the results of these meta-analyses differ from each other, the common point is that the prolonged DAPT time increases the risk of bleeding. Ischemic complications (MI, ST, stroke) risks vary according to the stent type used (Table 1). The data obtained from these meta-analyses roughly give the impression that the use of DAPT for 3 or 6 months is effective in patients who are stable after the 2nd generation or new generation DES implantation, and the use of DAPT for more than 12 months will benefit patients with high-risk and MI history. In addition, validation of subgroup analyses should be provided as the stable patient population in studies can directly affect the risk of ischemic complications. Also, randomized studies and meta-analysis that summarize the benefits of prolonged use of DAPT for more than 12 months should not be neglected.

Table 1. Meta-Analysis study-related DAPT (dual antiplatelet therapy) duration. Myocardial infarction (MI), stent thrombosis (ST), cerebrovascular accidents (CVAs), first-generation paclitaxel-eluting stent (PES), sirolimus-eluting stent (SES), the second-generation zotarolimus-eluting stent (ZES), everolimus-eluting stent (EES), Bleeding Academic Research Consortium(BARC), Global Use of Strategies to Open Occluded Coronary Arteries (GUSTO) bleeding, Safety and Efficacy of Enoxaparin in PCI Patients (STEEPLE).

Authors	Year	Number Of Randomized Controlled Trials (RCTs)	Number of Patients	Patients Characteristics and DES Qualification	Bleeding Score	DAPT Durations	Main Outcomes
Cassese *et al.* [73]	2012	4 RCTs	8158	●PCI with DES (ACS or Stable angina regardless) ● DES qualification: first and second-generation DESs (PES, SES, ZES, EES)	TIMI criteria	6.2-16.8 month	●Prolonged DAPT →Bleeding risks ↑ ● Prolonged DAPT does not diminish the risk of MI, ST, and CVAs related deaths

(Table 1) cont.....

Authors	Year	Number Of Randomized Controlled Trials (RCTs)	Number of Patients	Patients Characteristics and DES Qualification	Bleeding Score	DAPT Durations	Main Outcomes
Giustino *et al.* [74]	2015	10 RCTs	32,135	• PCI with DES (ACS or Stable angina regardless) • DES qualification: first and second-generation DESs(PES, SES, ZES, EES)	•TIMI •BARC •GUSTO •STEEPLE	•S-DAPT: shorter dual antiplatelet therapy: 3-6 month •L-DAPT: ¼ longer dual antiplatelet therapy: 12months or longer DAPT usage	•L-DAPT→Lower MI and ST risks •L-DAPT →Bleeding risks↑ • The benefit of L-DAPT in ST has decreased with the use of second-generation DES.
Bulluck *et al.* [75]	2014	8 RCTs	16,318	• PCI with DES and BMS (ACS or Stable angina regardless) •Stent qualification: first and second-generation DESs(PES, SES, ZES, EES) and BMS	•TIMI •BARC •STEEPLE	•3 *vs.* 12-month DAPT duration •6 *vs.* 12-month DAPT duration •6 *vs.* 24-month DAPT duration •12 *vs.* 24-month DAPT duration	•Prolonged DAPT →Bleeding risks ↑ • Prolonged DAPT does not diminish thrombotic complications and mortality •3-6 months DAPT duration lower bleeding risks •There was no additional benefit from DAPT death, or MI extended to 24 months.
Valgimigli *et al.* [76]	2012	3 RCTs	5622	•PCI with DES (ACS or Stable angina regardless) •DES qualification: first and second-generation DESs (PES, SES, ZES, EES)	•TIMI •BARC	•S-DAPT: shorter dual antiplatelet therapy: 3-12 month •L-DAPT: longer dual antiplatelet therapy: 12-24 months DAPT usage	•Prolonged DAPT ≥ 12 months→Bleeding and stroke risks 2-fold↑ •There was no additional benefit from prolonged DAPT death or MI.
Navarese *et al.* [77]	2015	10 RCTs	32,287	• PCI with DES (ACS or Stable angina regardless) •Stent qualification: first and second-generation DESs (PES, SES, ZES, EES) and BMS	•TIMI •BARC •GUSTO •STEEPLE	•S-DAPT: shorter dual antiplatelet therapy: <12 month •L-DAPT: longer dual antiplatelet therapy:≥ 12 month •Standard 12 month therapy (N-DAPT)	•S-DAPT and N-DAPT similar rate of MI and ST risks •L-DAPT (*versus* N-DAPT) reduced ST, MI but increased bleeding.

(Table 1) cont.....

Authors	Year	Number Of Randomized Controlled Trials (RCTs)	Number of Patients	Patients Characteristics and DES Qualification	Bleeding Score	DAPT Durations	Main Outcomes
Elmariah *et al.* [78]	2015	14 RCTs	69,644	• PCI with DES (ACS or Stable angina regardless) •Stent qualification: first and second-generation DESs (PES, SES, ZES, EES) and BMS	•TIMI •BARC •GUSTO •STEEPLE	•Monotherapy aspirin •S-DAPT: shorter dual antiplatelet therapy: ≤6 months • L-DAPT: longer dual antiplatelet therapy >6 months	• There is no relationship between L-DAPT and coronary or non-coronary death
Rozemeijer *et al.* [69]	2018	9 RCTs	19,099	• PCI with DES (ACS or Stable angina regardless) •Stent qualification: first and second-generation DESs (PES, SES, ZES, EES) and BMS	•TIMI •BARC •GUSTO/REPLACE-2	•S-DAPT: shorter dual antiplatelet therapy: 3-6 month •L-DAPT: longer dual antiplatelet therapy: 12-24 months DAPT	•S-DAPT associated with a 50% reduction in major bleeding risk •S-DAPT was not associated with ischemic complications.
Cassese *et al.* [79]	2015	10 RCTs	32,194	• PCI with DES (ACS or Stable angina regardless) •Stent qualification: first and second generation DESs(PES,SES,ZES,EES) and BMS	•TIMI •BARC	•Control DAPT: 6 (6–12) months • L-DAPT: longer dual antiplatelet therapy: 15 (12–24) months	•Prolonged DAPT →Bleeding risks ↑ and ST, MI ↓

• De-Escalation with Switching Monotherapy Antiplatelet Treatment.

Ensuring the appropriate DAPT duration is valuable in order to balance the bleeding complications and the risk of ischemic complications. For this reason, risk scores can be used while evaluating the DAPT duration. Although many bleeding scoring studies have been carried out so far, PRECISE-DAPT [71] and the DAPT scores [72] are the two essential scoring tools to estimate the DAPT duration.

The PRECISE-DAPT score is a 100-point scoring system consisting of 5 items that have been used to evaluate post-discharge bleeding complications in patients who have undergone coronary stents and have used DAPT. According to this scoring system, patients with a score of ≥25 are considered as having a high risk of bleeding, and it is recommended that DAPT treatment is continued for 3 or 6 months. Patients with a PRECISE-DAPT score of <25 were identified as a group of patients without high bleeding risk, and a standard (12 months) or prolonged (12-24 month) DAPT period is recommended [71].

The DAPT score provides information on the risk-benefit balance for patients that have been under the DAPT regimen for more than 12 months through a scale ranging from -2 to 10. The risk of bleeding is described as low in patients with a DAPT score of ≥ 2, and a long DAPT regimen is recommended, but not to exceed 30 months. For patients with DAPT score of <2, the risk of bleeding is defined as high, and 12 months of standard treatment was recommended for this group [72].

The transition to monotherapy has primarily cost-effective benefits as well as constructive effects in terms of decreasing the drug density used by the patients.

In the recent TWILIGHT study, in which the de-escalation strategy has been applied, patients with a high risk of bleeding or ischemic events after a three-month ticagrelor+aspirin regime have been randomized for 12 months to receive ticagrelor or ticagrelor + aspirin. Ticagrelor monotherapy was associated with 44% less bleeding than dual therapy and increased neither the risk of death, MI, nor stroke [80].

Deferring from the TWILIGHT study, in GLOBAL LEADERS, another critical study in which de-escalation strategies have been applied, treatment with Ticagrelor has been continued for 23 months, after one month of DAPT treatment (Ticagrelor + aspirin) of the experimental group. The 23-month ticagrelor monotherapy regimen administered after a one-month dual treatment has not been found to be superior in terms of mortality to the 12 months DAPT regimen determined in the international guidelines, and ticagrelor monotherapy has not provided any advantage in terms of ST and bleeding risk [81]. Since only patients using new polymer-based stents (BES) have been included in this study, it sheds light on patient management after using modern stents in PCI today. Although the GLOBAL LEADERS and TWILIGHT studies do not overlap, it should not be overlooked that DAPT durations and monotherapy durations have been varied in both studies. Likewise, in STOPDAPT-2 and SMART-CHOICE studies, clopidogrel monotherapy has been given after 1 and 3 months of dual treatment, respectively, and have been found to be superior, in terms of bleeding without increasing ischemic risk, to 12 months of classic DAPT [82, 83].

De-Escalation with Switching Between P2y$_{12}$ Inhibitors Drugs

This de-escalation strategy between the two different P2Y$_{12}$ inhibitor drugs generally refers to switching from a more potent inhibitor such as Prasugrel or Ticagrelor to clopidogrel. Side effects such as bleeding, dyspnea, as well as the need for anticoagulants and cost-effective causes, which develop due to conditions such as atrial fibrillation (AF), and stroke, the incidences of which increase with age, often mediate these switching strategies. The results of randomized and clinical studies are generally interpreted according to bleeding scores and platelet function tests. Therefore, in order to understand the studies, concepts such as high platelet reactivity and low platelet reactivity should be clarified.

Ischemic events following antiplatelet loading dose have been attributed to high on-treatment platelet reactivity (HTPR); therefore, HTPR reflects a weak antiplatelet effect. In addition, the definition of low on-treatment platelet reactivity (LTPR) is used to describe the extreme response to P2Y$_{12}$ blockers [84]. Clopidogrel has been associated with more HTPR than ticagrelor or prasugrel [85]. Therefore, platelet inhibition is provided in PCIs following ACS *via* a more intense P2Y$_{12}$ inhibitor such as ticagrelor or prasugrel [86]. However, following ticagrelor or prasugrel, it is possible to switch to clopidogrel after a while due to possible side effects and cost-effective problems [87, 88].

The SCOPE study has examined switching strategies, including post-intervention escalation and de-escalation in 1363 ACS patients that had undergone PCI, and switching from new P2Y$_{12}$ inhibitors to clopidogrel has been associated with an increased risk of recurrent ischemic events [89]. In the TOPIC study, the transition to a less concentrated DAPT regimen has been associated with minor bleeding complications [90].

Switching to a less dense P2Y$_{12}$ inhibitor agent usually occurs during discharge from the hospital [91]. ANTARCTIC [92] and TROPICAL-ACS [93], which are switching studies to a less dense P2Y$_{12}$ inhibitor, de-escalated with a platelet function tested (PFT) approach. In the ANTARCTIC study, a safer 5 mg prasugrel dose has been aimed to be adjusted according to the platelet response, whereas the TROPICAL-ACS study has aimed to select the appropriate P2Y$_{12}$ inhibitor (prasugrel or clopidogrel), according to the results of the platelet function test (HPR). Therefore, the method to be used in the P2Y$_{12}$ density reduction strategy is essential.

In the TOPIC-VASP study, 646 patients, in addition to 75 mg aspirin, the ticagrelor (MD: 180mg) or prasugrel (MD: 10mg) treatment regimen have been randomized as the unchanged treatment group, and the de-escalation (75 mg aspirin + 75 mg clopidogrel) group and patients have been followed for approximately one year [94]. In this study, it is valuable that all randomizations have been done independent of PFT, and the results of the study have been interpreted according to the distribution of patients without basal LTPR or LTPR in different groups. In this study, cardiovascular death, emergency coronary revascularization, stroke, and bleeding events were found to be significantly lower in LTPR patients in the de-escalation group. The number of cardiovascular mortality, emergency coronary revascularization, stroke, and bleeding events seen in non-LTPR (HTPR or normal) patients in the de-escalation group was found to be low, although the treatment regimen was not statistically significant compared to the control group. The most crucial finding in this study is that the de-escalation strategy administered regardless of the $P2Y_{12}$ inhibitor response is useful in terms of cardiovascular death, emergency coronary revascularization, stroke, and bleeding events. In addition, the benefit of de-escalation has been observed more in LTPR patients.

De-escalation, with a less intense $P2Y_{12}$ inhibitor, has been evaluated in several randomized and prospective-observational clinical trials. Randomized and other clinical studies involving prasugrel to clopidogrel de-escalation are summarized in Table **2**.

Table 2. De-escalation with switching from Prasugrel to clopidogrel; P: Prasugrel, C: clopidogrel, LD: loading dose, MD: maintenance dose, HTPR: High on-treatment platelet reactivity, HPR: high on-clopidogrel platelet reactivity, CAD: Coronary artery disease, ACS: Acute coronary syndrome, PCI: Percutan coronary intervention, UA/NSTEMI: unstable angina/non-ST elevation myocardial infarction Inhibition of platelet aggregation (IPA), PRU: $P2Y_{12}$ reaction unit, PFT: Platelet function testing, VLTPR: very low on-treatment platelet reactivity, RI-VASP: platelet reactivity index-vasodilator-stimulated phosphoprotein.

De-escalation with switching from Prasugrel to clopidogrel *Patients in all studies received aspirin concomitantly.*			
Study Design and Study Name	**Study Population**	**Switching Protocol**	**Clinical Outcomes**
RESET GENE *Trial [111] - Open-label, crossover randomized	Stable CAD patients undergoing PCI with DES	In the study, stable 32 CAD patients with HTPR> 450 AUC were included *via* $P2Y_{12}$ assay and were crossed-over to after 15 days P (10 mg / day) → C (150 mg / day) or C (150 mg / day) → P (10 mg / day)	In the HTRP patient group, P was more effective than C. 3 minor bleeding in the P group 1 minor bleeding in the C group
ACAPULCO* study [112] - Open-label, crossover randomized	UA/NSTEMI ACS patients	All patients were assigned to the P or C arm after taking 900 mg of C-LD. 54 UA / NSTEMI patients were included in the study, 27 of which were crossed-over to after 15 days P (10 mg / day) → C (150 mg / day) and 24 patients C (150 mg / day) → P (10 mg / day).	P 10 mg provided better platelet inhibition than C 150 mg. There were no differences in any non-CABG-related TIMI major or GUSTO severe/life-threatening bleeding events. Five subjects (3 P and 2 C) experienced bleeding during MD treatment.

(Table 2) cont.....

De-escalation with switching from Prasugrel to clopidogrel		
Patients in all studies received aspirin concomitantly.		
EPIPHANY [113]- Open-label, randomized	429 Patients PCI with DES	Treatment randomization was performed according to HTPR (PRU> 230) status. Patients were classified according to whether they received thienopyridine treatment before and thienopyridine naïve patients (n: 180) were randomized to P (60mg) or C (600mg). Switching was performed in patients with HTPR (P → C or C → P)	Regardless of whether patients have previously received thienopyridine therapy, alternative thienopyridine regimens can be selected in patients with HTPR. In addition, HTPR was lower in the study than P group C.
TROPICAL-ACS [93]- Open-label , parallel-group, randomized	2106 ACS patients undergoing PCI (STEMI and NSTEMI)	During discharge after ACS-PCI, patients were randomized 1:1 guided by PFT to standard P or P one week→ C HPR: ≥ 46U switched back to prasugrel, whereas those without HPR (<46 U) continued clopidogrel treatment.	The clinical benefit of the DAPT De-escalation strategies under the guidance of PFT in ACS-PCI patients is emphasized.
ANTARCTIC [92] – Open-label, randomized study	≥75 age 877 patients with ACS undergo PCI	Patients ≥75 years old; Randomization (1: 1) was performed to receive P (5mg) or P (5mg) and individual treatment adjusted to PFT after 14 days. ≥208 PRU→ P increased to 10 mg, ≤85 PRU→ P replaced to C (75mg)	Although the primary purpose of the study was PFT-guided dose adjustment in the elderly ACS-PCI population, the number of P (5mg) → C (75mg) patients with ≤85 PRU was 171. Safety did not improve significantly in patients switching to C, according to the PRU. PFT guided dose adjustment was not found to be superior in efficacy and safety in the aged ACS-PCI population.

(Table 2) cont.....

De-escalation with switching from Prasugrel to clopidogrel *Patients in all studies received aspirin concomitantly.*			
PRINCIPLE-TIMI 44 [114] randomized, double-blind, double-dummy, active comparator-controlled, crossover	201 planned PCI patients	Patients were randomized in 2 groups, either P (60mg) or C (600mg), and received a loading dose, and then received MD for 15 days (either P (10mg) or C (150mg) corresponding to the LD assignment, and crossover directly P (10mg) or C (150mg).	53 patients switched to P → C. 1 patient in P→ C crossover group had a myocardial infarction. No TIMI major or minor bleeds were observed in P→ C crossover group.
POBA study- [115] Prospective, observational	20 ACS patients with VLTPR (PRU≤ PRI VASP b 10%)	P(LD: 60 mg) and after P(10 mg ML) for 1 month, and defined as 20 VLTPR patients switched to C(75 mg) end of the 1st month.	No bleeding event was observed after switching to C with adequate platelet inhibition.
[116]- an open-label, randomized, parallel-group comparison study	136 patients with ACS undergo PCI, 36 patients with CAD requiring elective coronary stenting	P 20 mg LD → P 3.75 mg from day 2 and remained until 6 week P 20 mg LD → P 3.75 mg from day 2 and → C 75 mg at 2 weeks and continued until 6 weeks.	Although PRU decreased in all patients in the 2nd week, the PRU increased significantly in the switching group that was switched to C in the 6th week.
[117]- Prospective, observational registry	300 patients with ACS undergo PCI	Of the patients who received P (10mg) for 15 days after discharge and platelet reactivity test was done on 15th day, 31 of them switched to C (75mg) at the clinician's decision. Second PFT was performed in the C group 15 days later.	Switching to P → C provided platelet inhibition at a suitable and desired range according to the PRU and no major bleedings.
[95]- Prospective, open-label observational registry	45 ACS patients undergo PCI	P (LD: 20 mg and MD: 3.75 mg) for 7 days and after switched to C(75), and followed up 28 days. A total of 7 PRU values were measured, including basal PRU and the first day after PCI.	Maintaining the P→C switching strategy with the maintenance dose of C did not create an efficacy gap.

Prasugrel and clopidogrel both represent the same pharmacological subgroup of $P2Y_{12}$ inhibitors, as they are indirectly effective prodrugs. Therefore, there is no risk of drug-drug interaction in escalation regimens, from prasugrel to clopidogrel or *vice versa*. In studies performed, administration of 75 mg clopidogrel follow-up dose from prasugrel to clopidogrel has not created a gap in platelet inhibition [95], and therefore loading dose is not recommended in prasugrel to clopidogrel de-escalation to avoid the risk of bleeding. However, due to the rapid platelet turnover in the early phase of ACSs, clopidogrel may not adequately demonstrate its inhibitory effects on the receptor. Therefore, a loading dose of 600 mg of clopidogrel is recommended for de-escalation from Prasugrel to clopidogrel in ACS-acute periods [96]. Ticagrelor and cangrelor are direct-acting reversible agents, and in de-escalation strategies, the switching from these agents to clopidogrel or prasugrel can mediate possible drug-drug interactions and cause increased platelet reactivity through the blockade of binding of active metabolites to purigenic receptors [97, 98]. Although Ticagrelor has a fast offset time compared to clopidogrel, greater inhibition of platelet aggregation (IPA) is observed in the first 24 hours, and it is synchronized with clopidogrel at the 24th hour, and it progresses in less than 3-5 days after the last dose [99]. Therefore, this rapid offset time could create a deficit in platelet inhibition. In patients who do not risk being put on the expert opinion with switching strategies, it is recommended to administer clopidogrel loading dose at the 24th hour after the last dose of ticagrelor (when the IPAs are equal) considering the changes in the offset pharmacokinetics [96]. In the SWAP-4 study, no significant difference has been found on the platelet reactivity of the clopidogrel loading dose regimen (12-24h) administered at different times after ticagrelor [100]; however, in observational studies [89, 101], an increase in the risk of ischemic adverse events have been observed, due to an increase in platelet reactivity.

Switching from the Ticagrelor regimen to clopidogrel may occur during hospital discharge [102], or switching to clopidogrel therapy is possible after the hospital discharge [103]. Side effects and oral anticoagulants need developing under ticagrelor treatment are the significant causes of switching to clopidogrel [103]. The association of chronic obstructive pulmonary disease (COPD), female gender, and age with ticagrelor-associated dyspnea may require such a de-escalation strategy [104]. Studies involving the transition regimes from ticagrelor to clopidogrel are presented in Table **3**. As shown in the tables, there are very few studies on de-escalation strategies from ticagrelor to clopidogrel, due to the drug's interaction risk.

Patients who are under active oral antiplatelet therapy during the preoperative period (usually 5-7 days before surgery), a gap occurs in platelet inhibition by discontinuation of antiplatelet therapy. In order to minimize this unprotected period, intravenous (IV) P2Y₁₂ (cangrelor) inhibitors are administered to patients to provide rapid platelet inhibition preoperatively, and this switching therapy is called bridging. After the preoperative processes, patients should be re-switched from IV cangrelor to oral P2Y$_{12}$ inhibitors, and this de-escalation strategy is defined as a transition [96]. Since cangrelor provides a rapid and highly potent platelet inhibition and also following the procedure, there is a transition to oral P2Y$_{12}$ inhibitors in all patients; this time frame is called the transition.

Table 3. T: Ticagrelor, C: Clopidogrel, LD: loading dose, MD: maintenance dose, PFT: platelet function test, DAPT: Dual antiplatelet therapy, CAD: Coronary artery disease, ACS: Acute coronary syndrome.

De-escalation with switching from Ticagrelor to clopidogrel *Patients in all studies received aspirin concomitantly.*			
Study Design and Study Name	**Study Population**	**Switching Protocol**	**Clinical Outcomes**
RESPOND Study [118] Randomized, double-blind, double-dummy crossover	98 stable CAD patients	Responders and nonresponders groups were randomized to C (LD: 600 mg after MD: 75 mg) or T (LD: 180 mg after 90mg twice daily) for 14 days, and crossed-over to being T → C or C → T	The antiplatelet effect of T was not affected by the response state of C. More consistent IPA was observed in the nonresponders group with the transition to the T regimen. All serious adverse events and bleeding events were observed in the T regime.
CAPITAL OPTICROSS Study Prospective, randomized, open-label	60 ACS patients who were decided to switch from T to C	60 patients were equally randomized to two groups, with maintenance dose and bolus dose followed by a maintenance dose. For bolus group, T→C (LD:600 mg) 12 h after last T, and then C (MD: 75mg), Instead of the last dose of T → C (75 mg) and on the following days, C (75 mg). PFT measurements were collected 7 times, including basal (72 hours after last sample C).	T → C Bolus and MD dose strategies were not different in 72 hours for platelet inhibition. The incidence of HPR is higher in the MD dose strategy than in the bolus.

De-escalation with switching from Ticagrelor to clopidogrel *Patients in all studies received aspirin concomitantly.*			
SWAP-4 [100] Prospective, randomized, open-label	80 CAD patients	Patients receiving 80 DAPT (C + aspirin) were administered T (LD: 180 mg, then MD: 90 mg) for 7 days and then randomized into four groups. Two groups of LD strategies, C (LD: 600 mg) followed by C (MD: 75mg), were applied 12, 24 h after the last T dose, respectively. C (MD:75 mg 24 h after the last T) was administrated for one group, and the last group continued to receive T.	In the C-LD strategies, better platelet inhibition was observed in the first 48 hours compared to the C-MD approach, and there was no pharmacodynamic difference between the times of LD administration.

In the cangrelor bridging strategy of patients taking oral P2Y$_{12}$ inhibitors, a 3, 5 or 7 day P2Y$_{12}$, the inhibitor-free period is recommended. However, this may not always be achieved in situations that require urgent surgery. In such cases, cangrelor infusion (0.75 µg / kg/min) that does not require bolus application can be administered 3-4 days after prasugrel cessation and 2-3 days after clopidogrel or ticagrelor cessation [96].

Even if there is no platelet inhibition gap during the transition from oral P2Y$_{12}$ inhibitors to cangrelor, cangrelor prevents the active metabolite of clopidogrel from forming a disulfide bridge with cysteine residues, causing drug-drug interaction (DDI) [97, 105]. This transition-induced DDI, which has an even greater effect with concomitant administration, can be removed by clopidogrel administered after the cangrelor infusion and at the loading dose [96, 97]. Co-administration of prasugrel with cangrelor infusion has been associated with different clinical outcomes in cangrelor to prasugrel transition studies [106, 107]. Therefore, prasugrel is recommended after the cangrelor infusion due to insufficient data [96]. However, according to the European Medical Agency, prasugrel can be administered 30 minutes before the end of the cangrelor infusion [108].

Unlike prasugrel and clopidogrel, there has been no significant interaction during the transition from cangrelor to ticagrelor [109].

In the CANTIC study, in STEMI patients undergoing PCI, simultaneous application of ticagrelor and IV cangrelor in the form of crushed and suspension has been predicted to provide higher platelet inhibition than the crushed ticagrelor application alone (starting at 5 minutes and continued for 2 hours) [28]. Although the antiplatelet effects in patients in need of nasogastric tube have not been foreseen in this study, considering other studies with crushed ticagrelor, valuable data could have been provided with this patient population [110]. Transition strategies are summarized in Fig. (**5**).

Table 4. CAN: Cangrelor, T: Ticagrelor, P: Prasugrel, LD: loading dose, MD: maintenance dose, PFT: platelet function test, DAPT: Dual antiplatelet therapy, CAD: Coronary artery disease, ACS: Acute coronary syndrome, HTPR: High on-treatment platelet reactivity.

De-escalation with switching from Cangrelor to → Oral thienopyridine *Patients in all studies received aspirin concomitantly.*			
Study Design and Study Name	**Study Population**	**Switching Protocol**	**Clinical Outcomes**
[97] **Randomized, open-label**	20 Healthy volunteers	First group received CAN (LD: 30μg and after MD: 4.0 μg / kg / min for 1h) → C (LD: 600 mg). Second group received C (600 mg) and after 2 weeks received C (600 mg) +CAN (LD: 30μg and after MD: 4.0 μg / kg / min for 2h) concomitantly.	Although platelet inhibition was achieved within 2h by giving C alone, platelet inhibition was achieved at 3h by giving CAN immediately after C. With the simultaneous administration of C and CAN, platelet inhibition was similar to baseline, so adequate platelet inhibition was not achieved.
[109] **Prospective Non-randomized**	12 Patients with stable CAD	On the first day of study, patients received CAN (LD: 30μg and after MD: 4.0 μg / kg/min for 2h) and after T (LD: 180 mg). On 2-5 study days, he was randomized to receive six or seven doses of T (MD: 90 mg). On the 5th study day, it continued to be T → CAN (LD: 30μg and after MD: 4.0 μg / kg/min for 2h).	T did not alter the antithrombotic effects of CAN during CAN treatment or prior to CAN treatment. In concomitant CAN and T application, antithrombotic effects of T were preserved. Since T and CAN are both reversible agents, T can be given either before or during CAN application.

| **De-escalation with switching from Cangrelor to → Oral thienopyridine** | | | |
Patients in all studies received aspirin concomitantly.			
[106] **Prospective** **Non-randomized**	15 Patients with stable CAD	On the first day of study, patients received CAN (LD: 30µg and after MD: 4.0 µg / kg/min for 2h) and after P (LD: 60 mg). On 2-7 study days, he was randomized to receive five or six doses of P (MD: 10 mg). On the 8th study day, it continued to be P → CAN (LD: 30µg and after MD: 4.0 µg / kg/min for 2h) after 24 or 48 hours.	P did not alter the antithrombotic effects of CAN during CAN treatment or before CAN treatment. Significant platelet reactivity was observed during CAN → P transition. The interaction between P-CAN was minimal when P was administered 30 minutes before the cessation of CAN therapy.
BRIDGE Study [105] **Prospective,** **randomized,** **double-blind,** **placebo** **controlled**	210 ACS patients requiring bridging CAN→ Oral thienopyridine undergo CABG surgery	Patients were randomized to CAN (0.75 µg / kg/min) and Placebo infusion before CABG surgery. All patients received CAN or placebo infusions after oral P2Y₁₂ in discontinuation and 1-6 hours before surgery.	CAN (0.75 µg / kg / min) maintained the low antithrombotic risk level (PRU <240). Surgical bleeding was not significantly different in the CAN and placebo groups. Preoperative ischemic events were less common in the CAN group.
The ExcelsiorLOAD2 study [107] **Prospective** **Open,** **Blinded** **randomized**	110 CAD Patients undergo PCI 10 PCI patients	CAN (LD: 30µg and after MD: 4.0 µg / kg/min) started all patients just before the PCI procedure and continued through the PCI procedure for at least 2h. Patients were randomized to receiving T (180mg) and P (60mg) at the start of CAN infusion or C (LD: 600 mg) at the end of CAN infusion.	The highest platelet reactivity was seen in group C. The P administered at the beginning of the CAN infusion provided sufficient platelet inhibition, even 1h after the CAN infusion was stopped.

(Table 4) cont.....

De-escalation with switching from Cangrelor to → Oral thienopyridine			
Patients in all studies received aspirin concomitantly.			
CHAMPION Trials Substudy group [109] **The substudy group of the randomized CHAMPION-PCI and CHAMPION-PLATFORM studies**	167 CAD Patients undergo PCI	CAN be administered 30 minutes before the PCI procedure and continued for 2-4 h after PCI. After CAN discontinuation, patients were randomized to receive either C or placebo.	No pharmacodynamic interaction was observed with C administered 10 h after CAN cessation in HTPR patients.

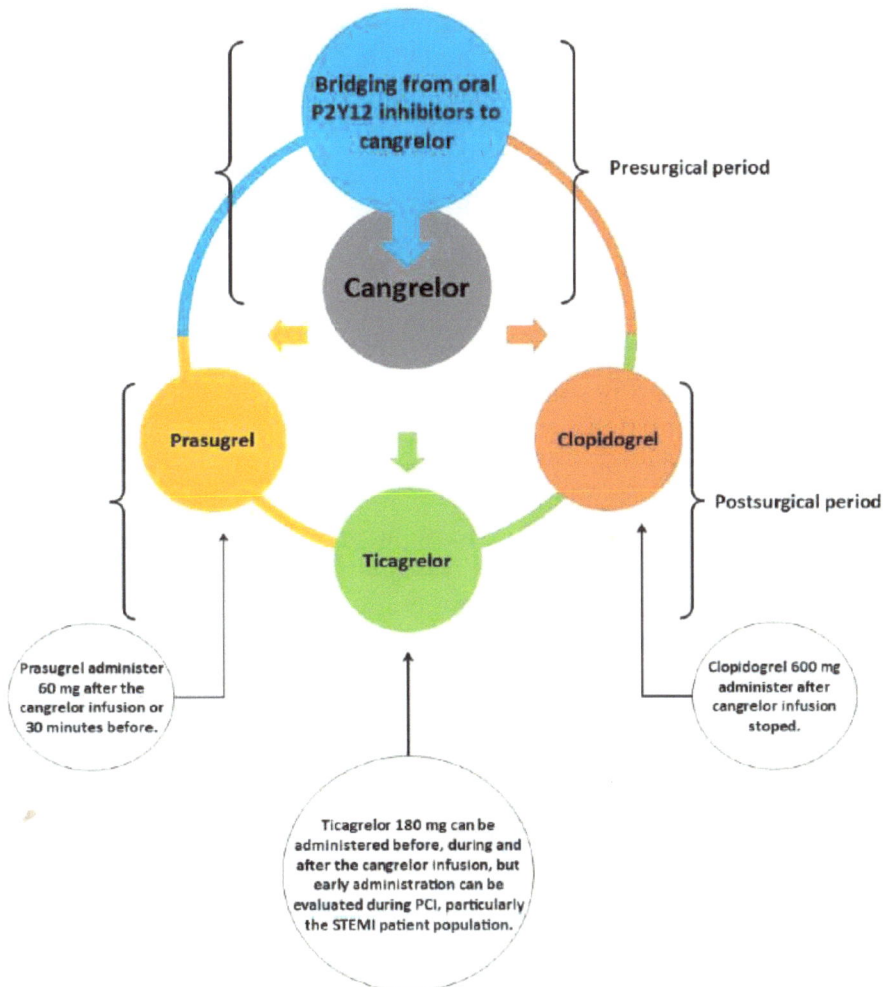

Fig. (5). Transition strategies from Cangrelor to oral $P2Y_{12}$ inhibitors.

De-escalation with Dose Reduction

Ticagrelor is recommended for ACS in both European and American guidelines. In the PEGASUS-TIMI 54 study, the Ticagrelor dose has been randomized and followed-up for approximately 33 months in patients who had undergone MI 1-3 years ago, including 60 mg, 90 mg and placebo, and at least one antithrombotic risk factor. All patients were given low-dose aspirin during the study period. This three-arm randomized study involved the reduction of ticagrelor dose from 90 to 60 reduced platelet inhibition intensity, but a more potent platelet inhibition than 75 mg of clopidogrel has been achieved [119]. In the ELECTRA study, which has aimed to measure platelet activity for 45 days after AMI, patients have been randomized to receive 90 mg bid of ticagrelor for the first 30 days and 60 mg bid of ticagrelor for the following 15 days and 90 mg bid of ticagrelor for 45 days and provided equal platelet inhibition in all patients [120]. All these studies shed light on the regulation of maintenance ticagrelor dose.

Escalation

Escalation refers to the transition from a low-density P2Y$_{12}$ inhibitor, such as clopidogrel, to a higher-density P2Y$_{12}$ inhibitor, such as ticagrelor or prasugrel. Escalation data can be obtained from cross-design studies evaluating platelet reactivity, such as ACAPULCO, RESPOND, EPIPHANY, as well as studies comparing clopidogrel to prasugrel or ticagrelor. Besides, the platelet reactivity [121], which is increased by the nature of the diabetes population, and thus contribute to the acquisition of data by the escalation in the pharmacodynamic studies in the diabetes population [122]. It has been shown that the platelet reactivity was increased in the ≥75 age population as in the diabetes population [123]. Escalation is generally preferred in high-risk ACS patients or patients with ACS when under clopidogrel + aspirin therapy, in clinical conditions associated with high platelet reactivity (diabetes, elderly population) or in other patients with high platelet reactivity. In addition, ACS patients undergoing fibrinolysis treatment may require escalation after standard clopidogrel treatment [124].

In the TRANSLATE-ACS study, where huge amount of data on escalation strategy has been obtained, and the switching from clopidogrel to prasugrel has been evaluated before discharge in HPR patients, the risk of ischemic events was reduced in the first year [125].

The crucial points in determining the escalation dose (LD or MD) and duration (before or after discharge) are the patient's anamnesis and drug history. In studies, the loading dose of Ticagrelor or Prasugrel has provided a more potent platelet inhibition than the maintenance dose [126, 127]. Providing adequate platelet inhibition in the acute phase of ACS is vital. For this reason, in the consensus of the experts, the escalation with the loading dose is recommended regardless of the duration of the last clopidogrel dose [96]. However, taking into account the risk of bleeding while escalating, there are individual cases that different dosing strategies are administered, which are:

- The escalation strategy to be administered in the late phase of acute coronary syndromes should be carried out at the next dosing period (≈24 hours later) at a maintenance dose.
- In patients aged ≥75 years, 5 mg maintenance dose provides sufficient platelet inhibition to prasugrel [128].
- Prasugrel provides sufficient platelet inhibition in patients with low body weight(≤60 kg) [129].
- In patients with a high risk of bleeding, escalation in the acute period of ACS, Prasugrel 30 mg loading dose or Ticagrelor 120 mg loading dose and after a maintenance dose of 60mg bid, can be considered as an alternative [130, 131].

Change Between Prasugrel and Ticagrelor

Side effects, contraindications, and cost-effective causes are the leading causes of the change strategy between ticagrelor and prasugrel. Although prasugrel is not recommended in the medical management of ACS, ticagrelor-related contraindications (previous intracranial hemorrhage or ongoing bleeds) or side effects (dyspnea) force the healthcare professional to change [68]. Pharmacodynamic data, including the strategies for change between prasugrel and ticagrelor, are not comprehensive. Therefore, the change is routinely carried out in practice for reasons such as side effects or contraindications.

SWAP-2 [132] and SWAP-3 [133] studies are the two crucial randomized clinical trials providing pharmacodynamic data on the strategy of change from ticagrelor to prasugrel or prasugrel to ticagrelor, respectively. In the SWAP-2 study, in stable CAD patients, the patients have been divided to change from ticagrelor to prasugrel, or to continue the ticagrelor regimen. Some patients have received a loading dose 60 mg prasugrel 12 h after the last dose of ticagrelor, and some patients have not received a loading dose, so the study patients have been randomized into three groups [133]. Platelet reactivity at the 7th day has been higher in patients randomized to prasugrel, and the enormous increase in platelet reactivity has occurred between 2-3 days, with less in the loading dose group. In this study, the increase in platelet reactivity has been seen in the early period of the change strategy, although it has occurred in the stable patient population, supporting the dose application in the change strategy (especially in patients who have developed ticagrelor side effects after ACS-PCI). The results of this study also draw attention to the interaction of ticagrelor and prasugrel, especially in the first three days due to prolonged platelet inhibition. Consequently, the loading dose should be preferred in patients who will have a strategy to switch from ticagrelor to prasugrel, since the increment in PRU may enhance the risk of ischemic events and cause possible DDI.

In the SWAP-3 study conducted in patients who have received aspirin and 10 mg prasugrel after ACS-PCI, the pharmacodynamic effects of the transition from prasugrel to ticagrelor have been investigated. Patients have been randomized to receive or not receive ticagrelor loading dose 24 h after the last dose of prasugrel [133]. In this study, unlike SWAP-2, no DDI was shown in the regimen with or without a loading dose in the transition from prasugrel to ticagrelor. However, higher platelet inhibition was observed in patients who switched to the ticagrelor regimen.

Although the SWAP-2 study has been conducted in a stable patient population, the SWAP-3 study has been held in stable ACS patients with PCI. For this reason, in patients who have switched from prasugrel to ticagrelor in the acute phase of ACS, a loading dose of ticagrelor 180 mg has been administered after the last prasugrel dose, and later a maintenance dose of ticagrelor 90mg bid was recommended. However, in stable CAD patients in the late phase of ACS, platelet inhibition could be maintained with the maintenance dose of 90 mg ticagrelor at the next P2Y$_{12}$ inhibitor dose schedule. In patients switching from ticagrelor to prasugrel, to prevent possible DDI, the loading dose suggested was 60 mg of prasugrel for patients in the ACS-early phase, and 10 mg of prasugrel for the stable patient population, 24 hours after the last ticagrelor dose [96].

The escalation, de-escalation and change strategies of P2Y12 inhibitors are summarized in Fig. (**6**).

Triple Antithrombotic Therapy

Triple antithrombotic therapy means the use of oral anticoagulants and the DAPT regimen [134]. This combination is generally preferred in patients undergoing elective ACS-PCI in addition to the need for long-term anticoagulation (with a history of AF, mechanical heart valve or venous thromboembolism). AF is a common cardiac arrhythmia, and its increased prevalence with age can cause patients to go to elective PCI, as it increases the risk of ischemic stroke and other cardiovascular events [135].

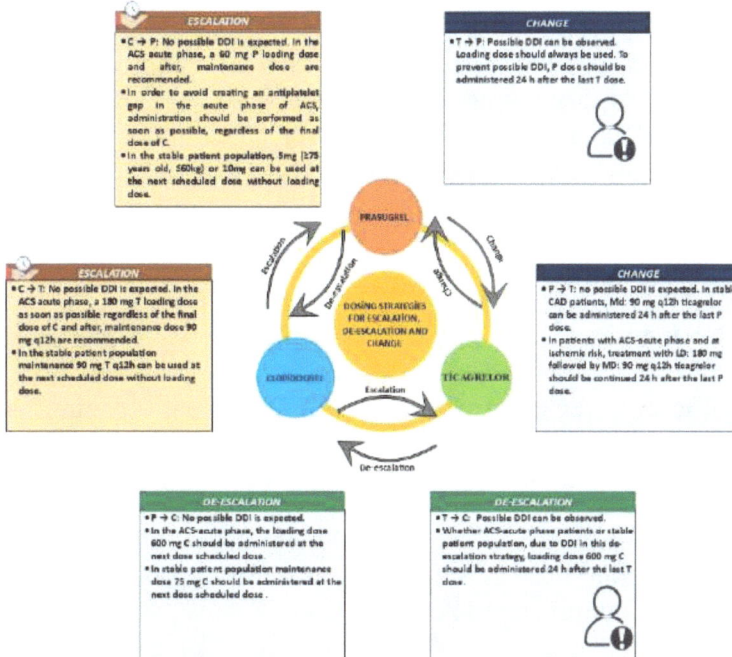

Fig. (6). Dosing strategies of $P2Y_{12}$ inhibitors in escalation, de-escalation and change modalities. C: Clopidogrel, P: Prasugrel, T: Ticagrelor, DDI: Drug-drug interaction, q12h: every 12 hours or twice a day.

Different strategies have been evaluated and proposed in the guidelines published to date [136, 137]. In the guidance for the 2015 ECS-NSTEMI, prasugrel and ticagrelor are recommended not to be used as part of triple therapy, as there is an insufficient level of evidence [46]. According to the 2017 ESC update, if the triple treatment is provided with vitamin K antagonists (VKA) such as warfarin, the international normalized ratio (INR) should be kept between 2-2,5. In the case of direct-effect oral anticoagulants such as factor Xa or thrombin inhibitors, the lowest possible dose should be used [68]. The current guidelines include the term peri-procedural PCI (peri-PCI) and refer to the period the patient is hospitalized for PCI. In these guidelines, in summary, it is recommended to use triple therapy during the hospital stay for PCI and then to switch to dual therapy with $P2Y_{12}$ + oral anticoagulant (OAC) [138, 139]. In the last guidelines, it has been suggested that ticagrelor and clopidogrel were suitable for triple therapy, but after 4-6 weeks, double treatment should be started [140].

The main point here is that a delicate balance between the ischemic risk and bleeding risk can be provided for the patient. In 2 different meta-analyses addressing four current randomized controlled studies, it has been demonstrated that triple therapy, including VKA, increased the risk of bleeding compared to dual therapy maintained with non-aspirin with non-Vitamin K antagonist drugs

(NVKA) + P2Y$_{12}$ inhibitors [141, 142]. In both randomized studies and meta-analyses, the data to be interpreted by classifying subgroup patient populations such as stable CASD population, ST-elevated ACS population, and NSE-ACS have been limited. In addition, since serious complications such as stent thrombosis are less common in the stable patient population, it is difficult to make a righteous interpretation of ischemic risk management. Therefore, a decision should be made according to the intensity of ischemia-bleeding balance with validated scoring tools.

Although NVKAs in AF patients have not been shown to be superior or less safe than VKAs in ACS with AF [143, 144], direct-acting agents in AF patients have been shown to be safer in terms of risk of intracranial bleeding, ischemic stroke and thromboembolism than warfarin [145]. Besides, there have been no head-t--head randomized data comparing different NVKAs with different PCI and AF coexistence.

The current guideline-based treatment approaches are summarized in Fig. (7) for patients with PCI-administered AF.

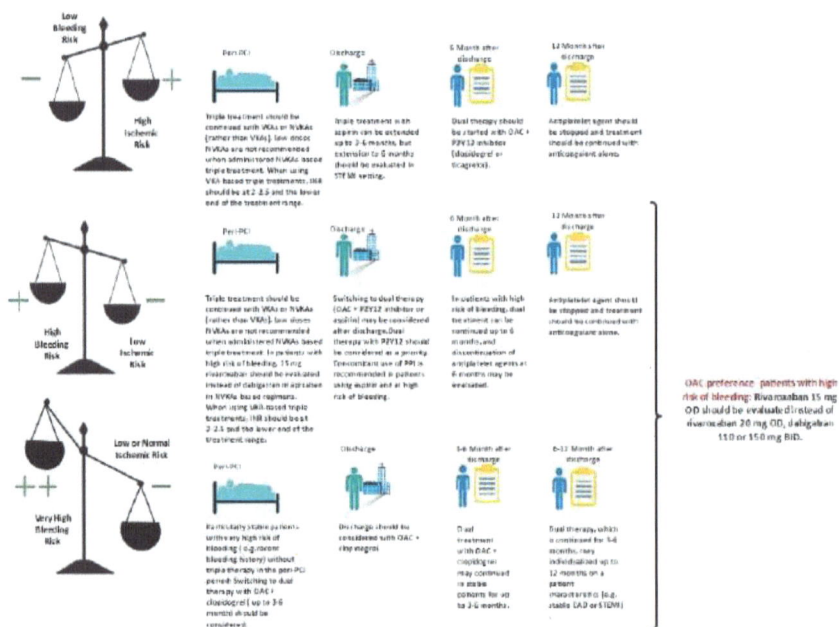

Fig. (7). Antithrombotic management in patients with AF undergo PCI, PCI: Percutaneous coronary intervention, VKA: Vitamin K antagonists, NVKA: non-vitamin K antagonist, OAC: Oral anticoagulant, CAD: Coronary artery disease, STEMI: ST-elevation myocardial infarction, OD: Once daily, BID: twice daily.

PRECISION MEDICINE ON P2Y$_{12}$ INHIBITORS WITH GENE TESTING APPROACH AND CLOPIDOGREL RESISTANCE

The fact that some patients treated with traditional doses of clopidogrel have not shown an adequate antiplatelet response revealed the definition of "clopidogrel resistance". Approximately 50% of the absorbed clopidogrel as a pro-drug, about 85% is hydrolyzed with carboxylesterase-1, only 15% can be used for active metabolite formation. The remaining 15% of clopidogrel undergo oxidative biotransformation with Cytochrome p450 enzymes such as Cyp1A2, Cyp2B6, Cyp 3A4, CYP2C9 and CYP2C19 in two consecutive steps [146]. Once converted to its active metabolite by hepatic cytochrome P450 enzymes, clopidogrel binds to the P2Y12 receptor on platelets, thereby irreversibly inhibiting platelet aggregation (Fig. **8**). CYP2C19 is the CYP450 enzyme that contributes 45% and 21% respectively in both steps of this oxidative process. However, it has been demonstrated by platelet function tests that some patients respond poorly to clopidogrel, but not to prasugrel or ticagrelor [147]. Studies have shown that the cause of this reduced response is genetic variations in the enzyme CYP2C19, which is responsible for most of the active metabolite formation [148].

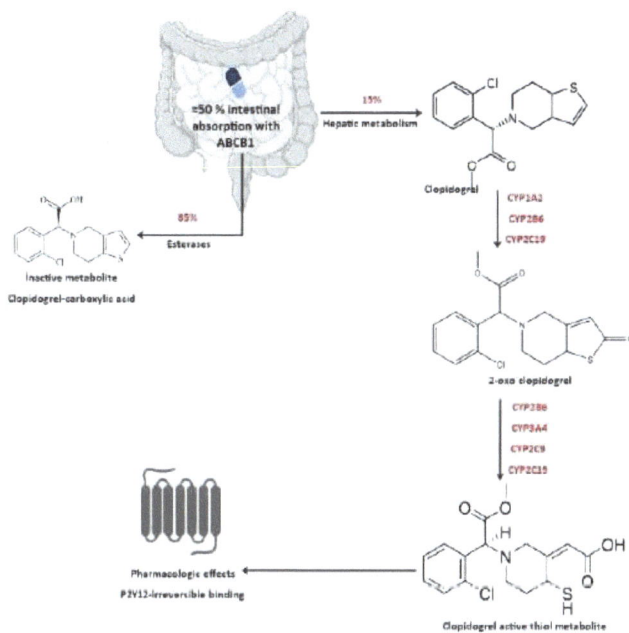

Fig. (8). Clopidogrel metabolism pathway.

More than 2000 genetic variants of CYP2C19, mostly intronic, have been identified. However, CYP2C19 * 2 and * 3 variant alleles, which are among the few variants in coding regions, result in dysfunctional proteins. CYP2C19 * 2 and CYP2C19 * 3 haplotypes contain variants that lead to dysfunctional protein production *via* splicing defect and an early stop codon that completes protein synthesis, respectively [149]. Although different CYP2C19 LOF loss of function (null allele, LOF allele) alleles are also present, CYP2C19 *2 (rs4244285, c.681G> A) and *3 (rs4986893, c.636G> A) comprise more than 99% of CYP2C19 alleles [150]. CYP2C19 *3 haplotype is more common in East Asians (6.3%) and less common in South Asians (0.4%) [151]. Other less common LOF alleles include CYP2C19 *4, *5, *6, *7 and *8 [152]. Depending on the test method and the definition of the response, 4% to 34% of patients have been shown not to respond to clopidogrel [153]. When the effect of the variations in the cytochrome p450 genes (CYP2C19 *2 and *3, CYP2C9 * 2 and * 3, CYP3A4 * 1B and CYP3A5 * 3) have been associated with the metabolism of clopidogrel, it has been observed that the carrying of LOF alleles of CYP2C19 *2 and CYP2C9 *3 increased the risk of stent thrombosis after PCI [154]. Various data have shown that CYP2C19 *2 loss-of-function allele is associated with decreased clopidogrel platelet response and poor prognosis [111, 155]. In patients without dysfunctional alleles, the activity of clopidogrel has been shown to be similar to that of other P2Y$_{12}$ receptor inhibitors. On the other hand, alternative treatment options have been tried in patients with cardiovascular disorder and have been found to respond poorly to clopidogrel by genotyping and platelet function testing (PFT). In a study, the functional loss allele has been observed in 572 of 1,815 PCI patients, and alternative antiplatelet therapy (prasugrel, ticagrelor) was recommended. The risk of major adverse cardiovascular events has been found to be significantly higher in patients with dysfunctional allele prescribed clopidogrel against alternative therapy. In addition, no difference has been observed in the major adverse cardiovascular events when alternative therapy was given to patients without functional loss allele and non-functional loss allele carriers [156]. In another study, the effect of prasugrel on the incidence of peri-procedural myocardial damage in patients undergoing elective PCI with clopidogrel resistance has been studied, and patients who have had a poor response to CYP2C19 allele genotyping and PFT with clopidogrel have been loaded with 60 mg prasugrel before PCI. As a consequence of the study, it has been found that the incidence of peri-procedural myocardial damage tended to be lower in patients with weak clopidogrel response treated with prasugrel, and it was suggested that early prasugrel administration might decrease the degree of peri-procedural myocardial damage during PCI in stable CAD patients [157]. A meta-analysis in 2014 was carried out due to the lack of a clear conclusion from studies on the relationship between CYP2C19 *2 gene polymorphism and clopidogrel resistance

[158]. Eight independent studies with a total of 2,331 individuals, including 1,066 clopidogrel resistance and 1,265 clopidogrel resistance patients were included, and the analysis concluded that CYP2C19 *2 gene polymorphism might be related to clopidogrel resistance. In another meta-analysis, the results of 36 studies conducted on Westerners and Asians on CYP2C19 polymorphism and clopidogrel resistance have been evaluated. The results of 44655 CAD patients who had received the percutaneous coronary intervention (PCI) and treated with clopidogrel have been included in the study. As a result of the analysis, it was determined that the reduced function CYP2C19 allele distribution varied between Western and Asians, and the ratio of 1 and 2 reduced-functional CYP2C19 mutant allele carriers in Asians was 42.5% and 10%, respectively, and 25.5% and 2.4% respectively in Westerners [159]. In relation to this, only 2-diminished function CYP2C19 mutant allele carriers among Asians had decreased clopidogrel effect, while among Westerners, both 1 and 2 diminished function CYP2C19 allele carriers had reduced effect. According to the results of the analysis, it has been suggested that CYP2C19 polymorphism affected the effectiveness of clopidogrel differently between Westerners and Asians. In a recent meta-analysis study evaluating the effect of CYP2C19 gene polymorphism on the clinical outcomes of Asian patients that had undergone PCI and treated with clopidogrel, 20 studies involving 13056 cardiovascular events have been evaluated [160]. Among the Asian populations, studies reporting clopidogrel treatment, clinically significant results (adverse cardiovascular events, stent thrombosis and bleeding), and studies reporting CYP2C19 genotypes have been included. The primary outcome was the recurrence of major adverse cardiovascular events (MACE), defined as a combination of cardiovascular death and myocardial infarction, and those carrying at least one of CYP2C19 *2 and / or *3 LOF alleles were shown to have an increased risk of MACE compared to non-carrier. When China, Korea and Japan have been evaluated together, the ethnic group with the highest MACE risk has been shown to be the Chinese LOF allele carriers. Also, Stent thrombosis was more common in LOF allele carriers, but the risk of bleeding was lower. As a result of this meta-analysis, it has been suggested that CYP2C19 gene test could help to personalize antiplatelet therapy, especially in the Asian population.

The association of genetic polymorphisms with clopidogrel activity in patients with ischemic stroke or TIA is controversial. In a meta-analysis study examining the relationship between CYP2C19 genotype and clopidogrel efficacy for ischemic stroke or TIA, 15 studies involving 4762 stroke or TIA patients treated with clopidogrel have been evaluated [161]. In patients with ischemic stroke or TIA patients treated with clopidogrel, the carriers of CYP2C19 *2, *3 and *8 dysfunctional alleles have been observed to be at increased risk of stroke compared to non-carriers (12.0% *vs.* 5.8%). Although the bleeding rates are not different in general, the frequency of composite vascular events has been found to be higher in the carriers of CYP2C19 dysfunctional alleles.

Current guidelines suggest dysfunctional CYP2C19 genotyping in a stable patient population, except for high-risk cases.

P2Y$_{12}$ Receptor Gene Polymorphisms

Genetic polymorphisms of the platelet surface receptors are also suggested to affect susceptibility to clopidogrel. Five polymorphisms of the P2Y$_{12}$ gene (T744C, C34T, G52T, ins801A and C139T) have been identified [162], and T744C (rs2046934), G52T (rs6809699) and C34T (rs6785930) polymorphisms have contributed to clopidogrel resistance [163 - 165]. However, studies claim that the relationship between P2Y$_{12}$ gene polymorphisms and weak clopidogrel response is not significant. To clarify whether there is a relationship between these three different P2Y$_{12}$ gene polymorphisms and clopidogrel resistance, a meta-analysis involving 5769 CVD patients from 15 separate studies has been performed [166]. As a result of the evaluations, a significant relationship between G52T and C34T polymorphism and clopidogrel resistance has been observed, while a lack of association has been found for the T744C polymorphism. Accordingly, it has been suggested that C34T and G52T polymorphisms at the P2Y$_{12}$ receptor gene might be a risk for platelet-poor response in patients receiving clopidogrel therapy. In another meta-analysis study examining 14 studies involving 8698 patients to evaluate the relationship between P2Y$_{12}$ polymorphisms and the risk of adverse clinical events in patients treated with clopidogrel, the T744C and C34T polymorphisms of the P2Y$_{12}$ gene have been associated with ischemic events in Han Chinese patients treated with clopidogrel and P2Y$_{12}$ G52T polymorphism has been found to have no significant effect on ischemic events [167]. However, it has been found that the risk of clinical ischemic events in the Caucasian population was not related to the T744C, G52T and C34T polymorphisms of the P2Y$_{12}$ gene. No significant relationship has been found between bleeding and P2Y$_{12}$ - C34T polymorphism in the Han Chinese population.

Dysfunctional CYP2C19 gene testing is not recommended routinely in escalation or de-escalation in stable CAD and ACS in the last updated expert consensus; however, it has been emphasized that it has prognostic significance to assess cardiovascular risk in patients with strategic conditions or on ongoing clopidogrel treatment [168]. In a recent randomized study of STEMI patients, the test guided dose adjustment was not superior in terms of thrombotic event risk, but genotyping guided dosing showed lower bleeding incidence [169]. In patients at risk of bleeding with randomized studies in subgroup populations, there is a need to clarify the effects of a genotyping-guided approach. It is not routinely recommended for treatment changes due to current data deficiency.

CONCLUSION

Cardiovascular disease-related mortality and the required antiplatelet therapies create an economic burden worldwide, and studies supporting the rational drug approach on the subject are increasing day by day. $P2y_{12}$ inhibitors are a fundamental drug group that constitutes the framework of antiplatelet therapy. Although $P2Y_{12}$ inhibitors have been used for about half a century, studies on their current use and duration are still needed. In the use of P2Y12 inhibitors, the precision medicine approach expresses all the strategies of escalation, de-escalation, change and transition. As in every field, there is a need for precision medicine in antiplatelet drug management, individual medical needs developed during the drug use period, or the requirements of the patient and disease when starting the first treatment. Besides these, mortality is a product of need to minimize hospitalization.

The highly heterogeneous patient population and diverse clinical uses justify the up-to-date requirements. Although it has been used in patients with acute coronary syndrome for years, the accompanying conditions support the need for individualization of treatment even in this patient population to establish a delicate balance between ischemic-bleeding risks. The rational management of ischemia-bleeding risk is quite complex in terms of both patient compliance and appropriate treatment due to periodic timed follow-ups. In this context, it would be a rational choice to use validated scoring methods to balance the ischemic-bleeding risk of patients.

Studies on the secondary prevention use of P2Y12 inhibitors are not as comprehensive as in acute coronary syndromes. Therefore, the relevant guides are more rigid in this regard. Appropriate treatment should be provided in the light of pertinent guidelines of secondary prevention use, but current studies evaluating specific patient populations should not be ignored. In particular, valvular valve diseases and stroke require precise management because of their heterogeneous nature. The multidisciplinary approach will guide in terms of treatment management in all areas of rational drug use.

The use of concomitant anticoagulants may complicate medical management due to increased diabetes with age, atrial fibrillation and acute coronary syndromes requiring percutaneous coronary intervention. In this case, current randomized studies, as well as current guidelines, can shed light on the management of the treatment. Although genetic sampling for clopidogrel resistance does not lead to treatment escalation or de-escalation, current studies evaluating specific patient populations may provide different data from these current treatments. In addition to the prognostic value of testing, subgroup population studies are needed to be used predictively.

CONSENT FOR PUBLICATION

Not applicable.

CONFLICT OF INTEREST

The author declares no conflict of interest, financial or otherwise.

ACKNOWLEDGEMENTS

Declared none.

REFERENCES

[1]   Vorchheimer DA, Becker R, Eds. Platelets in atherothrombosis. Mayo Clin Proc. Elsevier 2006; 81: pp. (1)59-68.

[2]   Hosseinzadegan H, Tafti DK. Modeling thrombus formation and growth. Biotechnol Bioeng 2017; 114(10): 2154-72.
[http://dx.doi.org/10.1002/bit.26343] [PMID: 28542700]

[3]   Paul BZ, Daniel JL, Kunapuli SP. Platelet shape change is mediated by both calcium-dependent and - independent signaling pathways. Role of p160 Rho-associated coiled-coil-containing protein kinase in platelet shape change. J Biol Chem 1999; 274(40): 28293-300.
[http://dx.doi.org/10.1074/jbc.274.40.28293] [PMID: 10497186]

[4]   Rana A, Westein E, Niego BE, Hagemeyer CE. Shear-dependent platelet aggregation: mechanisms and therapeutic opportunities. Front Cardiovasc Med 2019; 6: 141.

[5]   Jenne CN, Urrutia R, Kubes P. Platelets: bridging hemostasis, inflammation, and immunity. Int J Lab Hematol 2013; 35(3): 254-61.
[http://dx.doi.org/10.1111/ijlh.12084] [PMID: 23590652]

[6]   Suzuki H, Murasaki K, Kodama K, Takayama H. Intracellular localization of glycoprotein VI in human platelets and its surface expression upon activation. Br J Haematol 2003; 121(6): 904-12.
[http://dx.doi.org/10.1046/j.1365-2141.2003.04373.x] [PMID: 12786802]

[7]   Jackson SP. The growing complexity of platelet aggregation. Blood 2007; 109(12): 5087-95.
[http://dx.doi.org/10.1182/blood-2006-12-027698] [PMID: 17311994]

[8]   Nieswandt B, Offermanns S. Pharmacology of platelet adhesion and aggregation. In: Behrens J, Nelson WJ, Eds. Cell Adhesion. Springer 2004; pp. 437-71.

[9]   Trifiro E, Williams SA, Cheli Y, *et al.* The low-frequency isoform of platelet glycoprotein VIb attenuates ligand-mediated signal transduction but not receptor expression or ligand binding. Blood 2009; 114(9): 1893-9.
[http://dx.doi.org/10.1182/blood-2009-03-209510] [PMID: 19465689]

[10]   Razzuk MA, Pierce TB, Razzuk AM, Eds. Platelets and hemostasis: the role of glycoprotein IIb/IIIa in platelet aggregation. Baylor University Medical Center Proceedings. Taylor & Francis 1997; 10: pp. (1)21-6.

[11]   Gale AJ. Continuing education course #2: current understanding of hemostasis. Toxicol Pathol 2011; 39(1): 273-80.
[http://dx.doi.org/10.1177/0192623310389474] [PMID: 21119054]

[12]   Borea PA, Gessi S, Merighi S, Vincenzi F, Varani K. Pharmacology of adenosine receptors: the state of the art. Physiol Rev 2018; 98(3): 1591-625.
[http://dx.doi.org/10.1152/physrev.00049.2017] [PMID: 29848236]

[13]   Gachet C, Léon C, Hechler B. The platelet P2 receptors in arterial thrombosis. Blood Cells Mol Dis 2006; 36(2): 223-7.
[http://dx.doi.org/10.1016/j.bcmd.2005.12.024] [PMID: 16466948]

[14]   Junker A, Balasubramanian R, Ciancetta A, *et al*. Structure-based design of 3-(4-aryl-1 H-1, 2, 3-triazol-1-yl)-biphenyl derivatives as P2Y14 receptor antagonists. J Med Chem 2016; 59(13): 6149-68.
[http://dx.doi.org/10.1021/acs.jmedchem.6b00044] [PMID: 27331270]

[15]   Sarikaya E. Functions of purinergic receptors. In: Robson F, Ed. Receptors P1 and P2 as targets for drug therapy in humans: intechopen. Intechopen 2019; pp. 1-18.

[16]   Ohlmann P, de Castro S, Brown GG Jr, Gachet C, Jacobson KA, Harden TK. Quantification of recombinant and platelet P2Y(1) receptors utilizing a [(125)I]-labeled high-affinity antagonist 2-iod-N(6)-methyl-(N)-methanocarba-2′-deoxyadenosine-3′,5′-bisphosphate ([(125)I] MRS2500). Pharma col Res 2010; 62(4): 344-51.
[http://dx.doi.org/10.1016/j.phrs.2010.05.007] [PMID: 20594939]

[17]   Fabre J-E, Nguyen M, Latour A, *et al*. Decreased platelet aggregation, increased bleeding time and resistance to thromboembolism in P2Y1-deficient mice. Nat Med 1999; 5(10): 1199-202.
[http://dx.doi.org/10.1038/13522] [PMID: 10502826]

[18]   Hechler B, Zhang Y, Eckly A, Cazenave JP, Gachet C, Ravid K. Lineage-specific overexpression of the P2Y1 receptor induces platelet hyper-reactivity in transgenic mice. J Thromb Haemost 2003; 1(1): 155-63.
[http://dx.doi.org/10.1046/j.1538-7836.2003.00003.x] [PMID: 12871553]

[19]   Yang D, Chen H, Koupenova M, *et al*. A new role for the A2b adenosine receptor in regulating platelet function. J Thromb Haemost 2010; 8(4): 817-27.
[http://dx.doi.org/10.1111/j.1538-7836.2010.03769.x] [PMID: 20102488]

[20]   Ohlmann P, Lecchi A, El-Tayeb A, Müller CE, Cattaneo M, Gachet C. The platelet P2Y(12) receptor under normal and pathological conditions. Assessment with the radiolabeled selective antagonist [(3)H]PSB-0413. Purinergic Signal 2013; 9(1): 59-66.
[http://dx.doi.org/10.1007/s11302-012-9329-0] [PMID: 22892887]

[21]   Gachet C. P2Y(12) receptors in platelets and other hematopoietic and non-hematopoietic cells. Purinergic Signal 2012; 8(3): 609-19.
[http://dx.doi.org/10.1007/s11302-012-9303-x] [PMID: 22528678]

[22]   Hechler B, Gachet C. The P2 Receptors. In: Gresele P, Kleiman N, Lopez J, Page C, Neal SK, Eds. Platelets in Thrombotic and Non-Thrombotic Disorders. 1st edition. Springer International Publishing 2017; pp. 187-97.
[http://dx.doi.org/10.1007/978-3-319-47462-5_14]

[23]   Gratacap M-P, Guillermet-Guibert J, Martin V, *et al*. Regulation and roles of PI3Kβ, a major actor in platelet signaling and functions. Adv Enzyme Regul 2011; 51(1): 106-16.
[http://dx.doi.org/10.1016/j.advenzreg.2010.09.011] [PMID: 21035500]

[24]   Lova P, Paganini S, Hirsch E, *et al*. A selective role for phosphatidylinositol 3,4,5-trisphosphate in the Gi-dependent activation of platelet Rap1B. J Biol Chem 2003; 278(1): 131-8.
[http://dx.doi.org/10.1074/jbc.M204821200] [PMID: 12407113]

[25]   Stefanini L, Bergmeier W. RAP1-GTPase signaling and platelet function. J Mol Med (Berl) 2016; 94(1): 13-9.
[http://dx.doi.org/10.1007/s00109-015-1346-3] [PMID: 26423530]

[26]   Hashemzadeh M, Goldsberry S, Furukawa M, Khoynezhad A, Movahed MR. ADP receptor-blocker thienopyridines: chemical structures, mode of action and clinical use. A review. J Invasive Cardiol

2009; 21(8): 406-12.
[PMID: 19652255]

[27]   Husted S, Emanuelsson H, Heptinstall S, Sandset PM, Wickens M, Peters G. Pharmacodynamics, pharmacokinetics, and safety of the oral reversible P2Y12 antagonist AZD6140 with aspirin in patients with atherosclerosis: a double-blind comparison to clopidogrel with aspirin. Eur Heart J 2006; 27(9): 1038-47.
[http://dx.doi.org/10.1093/eurheartj/ehi754] [PMID: 16476694]

[28]   Franchi F, Rollini F, Rivas A, *et al.* Platelet inhibition with cangrelor and crushed ticagrelor in patients with ST-segment–elevation myocardial infarction undergoing primary percutaneous coronary intervention: results of the CANTIC Study. Circulation 2019; 139(14): 1661-70.
[http://dx.doi.org/10.1161/CIRCULATIONAHA.118.038317] [PMID: 30630341]

[29]   Farid NA, Kurihara A, Wrighton SA. Metabolism and disposition of the thienopyridine antiplatelet drugs ticlopidine, clopidogrel, and prasugrel in humans. J Clin Pharmacol 2010; 50(2): 126-42.
[http://dx.doi.org/10.1177/0091270009343005] [PMID: 19948947]

[30]   Jakubowski JA, Winters KJ, Naganuma H, Wallentin L. Prasugrel: a novel thienopyridine antiplatelet agent. A review of preclinical and clinical studies and the mechanistic basis for its distinct antiplatelet profile. Cardiovasc Drug Rev 2007; 25(4): 357-74.
[http://dx.doi.org/10.1111/j.1527-3466.2007.00027.x] [PMID: 18078435]

[31]   Hoffmann K, Lutz DA, Straßburger J, Baqi Y, Müller CE, von Kügelgen I. Competitive mode and site of interaction of ticagrelor at the human platelet P2Y12 -receptor. J Thromb Haemost 2014; 12(11): 1898-905.
[http://dx.doi.org/10.1111/jth.12719] [PMID: 25186974]

[32]   Fihn SD, Gardin JM, Abrams J, *et al.* 2012 ACCF/AHA/ACP/AATS/PCNA/SCAI/STS Guideline for the diagnosis and management of patients with stable ischemic heart disease: a report of the American College of Cardiology Foundation/American Heart Association Task Force on Practice Guidelines, and the American College of Physicians, American Association for Thoracic Surgery, Preventive Cardiovascular Nurses Association, Society for Cardiovascular Angiography and Interventions, and Society of Thoracic Surgeons. J Am Coll Cardiol 2012; 60(24): e44-e164.
[http://dx.doi.org/10.1016/j.jacc.2012.07.013] [PMID: 23182125]

[33]   Shah R. Optimal guideline-directed medical therapy for patients with stable ischemic heart disease. J Am Coll Cardiol 2018; 71(24): 2861-2.
[http://dx.doi.org/10.1016/j.jacc.2018.03.528]

[34]   Committee CS. CAPRIE Steering Committee. A randomised, blinded, trial of clopidogrel *versus* aspirin in patients at risk of ischaemic events (CAPRIE). Lancet 1996; 348(9038): 1329-39.
[http://dx.doi.org/10.1016/S0140-6736(96)09457-3] [PMID: 8918275]

[35]   Yuan J, Xu GM, Ding J. Aspirin *versus* clopidogrel monotherapy for the treatment of patients with stable coronary artery disease: a systematic review and meta-analysis. Adv Ther 2019; 36(8): 2062-71.
[http://dx.doi.org/10.1007/s12325-019-01004-6] [PMID: 31154631]

[36]   Bhatt DL, Fox KA, Hacke W, *et al.* Charisma Investigators. Clopidogrel and aspirin *versus* aspirin alone for the prevention of atherothrombotic events. N Engl J Med 2006; 354(16): 1706-17.
[http://dx.doi.org/10.1056/NEJMoa060989] [PMID: 16531616]

[37]   Dobesh P. Stable ischemic heart disease. In: Dipirio JT, Talbert RL, Yee GC, Matzke GR, Wells BG, Posey ML, Eds. Pharmacotherapy A Pathophysiologic Approach 10e. 10ᵗʰ edition. Newyork: McGraw-Hill Education 2017; pp. 385-512.

[38]   Saito Y, Kobayashi Y. Update on antithrombotic therapy after percutaneous coronary intervention. Intern Med 2020; 59(3): 311-21.
[http://dx.doi.org/10.2169/internalmedicine.3685-19] [PMID: 31588089]

[39]   Levine GN, Bates ER, Blankenship JC, *et al.* ACCF; AHA; SCAI. 2011 ACCF/AHA/SCAI Guideline for Percutaneous Coronary Intervention: executive summary: a report of the American College of

Cardiology Foundation/American Heart Association Task Force on Practice Guidelines and the Society for Cardiovascular Angiography and Interventions. Catheter Cardiovasc Interv 2012; 79(3): 453-95.
[http://dx.doi.org/10.1002/ccd.23438] [PMID: 22328235]

[40]   Levine GN, Bates ER, Bittl JA, *et al.* 2016 ACC/AHA guideline focused update on duration of dual antiplatelet therapy in patients with coronary artery disease: a report of the American College of Cardiology/American Heart Association Task Force on Clinical Practice Guidelines. J Am Coll Cardiol 2016; 68(10): 1082-115.
[http://dx.doi.org/10.1016/j.jacc.2016.03.513] [PMID: 27036918]

[41]   Ueno M, Miyazaki S. Acute coronary syndrome *vs.* stable angina pectoris: angioscopic point of view. In: Mizuno K, Takano M, Eds. Coronary Angioscopy. 1st ed., Tokyo, Japan: Springer 2015.
[http://dx.doi.org/10.1007/978-4-431-55546-9_10]

[42]   de Gaetano G, Cerletti C. Platelet adhesion and aggregation and fibrin formation in flowing blood: a historical contribution by Giulio Bizzozero. Platelets 2002; 13(2): 85-9.
[http://dx.doi.org/10.1080/09537100220122457] [PMID: 11897044]

[43]   Amsterdam EA, Wenger NK, Brindis RG, Casey DE, Ganiats TG, Holmes DR, *et al.* 2014 AHA/ACC guideline for the management of patients with non–ST-elevation acute coronary syndromes: executive summary: a report of the American College of Cardiology/American Heart Association Task Force on Practice Guidelines. J Am Coll Cardiol 2014; 64(24): 2645-87.
[http://dx.doi.org/10.1016/j.jacc.2014.09.016] [PMID: 25260718]

[44]   Steg PG, James SK, Atar D, *et al.* Task Force on the management of ST-segment elevation acute myocardial infarction of the European Society of Cardiology (ESC). ESC Guidelines for the management of acute myocardial infarction in patients presenting with ST-segment elevation. Eur Heart J 2012; 33(20): 2569-619.
[http://dx.doi.org/10.1093/eurheartj/ehs215] [PMID: 22922416]

[45]   Ibanez B, James S, Agewall S, *et al.* ESC Scientific Document Group. 2017 ESC Guidelines for the management of acute myocardial infarction in patients presenting with ST-segment elevation: The Task Force for the management of acute myocardial infarction in patients presenting with ST-segment elevation of the European Society of Cardiology (ESC). Eur Heart J 2018; 39(2): 119-77.
[http://dx.doi.org/10.1093/eurheartj/ehx393] [PMID: 28886621]

[46]   Roffi M, Patrono C, Collet J-P, *et al.* ESC Scientific Document Group. 2015 ESC Guidelines for the management of acute coronary syndromes in patients presenting without persistent ST-segment elevation: Task Force for the Management of Acute Coronary Syndromes in Patients Presenting without Persistent ST-Segment Elevation of the European Society of Cardiology (ESC). Eur Heart J 2016; 37(3): 267-315.
[http://dx.doi.org/10.1093/eurheartj/ehv320] [PMID: 26320110]

[47]   Patel MR, Calhoon JH, Dehmer GJ, *et al.* ACC/AATS/AHA/ASE/ASNC/SCAI/SCCT/STS 2016 appropriate use criteria for coronary revascularization in patients with acute coronary syndromes: a report of the american college of cardiology appropriate use criteria task force, american association for thoracic surgery, american heart association, american society of echocardiography, american society of nuclear cardiology, society for cardiovascular angiography and interventions, society of cardiovascular computed tomography, and the society of thoracic surgeons. J Am Coll Cardiol 2017; 69(5): 570-91.
[http://dx.doi.org/10.1016/j.jacc.2016.10.034] [PMID: 28012615]

[48]   Parmar P, Sumaria S, Hashi S. Stroke: classification and diagnosis. Pharm J 2011; 3: 200-4.

[49]   Association S. State of the Nation: stroke statistics 2017. Available from: https://www.stroke.org.uk/resources/state-nation-stroke-statistics

[50]   Diener H-C, Hankey GJ. Primary and Secondary Prevention of Ischemic Stroke and Cerebral Hemorrhage: JACC Focus Seminar. J Am Coll Cardiol 2020; 75(15): 1804-18.
[http://dx.doi.org/10.1016/j.jacc.2019.12.072] [PMID: 32299593]

[51]   National GCU. Stroke and transient ischaemic attack in over 16s: diagnosis and initial management. 2019.

[52]   Kernan WN, Ovbiagele B, Black HR, *et al.* American Heart Association Stroke Council, Council on Cardiovascular and Stroke Nursing, Council on Clinical Cardiology, and Council on Peripheral Vascular Disease. Guidelines for the prevention of stroke in patients with stroke and transient ischemic attack: a guideline for healthcare professionals from the American Heart Association/American Stroke Association. Stroke 2014; 45(7): 2160-236.
[http://dx.doi.org/10.1161/STR.0000000000000024] [PMID: 24788967]

[53]   Diener H-C, Bogousslavsky J, Brass LM, *et al.* MATCH investigators. Aspirin and clopidogrel compared with clopidogrel alone after recent ischaemic stroke or transient ischaemic attack in high-risk patients (MATCH): randomised, double-blind, placebo-controlled trial. Lancet 2004; 364(9431): 331-7.
[http://dx.doi.org/10.1016/S0140-6736(04)16721-4] [PMID: 15276392]

[54]   Benavente OR, Hart RG, McClure LA, Szychowski JM, Coffey CS, Pearce LA. SPS3 Investigators. Effects of clopidogrel added to aspirin in patients with recent lacunar stroke. N Engl J Med 2012; 367(9): 817-25.
[http://dx.doi.org/10.1056/NEJMoa1204133] [PMID: 22931315]

[55]   Wang Y, Wang Y, Zhao X, *et al.* CHANCE Investigators. Clopidogrel with aspirin in acute minor stroke or transient ischemic attack. N Engl J Med 2013; 369(1): 11-9.
[http://dx.doi.org/10.1056/NEJMoa1215340] [PMID: 23803136]

[56]   Wang Y, Pan Y, Zhao X, *et al.* CHANCE Investigators. Clopidogrel with aspirin in acute minor stroke or transient ischemic attack (CHANCE) trial: one-year outcomes. Circulation 2015; 132(1): 40-6.
[http://dx.doi.org/10.1161/CIRCULATIONAHA.114.014791] [PMID: 25957224]

[57]   Johnston SC, Easton JD, Farrant M, *et al.* Clinical Research Collaboration, Neurological Emergencies Treatment Trials Network, and the POINT Investigators. Clopidogrel and aspirin in acute ischemic stroke and high-risk TIA. N Engl J Med 2018; 379(3): 215-25.
[http://dx.doi.org/10.1056/NEJMoa1800410] [PMID: 29766750]

[58]   Johnston SC, Amarenco P, Albers GW, *et al.* SOCRATES Steering Committee and Investigators. Ticagrelor *versus* aspirin in acute stroke or transient ischemic attack. N Engl J Med 2016; 375(1): 35-43.
[http://dx.doi.org/10.1056/NEJMoa1603060] [PMID: 27160892]

[59]   Wang Y, Lin Y, Meng X, Chen W, Chen G, Wang Z, *et al.* Effect of ticagrelor with clopidogrel on high on-treatment platelet reactivity in acute stroke or transient ischemic attack (PRINCE) trial: Rationale and design. Int J Stroke 2017; 12(3): 321-25.
[http://dx.doi.org/10.1177/1747493017694390]

[60]   Iung B, Baron G, Butchart EG, *et al.* A prospective survey of patients with valvular heart disease in Europe: The Euro Heart Survey on Valvular Heart Disease. Eur Heart J 2003; 24(13): 1231-43.
[http://dx.doi.org/10.1016/S0195-668X(03)00201-X] [PMID: 12831818]

[61]   Applegate PM, Boyd WD, Applegate Ii RL, Liu H. Is it the time to reconsider the choice of valves for cardiac surgery: mechanical or bioprosthetic? J Biomed Res 2017; 31(5): 373-6.
[PMID: 28958994]

[62]   Carabello BA. Transcatheter aortic-valve implantation for aortic stenosis in patients who cannot undergo surgery. Curr Cardiol Rep 2011; 13(3): 173-4.
[http://dx.doi.org/10.1007/s11886-011-0173-6] [PMID: 21336623]

[63]   Mérie C, Køber L, Skov Olsen P, *et al.* Association of warfarin therapy duration after bioprosthetic aortic valve replacement with risk of mortality, thromboembolic complications, and bleeding. JAMA 2012; 308(20): 2118-25.
[http://dx.doi.org/10.1001/jama.2012.54506] [PMID: 23188028]

[64] Dvir D, Webb JG, Bleiziffer S, *et al.* Valve-in-Valve International Data Registry Investigators. Transcatheter aortic valve implantation in failed bioprosthetic surgical valves. JAMA 2014; 312(2): 162-70.
[http://dx.doi.org/10.1001/jama.2014.7246] [PMID: 25005653]

[65] Matiasz R, Rigolin VH. 2017 focused update for management of patients with valvular heart disease: summary of new recommendations. J Am Heart Assoc 2018; 7(1): e007596.
[http://dx.doi.org/10.1161/JAHA.117.007596]

[66] Han Y-L. De-escalation of anti-platelet therapy in patients with acute coronary syndromes undergoing percutaneous coronary intervention: a narrative review. Chin Med J (Engl) 2019; 132(2): 197-210.
[http://dx.doi.org/10.1097/CM9.0000000000000047] [PMID: 30614864]

[67] Yusuf S, Zhao F, Mehta SR, Chrolavicius S, Tognoni G, Fox KK. Clopidogrel in Unstable Angina to Prevent Recurrent Events Trial Investigators. Effects of clopidogrel in addition to aspirin in patients with acute coronary syndromes without ST-segment elevation. N Engl J Med 2001; 345(7): 494-502.
[http://dx.doi.org/10.1056/NEJMoa010746] [PMID: 11519503]

[68] Valgimigli M, Bueno H, Byrne RA, *et al.* ESC Scientific Document Group. 2017 ESC focused update on dual antiplatelet therapy in coronary artery disease developed in collaboration with EACTS. Eur J Cardiothorac Surg 2018; 53(1): 34-78.
[http://dx.doi.org/10.1093/ejcts/ezx334] [PMID: 29045581]

[69] Rozemeijer R, Voskuil M, Greving JP, Bots ML, Doevendans PA, Stella PR. Short *versus* long duration of dual antiplatelet therapy following drug-eluting stents: a meta-analysis of randomised trials. Neth Heart J 2018; 26(5): 242-51.
[http://dx.doi.org/10.1007/s12471-018-1104-6] [PMID: 29541996]

[70] Moon JY, Franchi F, Rollini F, Angiolillo DJ. Evolution of coronary stent technology and implications for duration of dual antiplatelet therapy. Prog Cardiovasc Dis 2018; 60(4-5): 478-90.
[http://dx.doi.org/10.1016/j.pcad.2017.12.004] [PMID: 29291426]

[71] Costa F, van Klaveren D, James S, *et al.* PRECISE-DAPT Study Investigators. Derivation and validation of the predicting bleeding complications in patients undergoing stent implantation and subsequent dual antiplatelet therapy (PRECISE-DAPT) score: a pooled analysis of individual-patient datasets from clinical trials. Lancet 2017; 389(10073): 1025-34.
[http://dx.doi.org/10.1016/S0140-6736(17)30397-5] [PMID: 28290994]

[72] Yeh RW, Secemsky EA, Kereiakes DJ, *et al.* DAPT Study Investigators. Development and validation of a prediction rule for benefit and harm of dual antiplatelet therapy beyond 1 year after percutaneous coronary intervention. JAMA 2016; 315(16): 1735-49.
[http://dx.doi.org/10.1001/jama.2016.3775] [PMID: 27022822]

[73] Cassese S, Byrne RA, Tada T, King LA, Kastrati A. Clinical impact of extended dual antiplatelet therapy after percutaneous coronary interventions in the drug-eluting stent era: a meta-analysis of randomized trials. Eur Heart J 2012; 33(24): 3078-87.
[http://dx.doi.org/10.1093/eurheartj/ehs318] [PMID: 23091199]

[74] Giustino G, Baber U, Sartori S, *et al.* Duration of dual antiplatelet therapy after drug-eluting stent implantation: a systematic review and meta-analysis of randomized controlled trials. J Am Coll Cardiol 2015; 65(13): 1298-310.
[http://dx.doi.org/10.1016/j.jacc.2015.01.039] [PMID: 25681754]

[75] Bulluck H, Kwok CS, Ryding AD, Loke YK. Safety of short-term dual antiplatelet therapy after drug-eluting stents: An updated meta-analysis with direct and adjusted indirect comparison of randomized control trials. Int J Cardiol 2015; 181: 331-9.
[http://dx.doi.org/10.1016/j.ijcard.2014.12.037] [PMID: 25555272]

[76] Valgimigli M, Park S-J, Kim H-S, *et al.* Benefits and risks of long-term duration of dual antiplatelet therapy after drug-eluting stenting: a meta-analysis of randomized trials. Int J Cardiol 2013; 168(3): 2579-87.

[http://dx.doi.org/10.1016/j.ijcard.2013.03.047] [PMID: 23590932]

[77]   Navarese EP, Andreotti F, Schulze V, *et al.* Optimal duration of dual antiplatelet therapy after percutaneous coronary intervention with drug eluting stents: meta-analysis of randomised controlled trials. BMJ 2015; 350: h1618.
       [http://dx.doi.org/10.1136/bmj.h1618] [PMID: 25883067]

[78]   Elmariah S, Mauri L, Doros G, *et al.* Extended duration dual antiplatelet therapy and mortality: a systematic review and meta-analysis. Lancet 2015; 385(9970): 792-8.
       [http://dx.doi.org/10.1016/S0140-6736(14)62052-3] [PMID: 25467565]

[79]   Cassese S, Byrne RA, Ndrepepa G, Schunkert H, Fusaro M, Kastrati A. Prolonged dual antiplatelet therapy after drug-eluting stenting: meta-analysis of randomized trials. Clin Res Cardiol 2015; 104(10): 887-901.
       [http://dx.doi.org/10.1007/s00392-015-0860-1] [PMID: 25903112]

[80]   Mehran R, Baber U, Sharma SK, *et al.* Ticagrelor with or without aspirin in high-risk patients after PCI. N Engl J Med 2019; 381(21): 2032-42.
       [http://dx.doi.org/10.1056/NEJMoa1908419] [PMID: 31556978]

[81]   Vranckx P, Valgimigli M, Jüni P, *et al.* GLOBAL LEADERS Investigators. Ticagrelor plus aspirin for 1 month, followed by ticagrelor monotherapy for 23 months *vs* aspirin plus clopidogrel or ticagrelor for 12 months, followed by aspirin monotherapy for 12 months after implantation of a drug-eluting stent: a multicentre, open-label, randomised superiority trial. Lancet 2018; 392(10151): 940-9.
       [http://dx.doi.org/10.1016/S0140-6736(18)31858-0] [PMID: 30166073]

[82]   Watanabe H, Domei T, Morimoto T, *et al.* STOPDAPT-2 Investigators. Effect of 1-month dual antiplatelet therapy followed by clopidogrel *vs* 12-month dual antiplatelet therapy on cardiovascular and bleeding events in patients receiving PCI: the STOPDAPT-2 randomized clinical trial. JAMA 2019; 321(24): 2414-27.
       [http://dx.doi.org/10.1001/jama.2019.8145] [PMID: 31237644]

[83]   Hahn J-Y, Song YB, Oh J-H, *et al.* SMART-CHOICE Investigators. Effect of P2Y12 inhibitor monotherapy *vs* dual antiplatelet therapy on cardiovascular events in patients undergoing percutaneous coronary intervention: the SMART-CHOICE randomized clinical trial. JAMA 2019; 321(24): 2428-37.
       [http://dx.doi.org/10.1001/jama.2019.8146] [PMID: 31237645]

[84]   Cuisset T, Grosdidier C, Loundou AD, *et al.* Clinical implications of very low on-treatment platelet reactivity in patients treated with thienopyridine: the POBA study (predictor of bleedings with antiplatelet drugs). JACC Cardiovasc Interv 2013; 6(8): 854-63.
       [http://dx.doi.org/10.1016/j.jcin.2013.04.009] [PMID: 23968703]

[85]   Gurbel PA, Bliden KP, Guyer K, *et al.* Platelet reactivity in patients and recurrent events post-stenting: results of the PREPARE POST-STENTING Study. J Am Coll Cardiol 2005; 46(10): 1820-6.
       [http://dx.doi.org/10.1016/j.jacc.2005.07.041] [PMID: 16286165]

[86]   Neumann F-J, Sousa-Uva M, Ahlsson A, *et al.* ESC Scientific Document Group. 2018 ESC/EACTS Guidelines on myocardial revascularization. Eur Heart J 2019; 40(2): 87-165.
       [http://dx.doi.org/10.1093/eurheartj/ehy394] [PMID: 30165437]

[87]   Alexopoulos D, Xanthopoulou I, Deftereos S, Sitafidis G, Kanakakis I, Hamilos M, *et al.* In-hospital switching of oral P2Y12 inhibitor treatment in patients with acute coronary syndrome undergoing percutaneous coronary intervention: prevalence, predictors and short-term outcome. Am Heart J 2014; 167(1): 68-76. e2.
       [http://dx.doi.org/10.1016/j.ahj.2013.10.010]

[88]   Clemmensen P, Grieco N, Ince H, *et al.* MULTIPRAC study investigators. MULTInational non-interventional study of patients with ST-segment elevation myocardial infarction treated with PRimary Angioplasty and Concomitant use of upstream antiplatelet therapy with prasugrel or clopidogrel--the European MULTIPRAC Registry. Eur Heart J Acute Cardiovasc Care 2015; 4(3): 220-9.

[http://dx.doi.org/10.1177/2048872614547449] [PMID: 25182465]

[89]   De LL, D'Ascenzo F, Musumeci G, Saia F, Parodi G, Varbella F, *et al*. Incidence and outcome of switching of oral platelet P2Y12 receptor inhibitors in patients with acute coronary syndromes undergoing percutaneous coronary intervention: the SCOPE registry. Euro Intervention: Journal of EuroPCR in collaboration with the Working Group on Interventional Cardiology of the European Society of Cardiology 2017; 13(4): 459-66.

[90]   Cuisset T, Deharo P, Quilici J, *et al*. Benefit of switching dual antiplatelet therapy after acute coronary syndrome: the TOPIC (timing of platelet inhibition after acute coronary syndrome) randomized study. Eur Heart J 2017; 38(41): 3070-8.
        [http://dx.doi.org/10.1093/eurheartj/ehx175] [PMID: 28510646]

[91]   Zettler ME, Peterson ED, McCoy LA, *et al*. TRANSLATE-ACS Investigators. Switching of adenosine diphosphate receptor inhibitor after hospital discharge among myocardial infarction patients: Insights from the Treatment with Adenosine Diphosphate Receptor Inhibitors: Longitudinal Assessment of Treatment Patterns and Events after Acute Coronary Syndrome (TRANSLATE-ACS) observational study. Am Heart J 2017; 183: 62-8.
        [http://dx.doi.org/10.1016/j.ahj.2016.10.006] [PMID: 27979043]

[92]   Cayla G, Cuisset T, Silvain J, *et al*. ANTARCTIC investigators. Platelet function monitoring to adjust antiplatelet therapy in elderly patients stented for an acute coronary syndrome (ANTARCTIC): an open-label, blinded-endpoint, randomised controlled superiority trial. Lancet 2016; 388(10055): 2015-22.
        [http://dx.doi.org/10.1016/S0140-6736(16)31323-X] [PMID: 27581531]

[93]   Sibbing D, Aradi D, Jacobshagen C, *et al*. TROPICAL-ACS Investigators. A randomised trial on platelet function-guided de-escalation of antiplatelet treatment in ACS patients undergoing PCI. Rationale and design of the Testing Responsiveness to Platelet Inhibition on Chronic Antiplatelet Treatment for Acute Coronary Syndromes (TROPICAL-ACS) Trial. Thromb Haemost 2017; 117(1): 188-95.
        [http://dx.doi.org/10.1160/TH16-07-0557] [PMID: 27652610]

[94]   Deharo P, Quilici J, Camoin-Jau L, *et al*. Benefit of switching dual antiplatelet therapy after acute coronary syndrome according to on-treatment platelet reactivity: the TOPIC-VASP pre-specified analysis of the TOPIC randomized study. JACC Cardiovasc Interv 2017; 10(24): 2560-70.
        [http://dx.doi.org/10.1016/j.jcin.2017.08.044] [PMID: 29268886]

[95]   Furuse E, Takano H, Yamamoto T, *et al*. Time course of the antiplatelet effect after switching to clopidogrel from initial prasugrel therapy in patients with acute coronary syndrome. Heart Vessels 2017; 32(12): 1432-8.
        [http://dx.doi.org/10.1007/s00380-017-1016-1] [PMID: 28685204]

[96]   Angiolillo DJ, Rollini F, Storey RF, *et al*. International expert consensus on switching platelet P2Y12 receptor–inhibiting therapies. Circulation 2017; 136(20): 1955-75.
        [http://dx.doi.org/10.1161/CIRCULATIONAHA.117.031164] [PMID: 29084738]

[97]   Steinhubl SR, Oh JJ, Oestreich JH, Ferraris S, Charnigo R, Akers WS. Transitioning patients from cangrelor to clopidogrel: pharmacodynamic evidence of a competitive effect. Thromb Res 2008; 121(4): 527-34.
        [http://dx.doi.org/10.1016/j.thromres.2007.05.020] [PMID: 17631948]

[98]   Dovlatova NL, Jakubowski JA, Sugidachi A, Heptinstall S. The reversible P2Y antagonist cangrelor influences the ability of the active metabolites of clopidogrel and prasugrel to produce irreversible inhibition of platelet function. J Thromb Haemost 2008; 6(7): 1153-9.
        [http://dx.doi.org/10.1111/j.1538-7836.2008.03020.x] [PMID: 18485086]

[99]   Gurbel P, Bliden K, Butler K, Tantry U, Teng R, Antonino M, *et al*. A randomized double-blind study to assess the onset and offset of the antiplatelet effects of ticagrelor *versus*. Clopidogrel in Patients With Stable Coronary Artery Disease. Am Heart Assoc 2009; 120: pp. 2577-585.

[100] Franchi F, Rollini F, Rivas Rios J, *et al.* Pharmacodynamic effects of switching from ticagrelor to clopidogrel in patients with coronary artery disease: results of the SWAP-4 study. Circulation 2018; 137(23): 2450-62.
[http://dx.doi.org/10.1161/CIRCULATIONAHA.118.033983] [PMID: 29526833]

[101] Wu H, Wang Q, Zhou J, Qian J, Ge J. First report of stent thrombosis after a switch therapy resulting from ticagrelor-related dyspnea. Int J Cardiol 2014; 176(3): e127-8.
[http://dx.doi.org/10.1016/j.ijcard.2014.07.216] [PMID: 25129304]

[102] Bagai A, Chua D, Cohen EA, *et al.* Pharmacodynamic and clinical implications of switching between P2Y12 receptor antagonists: considerations for practice. Crit Pathw Cardiol 2014; 13(4): 156-8.
[http://dx.doi.org/10.1097/HPC.0000000000000030] [PMID: 25396293]

[103] Biscaglia S, Campo G, Pavasini R, Tebaldi M, Tumscitz C, Ferrari R. Occurrence, causes, and outcome after switching from ticagrelor to clopidogrel in a real-life scenario: data from a prospective registry. Platelets 2016; 27(5): 484-7.
[http://dx.doi.org/10.3109/09537104.2015.1119815] [PMID: 27050796]

[104] Prosser AE, Dawson JL, Koo K, *et al.* Real-world incidence of patient-reported dyspnoea with ticagrelor. Ther Adv Drug Saf 2018; 9(10): 577-84.
[http://dx.doi.org/10.1177/2042098618788991] [PMID: 30283625]

[105] Angiolillo DJ, Firstenberg MS, Price MJ, *et al.* BRIDGE Investigators. Bridging antiplatelet therapy with cangrelor in patients undergoing cardiac surgery: a randomized controlled trial. JAMA 2012; 307(3): 265-74.
[http://dx.doi.org/10.1001/jama.2011.2002] [PMID: 22253393]

[106] Schneider DJ, Seecheran N, Raza SS, Keating FK, Gogo P. Pharmacodynamic effects during the transition between cangrelor and prasugrel. Coron Artery Dis 2015; 26(1): 42-8.
[http://dx.doi.org/10.1097/MCA.0000000000000158] [PMID: 25089928]

[107] Hochholzer W, Kleiner P, Younas I, *et al.* Randomized comparison of oral P2Y12-receptor inhibitor loading strategies for transitioning from cangrelor: the ExcelsiorLOAD2 trial. JACC Cardiovasc Interv 2017; 10(2): 121-9.
[http://dx.doi.org/10.1016/j.jcin.2016.10.004] [PMID: 28104204]

[108] Characteristics EMA-SOP. Summary of product characteristics-Kengrexal 2020. Available from: https://www.ema.europa.eu/en/documents/product-information/kengrexal-epar-product-information_en.pdf

[109] Schneider DJ, Agarwal Z, Seecheran N, Keating FK, Gogo P. Pharmacodynamic effects during the transition between cangrelor and ticagrelor. JACC Cardiovasc Interv 2014; 7(4): 435-42.
[http://dx.doi.org/10.1016/j.jcin.2013.08.017] [PMID: 24656538]

[110] Parodi G, Xanthopoulou I, Bellandi B, *et al.* Ticagrelor crushed tablets administration in STEMI patients: the MOJITO study. J Am Coll Cardiol 2015; 65(5): 511-2.
[http://dx.doi.org/10.1016/j.jacc.2014.08.056] [PMID: 25660931]

[111] Sardella G, Calcagno S, Mancone M, *et al.* Pharmacodynamic effect of switching therapy in patients with high on-treatment platelet reactivity and genotype variation with high clopidogrel Dose *versus* prasugrel: the RESET GENE trial. Circ Cardiovasc Interv 2012; 5(5): 698-704.
[http://dx.doi.org/10.1161/CIRCINTERVENTIONS.112.972463] [PMID: 23048056]

[112] Montalescot G, Sideris G, Cohen R, *et al.* Prasugrel compared with high-dose clopidogrel in acute coronary syndrome. The randomised, double-blind ACAPULCO study. Thromb Haemost 2010; 103(1): 213-23.
[http://dx.doi.org/10.1160/TH09-07-0482] [PMID: 20062936]

[113] Lee MS, Shlofmitz E, Haag E, *et al.* Optimal same-day platelet inhibition in patients receiving drug-eluting stents with or without previous maintenance thienopyridine therapy: from the Evaluation of Platelet Inhibition in Patients Having A VerifyNow Assay (EPIPHANY) trial. Am J Cardiol 2017;

119(7): 991-5.
[http://dx.doi.org/10.1016/j.amjcard.2016.11.057] [PMID: 28159194]

[114] Sd W, Trenk D, Al F, O'Donoghue M. FJ N, AD M. Prasugrel compared with high loading-and maintenance-dose clopidogrel in patients with planned percutaneous coronary intervention. Circulation 2007; 116: 2923-32.
[http://dx.doi.org/10.1161/CIRCULATIONAHA.107.740324]

[115] Deharo P, Pons C, Pankert M, *et al.* Effectiveness of switching 'hyper responders' from Prasugrel to Clopidogrel after acute coronary syndrome: the POBA (Predictor of Bleeding with Antiplatelet drugs) SWITCH study. Int J Cardiol 2013; 168(5): 5004-5.
[http://dx.doi.org/10.1016/j.ijcard.2013.07.121] [PMID: 23915522]

[116] Ueno T, Koiwaya H, Sasaki KI, *et al.* Changes in P2Y12 reaction units after switching treatments from prasugrel to clopidogrel in Japanese patients with acute coronary syndrome followed by elective coronary stenting. Cardiovasc Interv Ther 2017; 32(4): 341-50.
[http://dx.doi.org/10.1007/s12928-016-0417-x] [PMID: 27488859]

[117] Kerneis M, Silvain J, Abtan J, *et al.* Switching acute coronary syndrome patients from prasugrel to clopidogrel. JACC Cardiovasc Interv 2013; 6(2): 158-65.
[http://dx.doi.org/10.1016/j.jcin.2012.09.012] [PMID: 23428007]

[118] Gurbel PA, Bliden KP, Butler K, *et al.* Response to ticagrelor in clopidogrel nonresponders and responders and effect of switching therapies: the RESPOND study. Circulation 2010; 121(10): 1188-99.
[http://dx.doi.org/10.1161/CIRCULATIONAHA.109.919456] [PMID: 20194878]

[119] Bonaca MP, Bhatt DL, Cohen M, *et al.* PEGASUS-TIMI 54 Steering Committee and Investigators. Long-term use of ticagrelor in patients with prior myocardial infarction. N Engl J Med 2015; 372(19): 1791-800.
[http://dx.doi.org/10.1056/NEJMoa1500857] [PMID: 25773268]

[120] Kubica J, Adamski P, Buszko K, *et al.* Rationale and Design of the Effectiveness of LowEr maintenanCe dose of TicagRelor early After myocardial infarction (ELECTRA) pilot study. Eur Heart J Cardiovasc Pharmacother 2018; 4(3): 152-7.
[http://dx.doi.org/10.1093/ehjcvp/pvx032] [PMID: 29040445]

[121] Angiolillo DJ, Fernandez-Ortiz A, Bernardo E, *et al.* Variability in individual responsiveness to clopidogrel: clinical implications, management, and future perspectives. J Am Coll Cardiol 2007; 49(14): 1505-16.
[http://dx.doi.org/10.1016/j.jacc.2006.11.044] [PMID: 17418288]

[122] Cuisset T, Gaborit B, Dubois N, *et al.* Platelet reactivity in diabetic patients undergoing coronary stenting for acute coronary syndrome treated with clopidogrel loading dose followed by prasugrel maintenance therapy. Int J Cardiol 2013; 168(1): 523-8.
[http://dx.doi.org/10.1016/j.ijcard.2012.09.214] [PMID: 23084816]

[123] Gremmel T, Steiner S, Seidinger D, Koppensteiner R, Panzer S, Kopp CW. Adenosine diphosphate-inducible platelet reactivity shows a pronounced age dependency in the initial phase of antiplatelet therapy with clopidogrel. J Thromb Haemost 2010; 8(1): 37-42.
[http://dx.doi.org/10.1111/j.1538-7836.2009.03644.x] [PMID: 19818001]

[124] Chin CT, Wang TY, Anstrom KJ, *et al.* Treatment with adenosine diphosphate receptor inhibitors-longitudinal assessment of treatment patterns and events after acute coronary syndrome (TRANSLATE-ACS) study design: expanding the paradigm of longitudinal observational research. Am Heart J 2011; 162(5): 844-51.
[http://dx.doi.org/10.1016/j.ahj.2011.08.021] [PMID: 22093200]

[125] Bagai A, Peterson ED, McCoy LA, *et al.* Association of measured platelet reactivity with changes in P2Y$_{12}$ receptor inhibitor therapy and outcomes after myocardial infarction: Insights into routine clinical practice from the treatment with ADP receptor inhibitors: Longitudinal Assessment of

Treatment Patterns and Events after Acute Coronary Syndrome (TRANSLATE-ACS) study. Am Heart J 2017; 187: 19-28.
[http://dx.doi.org/10.1016/j.ahj.2017.02.003] [PMID: 28454802]

[126] Lhermusier T, Voisin S, Murat G, *et al.* Switching patients from clopidogrel to novel P2Y12 receptor inhibitors in acute coronary syndrome: comparative effects of prasugrel and ticagrelor on platelet reactivity. Int J Cardiol 2014; 174(3): 874-6.
[http://dx.doi.org/10.1016/j.ijcard.2014.04.208] [PMID: 24820749]

[127] Payne CD, Li YG, Brandt JT, *et al.* Switching directly to prasugrel from clopidogrel results in greater inhibition of platelet aggregation in aspirin-treated subjects. Platelets 2008; 19(4): 275-81.
[http://dx.doi.org/10.1080/09537100801891640] [PMID: 18569863]

[128] Capranzano P, Tamburino C, Capodanno D, *et al.* Platelet function profiles in the elderly: results of a pharmacodynamic study in patients on clopidogrel therapy and effects of switching to prasugrel 5 mg in patients with high platelet reactivity. Thromb Haemost 2011; 106(6): 1149-57.
[PMID: 22011914]

[129] Erlinge D, Ten Berg J, Foley D, Angiolillo D, Brown P, Wagner H, *et al.* Prasugrel 5 mg in low body weight patients reduces platelet reactivity to a similar extent as prasugrel 10 mg in higher body weight patients: results from the feather trial. J Am Coll Cardiol 2012; 59(13) (Suppl.): E341.
[http://dx.doi.org/10.1016/S0735-1097(12)60342-8]

[130] Kumari P, Ranwa BL. Comparison of lower loading dose of prasugrel with conventional loading dose of prasugrel in Indian patients undergoing percutaneous coronary interventions. Indian Heart J 2018; 70 (Suppl. 3): S319-22.
[http://dx.doi.org/10.1016/j.ihj.2018.08.004] [PMID: 30595283]

[131] Wang Y, Zhao HW, Wang CF, *et al.* Efficacy and safety of standard and low dose ticagrelor *versus* clopidogrel in east AsianPatients with chronic total occlusion undergoing percutaneous coronary intervention: a single center retrospective study. BMC Cardiovasc Disord 2020; 20(1): 109.
[http://dx.doi.org/10.1186/s12872-019-01307-0] [PMID: 32138662]

[132] Angiolillo DJ, Curzen N, Gurbel P, *et al.* Pharmacodynamic evaluation of switching from ticagrelor to prasugrel in patients with stable coronary artery disease: Results of the SWAP-2 Study (Switching Anti Platelet-2). J Am Coll Cardiol 2014; 63(15): 1500-9.
[http://dx.doi.org/10.1016/j.jacc.2013.11.032] [PMID: 24333493]

[133] Franchi F, Faz GT, Rollini F, *et al.* Pharmacodynamic effects of switching from prasugrel to ticagrelor: results of the prospective, randomized SWAP-3 study. JACC Cardiovasc Interv 2016; 9(11): 1089-98.
[http://dx.doi.org/10.1016/j.jcin.2016.02.039] [PMID: 27013060]

[134] Andrade JG, Verma A, Mitchell LB, *et al.* CCS Atrial Fibrillation Guidelines Committee. 2018 focused update of the Canadian Cardiovascular Society guidelines for the management of atrial fibrillation. Can J Cardiol 2018; 34(11): 1371-92.
[http://dx.doi.org/10.1016/j.cjca.2018.08.026] [PMID: 30404743]

[135] Connolly S, Pogue J, Hart R, *et al.* ACTIVE Writing Group of the active Investigators. Clopidogrel plus aspirin versus oral anticoagulation for atrial fibrillation in the Atrial fibrillation Clopidogrel Trial with Irbesartan for prevention of Vascular Events (ACTIVE W): a randomised controlled trial. Lancet 2006; 367(9526): 1903-12.
[http://dx.doi.org/10.1016/S0140-6736(06)68845-4] [PMID: 16765759]

[136] Lip GY, Huber K, Andreotti F, *et al.* Consensus Document of European Society of Cardiology Working Group on Thrombosis. Antithrombotic management of atrial fibrillation patients presenting with acute coronary syndrome and/or undergoing coronary stenting: executive summary--a Consensus Document of the European Society of Cardiology Working Group on Thrombosis, endorsed by the European Heart Rhythm Association (EHRA) and the European Association of Percutaneous Cardiovascular Interventions (EAPCI). Eur Heart J 2010; 31(11): 1311-8.
[http://dx.doi.org/10.1093/eurheartj/ehq117] [PMID: 20447945]

[137] January CT, Wann LS, Alpert JS, *et al.* ACC/AHA Task Force Members. 2014 AHA/ACC/HRS guideline for the management of patients with atrial fibrillation: executive summary: a report of the American College of Cardiology/American Heart Association Task Force on practice guidelines and the Heart Rhythm Society. Circulation 2014; 130(23): 2071-104.
[http://dx.doi.org/10.1161/CIR.0000000000000040] [PMID: 24682348]

[138] Lip GYH, Collet J-P, Haude M, *et al.* ESC Scientific Document Group. 2018 Joint European consensus document on the management of antithrombotic therapy in atrial fibrillation patients presenting with acute coronary syndrome and/or undergoing percutaneous cardiovascular interventions: a joint consensus document of the European Heart Rhythm Association (EHRA), European Society of Cardiology Working Group on Thrombosis, European Association of Percutaneous Cardiovascular Interventions (EAPCI), and European Association of Acute Cardiac Care (ACCA) endorsed by the Heart Rhythm Society (HRS), Asia-Pacific Heart Rhythm Society (APHRS), Latin America Heart Rhythm Society (LAHRS), and Cardiac Arrhythmia Society of Southern Africa (CASSA). Europace 2019; 21(2): 192-3.
[http://dx.doi.org/10.1093/europace/euy174] [PMID: 30052888]

[139] Angiolillo DJ, Goodman SG, Bhatt DL, *et al.* Antithrombotic therapy in patients with atrial fibrillation treated with oral anticoagulation undergoing percutaneous coronary intervention: a North American perspective–2018 update. Circulation 2018; 138(5): 527-36.
[http://dx.doi.org/10.1161/CIRCULATIONAHA.118.034722] [PMID: 30571525]

[140] January CT, Wann LS, Calkins H, *et al.* 2019 AHA/ACC/HRS Focused Update of the 2014 AHA/ACC/HRS Guideline for the Management of Patients With Atrial Fibrillation: A Report of the American College of Cardiology/American Heart Association Task Force on Clinical Practice Guidelines and the Heart Rhythm Society. J Am Coll Cardiol 2019; 74(1): 104-32.
[http://dx.doi.org/10.1016/j.jacc.2019.01.011] [PMID: 30703431]

[141] Khan SU, Osman M, Khan MU, *et al.* Dual *Versus* triple therapy for atrial fibrillation after percutaneous coronary intervention: a systematic review and meta-analysis. Ann Intern Med 2020; 172(7): 474-83.
[http://dx.doi.org/10.7326/M19-3763] [PMID: 32176890]

[142] Dahal K, Mosleh W, Almnajam M, Khaddr M, Adeel MY, Vashist A, *et al.* NOAC-based dual therapy *versus* warfarin-based triple therapy after percutaneous coronary intervention or acute coronary syndrome in patients with atrial fibrillation: A systematic review and meta-analysis. Cardiovasc Revasc Med 2020; 21(10): 1202-8.
[http://dx.doi.org/10.1016/j.carrev.2020.03.012]

[143] Connolly SJ, Ezekowitz MD, Yusuf S, *et al.* RE-LY Steering Committee and Investigators. Dabigatran *versus* warfarin in patients with atrial fibrillation. N Engl J Med 2009; 361(12): 1139-51.
[http://dx.doi.org/10.1056/NEJMoa0905561] [PMID: 19717844]

[144] Granger CB, Alexander JH, McMurray JJ, *et al.* ARISTOTLE Committees and Investigators. Apixaban *versus* warfarin in patients with atrial fibrillation. N Engl J Med 2011; 365(11): 981-92.
[http://dx.doi.org/10.1056/NEJMoa1107039] [PMID: 21870978]

[145] Ruff CT, Giugliano RP, Braunwald E, *et al.* Comparison of the efficacy and safety of new oral anticoagulants with warfarin in patients with atrial fibrillation: a meta-analysis of randomised trials. Lancet 2014; 383(9921): 955-62.
[http://dx.doi.org/10.1016/S0140-6736(13)62343-0] [PMID: 24315724]

[146] Ferri N, Corsini A, Bellosta S. Pharmacology of the new P2Y12 receptor inhibitors: insights on pharmacokinetic and pharmacodynamic properties. Drugs 2013; 73(15): 1681-709.
[http://dx.doi.org/10.1007/s40265-013-0126-z] [PMID: 24114622]

[147] Breet NJ, van Werkum JW, Bouman HJ, *et al.* Comparison of platelet function tests in predicting clinical outcome in patients undergoing coronary stent implantation. JAMA 2010; 303(8): 754-62.
[http://dx.doi.org/10.1001/jama.2010.181] [PMID: 20179285]

[148] Giusti B, Gori AM, Marcucci R, Saracini C, Vestrini A, Abbate R. Determinants to optimize response to clopidogrel in acute coronary syndrome. Pharm Genomics Pers Med 2010; 3: 33-50.
[http://dx.doi.org/10.2147/PGPM.S5056] [PMID: 23226041]

[149] de Morais SM, Wilkinson GR, Blaisdell J, Nakamura K, Meyer UA, Goldstein JA. The major genetic defect responsible for the polymorphism of S-mephenytoin metabolism in humans. J Biol Chem 1994; 269(22): 15419-22.
[PMID: 8195181]

[150] Scott SA, Sangkuhl K, Stein CM, *et al.* Clinical Pharmacogenetics Implementation Consortium. Clinical Pharmacogenetics Implementation Consortium guidelines for CYP2C19 genotype and clopidogrel therapy: 2013 update. Clin Pharmacol Ther 2013; 94(3): 317-23.
[http://dx.doi.org/10.1038/clpt.2013.105] [PMID: 23698643]

[151] Pereira NL, Rihal CS, So DYF, *et al.* Clopidogrel Pharmacogenetics. Circ Cardiovasc Interv 2019; 12(4): e007811.
[http://dx.doi.org/10.1161/CIRCINTERVENTIONS.119.007811] [PMID: 30998396]

[152] Wilber DJ, Pappone C, Neuzil P, *et al.* ThermoCool AF Trial Investigators. Comparison of antiarrhythmic drug therapy and radiofrequency catheter ablation in patients with paroxysmal atrial fibrillation: a randomized controlled trial. JAMA 2010; 303(4): 333-40.
[http://dx.doi.org/10.1001/jama.2009.2029] [PMID: 20103757]

[153] O'Donoghue M, Wiviott SD. Clopidogrel response variability and future therapies: clopidogrel: does one size fit all? Circulation 2006; 114(22): e600-6.
[http://dx.doi.org/10.1161/CIRCULATIONAHA.106.643171] [PMID: 17130347]

[154] Harmsze AM, van Werkum JW, Ten Berg JM, *et al.* CYP2C19*2 and CYP2C9*3 alleles are associated with stent thrombosis: a case-control study. Eur Heart J 2010; 31(24): 3046-53.
[http://dx.doi.org/10.1093/eurheartj/ehq321] [PMID: 20833683]

[155] Hulot J-S, Collet J-P, Silvain J, *et al.* Cardiovascular risk in clopidogrel-treated patients according to cytochrome P450 2C19*2 loss-of-function allele or proton pump inhibitor coadministration: a systematic meta-analysis. J Am Coll Cardiol 2010; 56(2): 134-43.
[http://dx.doi.org/10.1016/j.jacc.2009.12.071] [PMID: 20620727]

[156] Lee CR, Sriramoju VB, Cervantes A, *et al.* Clinical outcomes and sustainability of using CYP2C19 genotype–guided antiplatelet therapy after percutaneous coronary intervention. Circulation. Circ Genom Precis Med 2018; 11(4): e002069.
[http://dx.doi.org/10.1161/CIRCGEN.117.002069] [PMID: 29615454]

[157] Tomaniak M, Kołtowski Ł, Kochman J, *et al.* Can prasugrel decrease the extent of periprocedural myocardial injury during elective percutaneous coronary intervention? Pol Arch Intern Med 2017; 127(11): 730-40.
[PMID: 28817535]

[158] Hou X, Shi J, Sun H. Gene polymorphism of cytochrome P450 2C19*2 and clopidogrel resistance reflected by platelet function assays: a meta-analysis. Eur J Clin Pharmacol 2014; 70(9): 1041-7.
[http://dx.doi.org/10.1007/s00228-014-1714-x] [PMID: 24996381]

[159] Niu X, Mao L, Huang Y, *et al.* CYP2C19 polymorphism and clinical outcomes among patients of different races treated with clopidogrel: A systematic review and meta-analysis. J Huazhong Univ Sci Technolog Med Sci 2015; 35(2): 147-56. [Medical Sciences].
[http://dx.doi.org/10.1007/s11596-015-1404-7] [PMID: 25877345]

[160] Xi Z, Fang F, Wang J, AlHelal J, Zhou Y, Liu W. CYP2C19 genotype and adverse cardiovascular outcomes after stent implantation in clopidogrel-treated Asian populations: A systematic review and meta-analysis. Platelets 2019; 30(2): 229-40.
[http://dx.doi.org/10.1080/09537104.2017.1413178] [PMID: 29257922]

[161] Pan Y, Chen W, Xu Y, *et al.* Genetic polymorphisms and clopidogrel efficacy for acute ischemic

stroke or transient ischemic attack: a systematic review and meta-analysis. Circulation 2017; 135(1): 21-33.
[http://dx.doi.org/10.1161/CIRCULATIONAHA.116.024913] [PMID: 27806998]

[162] Fontana P, Dupont A, Gandrille S, *et al.* Adenosine diphosphate-induced platelet aggregation is associated with P2Y12 gene sequence variations in healthy subjects. Circulation 2003; 108(8): 989-95.
[http://dx.doi.org/10.1161/01.CIR.0000085073.69189.88] [PMID: 12912815]

[163] Galić E, Vrbanić L, Kapitanović S, *et al.* P2RY12 gene polymorphisms and effect of clopidogrel on platelet aggregation. Coll Antropol 2013; 37(2): 491-8.
[PMID: 23940995]

[164] Staritz P, Kurz K, Stoll M, Giannitsis E, Katus HA, Ivandic BT. Platelet reactivity and clopidogrel resistance are associated with the H2 haplotype of the P2Y12-ADP receptor gene. Int J Cardiol 2009; 133(3): 341-5.
[http://dx.doi.org/10.1016/j.ijcard.2007.12.118] [PMID: 18485500]

[165] Zoheir N, Abd Elhamid S, Abulata N, El Sobky M, Khafagy D, Mostafa A. P2Y12 receptor gene polymorphism and antiplatelet effect of clopidogrel in patients with coronary artery disease after coronary stenting. Blood Coagul Fibrinolysis 2013; 24(5): 525-31.
[http://dx.doi.org/10.1097/MBC.0b013e32835e98bf] [PMID: 23751603]

[166] Cui G, Zhang S, Zou J, Chen Y, Chen H. P2Y12 receptor gene polymorphism and the risk of resistance to clopidogrel: A meta-analysis and review of the literature. Adv Clin Exp Med 2017; 26(2): 343-9.

[167] Zhao K, Yang M, Lu Y, *et al.* P2Y12 Polymorphisms and the Risk of Adverse Clinical Events in Patients Treated with Clopidogrel: A Meta-Analysis. Drug Res (Stuttg) 2019; 69(1): 23-31.
[http://dx.doi.org/10.1055/a-0622-8110] [PMID: 29791922]

[168] Sibbing D, Aradi D, Alexopoulos D, *et al.* Updated expert consensus statement on platelet function and genetic testing for guiding P2Y12 receptor inhibitor treatment in percutaneous coronary intervention. JACC Cardiovasc Interv 2019; 12(16): 1521-37.
[http://dx.doi.org/10.1016/j.jcin.2019.03.034] [PMID: 31202949]

[169] Claassens DMF, Vos GJA, Bergmeijer TO, *et al.* A genotype-guided strategy for oral P2Y12 inhibitors in primary PCI. N Engl J Med 2019; 381(17): 1621-31.
[http://dx.doi.org/10.1056/NEJMoa1907096] [PMID: 31479209]

CHAPTER 5

Pathophysiological Links Between Diabetes and Cardiovascular Diseases: at the Biochemical and Molecular Levels

M.M. Towhidul Islam[1] and Yearul Kabir[1,*]

[1] *Department of Biochemistry and Molecular Biology, University of Dhaka, Dhaka-1000, Bangladesh*

Abstract: The cardiovascular system mainly involves blood circulation to transport oxygen, nutrients and metabolic compounds throughout the body. The blood is also used to transport different endocrine hormones (for example, insulin) from the pancreas to various cells in response to blood glucose levels. Unfortunately, any imbalance in glucose and insulin levels may help to develop diabetes mellitus (DM) and increase the risk of developing cardiovascular diseases (CVD) complications such as atherosclerosis, hypertension, and myocardial infarction. Obesity plays a crucial role in developing atherosclerotic plaques and other cardiovascular diseases. It is also responsible for the inappropriate secretion of endocrine factors, resulting in metabolic impairment of insulin target tissues and eventually failure of insulin-producing β-cells. It has been found that 65% of diabetic patients develop cardiovascular problems. Therefore, to know the underlying etiological factors, it is essential to study the molecular mechanisms behind cardiovascular complications from diabetes. Understanding the mechanisms and biomarkers of heart disease in diabetes research can bridge the knowledge gap between diabetes and cardiovascular diseases.

Keywords: Biomarkers, Cardiovascular Diseases, Diabetes, Dyslipidemia, Gene, Insulin, Single Nucleotide Polymorphisms.

INTRODUCTION

DM and CVD are multifactorial but interrelated non-communicable diseases (NCD) affecting a large population worldwide. Unfortunately, both DM and CVD significantly increase the risk of fatal outcomes like stroke. To prevent these deadly diseases, it is necessary to understand the reasons behind these diseases' exceptional growth in recent times. In this review, we are, therefore, trying to

* **Corresponding author:** Yearul Kabir, PhD; Professor, Department of Biochemistry and Molecular Biology, Faculty of Biological Sciences, University of Dhaka, Dhaka-1000, Bangladesh; Tel: +8801710327716; E-mail: ykabir@du.ac.bd

figure out the links between DM and CVD, exploring the fundamental changes responsible for this epidemic, evaluating the association of genes with these conditions, and lastly, current and possible future treatment options to control these diseases.

DM, also called diabetes, is a metabolic condition when the body has an impaired ability to process blood glucose. DM is of two major types: type 1 and type 2. Type 1 diabetes (T1DM) occurs due to genetic disorders when the body fails to produce insulin. On the other hand, type 2 diabetes mellitus (T2DM) happens due to diseases where beta-cell impairment and concomitant insulin resistance lead to hyperglycemia [1]. The prevalence of T2DM is much higher than T1DM, which is maybe due to the rise in life expectancy, increasing frequency of obesity, and westernization of lifestyles, etc [2, 3]. In the long run, both these DMs are the causes of morbidity, mortality, and exceptionally higher healthcare costs [4, 5]. Similar to diabetes mellitus, these factors are also responsible for CVD, which is the topmost health problem right now [6]. Several studies have revealed that diabetic patients have a higher, almost two- to fourfold, tendency to acquire coronary artery disease (CAD) and myocardial infarction (MI). This is similar to the fact that most T2DM patients at the age of $\geq$65 die from CVD [6]. Reports showed that T2DM patients with no CAD records have a comparable cardiovascular risk as patients with previous MI events [7], supporting the idea that T2DM is an independent risk factor for stroke and heart disease [8]. Several studies explain the relationship between poor glycemic control, insulin resistance markers, oxidative stress, and low-grade inflammation as putative factors linking these two conditions, which is summarized in Fig. (**1**).

EPIDEMIOLOGICAL STUDIES

Cardiovascular disease is responsible for 68% of all diabetic deaths and is therefore believed as the foremost reason for morbidity and mortality among individuals with T2DM [10]. In the USA, it has been found that the number of people aged $\geq$35 years with diagnosed T2DM who reported having CVD increased by 36% between 1997 and 2005 [11]. Another study showed that DM is associated with a 24% greater risk of atrial fibrillation (95% CI, 6%-44%) [12]. T2DM was associated with >2-fold risk (95% CI, 2.11–2.56) of death from vascular reasons [13]. Interestingly, among the participants, the females with T2DM having a much higher tendency to develop CVD [14]. Reports showed that women with T2DM have a 44% increased possibility of CAD and a 27% greater risk of stroke than men with T2DM [15, 16]. Although T2DM increases different vascular complications, venous thromboembolism (pooled hazard ratio, HR=1.35; 95% CI, 1.17–1.55) and sudden cardiac death (HR=2.18; 95% CI, 1.89–2.52) in individuals compared to non-T2DM patients, evidence found no significant difference of risk estimates between men and women [17, 18].

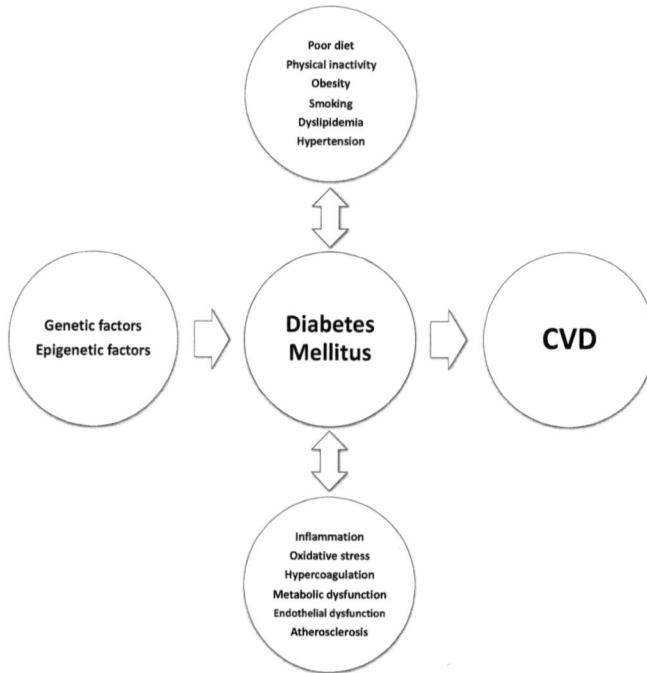

Fig. (1). Common pathophysiology of type 2 diabetes mellitus (DM) and cardiovascular disease (CVD) (modified from Brunetti *et al.* [9].

STRUCTURAL AND FUNCTIONAL CHANGES OF CARDIAC TISSUE DURING DIABETES

Echocardiographic studies have revealed a characteristic left ventricular concentric remodeling in diabetic myocardium [19]. Scientists believe myocardial triglyceride and collagen deposition followed by fibrosis is responsible for this hypertrophic remodeling in the diabetic heart [20] and/or increased extracellular volume of the heart [21]. This increased extracellular volume is the reason for the high frequency of heart failure, as well as mortality among different populations [22]. Besides, hyperinsulinemia due to insulin resistance may also promote this remodeling *via* exacerbating the hypertrophic process [23]. Others have reported a direct impairment of myocardial oxygen supply, energetics, tissue perfusion, systolic strain, and substrate obtainability in patients with diabetes, suggesting microcirculatory impairment is another causative factor for diabetic cardio-myopathy [19, 24].

Glucose, a reducing sugar, can bind nonenzymatically to proteins (like hemoglobin and albumin) and lipids *via* glycosylation reactions. Upon binding, it can cause structural and functional modifications of cellular macromolecules [25]. These reactions are getting even faster in hyperglycemia, oxidative stress, and inflammatory conditions. Upon production, these glycated adducts undergo complex reactions, for example, oxidation-reduction, dehydration, condensation, and form advanced glycation end products (AGEs), which are dim in appearance, have fluorescence and molecular cross-linking tendency. Reports indicated that DM patients have significantly higher skin autofluorescence values (which is an independent risk factor for carotid atherosclerosis) than healthy controls [26]. In DM, due to high blood glucose levels, AGEs cannot be metabolized and accumulated in the body. Excess AGEs then initiate molecular cross-linking and thus accelerate the progression of vascular disorders. In the body, AGEs are detected by receptors for the advanced glycation end product (RAGE), which are pattern recognition receptors of the immune globulin family. AGE-receptor interaction initiates further inflammatory signaling, induces apoptosis, fibrotic remodeling, and immune cell infiltration in cardiac tissue [27]. Accumulation of AGEs in the microvascular can potentiate further damage and has been associated with cardiomyocyte stiffness and accelerated collagen deposition in the heart [25]. The resulting increase in myocardial rigidity triggers diastolic dysfunction, decreased myocardial strain, and atrial expansion, which ultimately leads to atrial fibrillation in DM patients [28].

In T2DM, insulin resistance reduces cardiac glucose availability and shifts toward fatty acid oxidation [29]. However, high blood glucose and free fatty acids (FFA) resemble a state of energetic oversupply, which leads to inappropriate accumulation of lipid in extra-adipose tissues, including the heart [30]. This is connected to the functional mutilation of oxidative phosphorylation as an outcome of a disproportionate caloric supply in the absence of adequate energy utilization [31]. Unfortunately, cardiomyocytes are not appropriately designed to accumulate an excess amount of lipids, which may cause, in other cases, cardiomyocyte damage by lipotoxicity. Besides, inappropriately handled lipid fragments can initiate different inflammatory mechanisms, such as protein kinase C and nuclear factor kappa b (NF-kB) mediated pathways that ultimately affect insulin signaling as well as cardiac metabolism [32].

Excess glucose and fatty acids can also drain to the citric acid cycle to produce donors for the electron transport chain (ETC). However, the lack of energy requirement in an energetically saturated condition lowers the ATP requirement and causes an accumulation of electrons along with the ETC [33]. Excess electrons increase the probability of leakage and, therefore, reaction with molecular oxygen to generate Reactive Oxygen Species (ROS) (Fig. **2**).

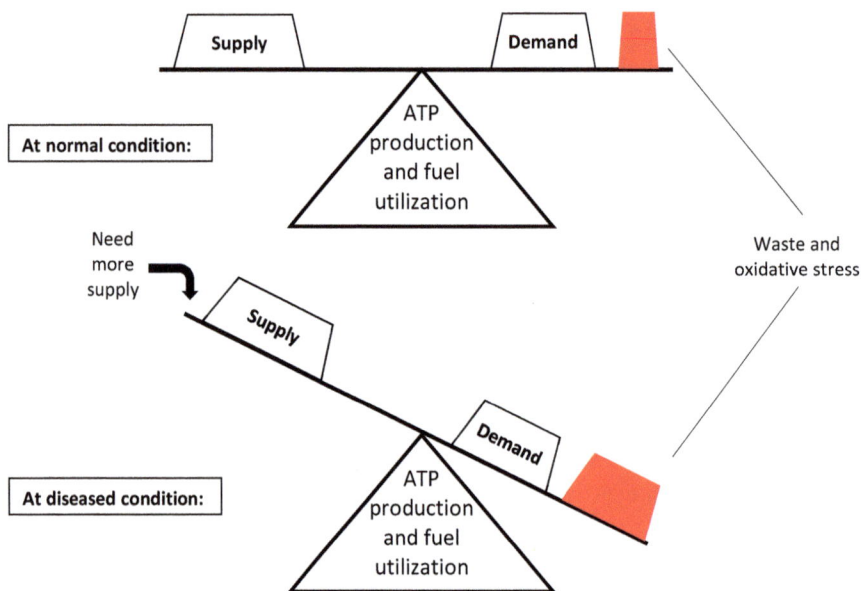

Fig. (2). Regulation of cellular bioenergetics under normal physiologic conditions of balanced nutrient availability and disease condition (modified from Lehrke *et al.* [34]) ATP = adenosine triphosphate.

In DM, hyperglycemia can lead to the instigation of hexosamine and aldose reductase signaling as alternative metabolic pathways. During the prolonged hyperglycemic situation, these pathways may also trigger a boosted synthesis of ROS as well as diminishes substrates for the antioxidant enzymes. *In vitro* study revealed that under hyperglycemia, human aortic endothelial cells produce ROS that can modify histone 3 *via* lysine monomethylation to increase the expression of the p65 subunit of NF-kB [35]. Upon activation, this NF-kB then increases the transcription of monocyte chemoattractant molecule 1 (MCP-1), vascular cell adhesion molecule 1 (VCAM- 1), and other inflammatory proteins like interleukin 6 (IL-6), intercellular adhesion molecule 1 (ICAM-1), and Nitric oxide synthase (Nos), which are directly connected to arterial pathophysiology. These effects even persist after six days of successive normoglycemia. Moreover, it is well documented that increased mitochondrial ROS production is the central pathology of both diabetes and cardiovascular complications [36]. Thus, many strategies are now aiming to avoid ROS production to metabolically reverse organ dysfunctions (Fig. **2**) [37].

During the heart failure condition, cardiac metabolism gets altered *via* changing the substrate preferences from fatty acids to glucose oxidation. In contrast, due to the lack of insulin, DM patient shows the opposite phenomenon, utilizing more fatty acids than glucose to fulfill its energy demand [38]. When advanced heart failure patients' cardiac tissue samples were used for metabolic profiling, a reduced amount of fatty acids, with the diminished activity of the fatty-acid oxidation machinery, was observed [39]. Thus, a failing heart is dependent on glucose metabolism to continue its function and pumping activity. Therefore, the coexistence of T2DM and heart failure in the same individual can limit the energetic supply and destroy cardiac function [40]. This is the reason why the heart failure condition has been believed as "an engine out of fuel" [41]. Recent reports showed the role of cardiac ketone bodies as an alternative energy supply for the failing heart. Due to the shortage of energy supply, ketone body concentrations get increased in the failing heart to provide enough energy in an insulin-independent manner. Supporting the idea, it was found that the expression of ketone body processing enzymes was increased in the hypertrophied as well as in the failing heart. These enzymes start energy production *via* ketone body oxidation instead of fatty acid oxidation [42, 43]. However, new understandings are required to figure out the impact of ROS production and fuel shifting, whether adaptive or maladaptive, in heart function and whether this concept can be utilized for different therapeutic approaches.

Role of Obesity in Diabetes and CVD

Abdominal obesity increases insulin resistance and is recognized as a risk factor for CVD [44]. In the disease condition, waist circumference increases despite a plateauing in general obesity. This is the same reason why obesity is the foremost threatening cause for T2DM [45] and why the pattern and frequency of occurrence of T2DM just reflected those of obesity. It was found T2DM is pronouncedly increased among those who were obese (Body mass index, BMI 18.0 to 20.1), suggesting that obesity has a significant contribution to T2DM development [46]. Reports also indicated that 85.2% of people with T2DM are overweight or obese [47]. Likewise, it is now well documented that the development of T2DM can be controlled by nonpharmacologic treatments, lifestyle changes, daily physical workout, decrease in salt intake (<1500 mg per day), reduction of alcohol consumption, and termination of smoking as well as *via* bodyweight reduction [48]. The Finish Diabetes Prevention Study Group found that intensive lifestyle changes can reduce the incidence of diabetes by 58% compared to placebo and remain lower by 34% after 10-years of follow-up [49]. Therefore, the importance of adopting a healthy lifestyle to combat the obesity epidemic is enormous.

Abdominal obesity is responsible for low-grade inflammation that plays a major role in the pathogenesis of T2DM and is associated with higher rates of morbidity and mortality due to CVD [50]. T2DM can induce adipose tissue, macrophages, and other cells to produce cytokines, for example, interleukin-1 (IL-1), IL-6, Tumor necrosis factor-alpha (TNF-alpha), leptin, MCP-1, C-reactive protein (CRP), plasminogen activator inhibitor-1 (PAI-1), fibrinogen, angiotensin, retinol-binding protein-4 (RBP), and adiponectin, that are responsible for the prolong subclinical inflammation [51]. These mediators may induce chronic inflammatory processes in the vessel wall at the molecular level, promoting lipid accumulation with consequent development of atherosclerosis and CVD [52]. Moreover, adipose tissue can lead to endothelial dysfunction with increased expression of adhesion molecules (ICAM-1, VCAM-1, P-selectin, and E-selectin) on neutrophils, migration of monocytes and T lymphocytes [53]. Likewise Insulin resistance stimulates a chronic increase of FFA in the plasma leading to increase storage of triglycerides in muscle, reducing glucose uptake by muscle and liver. At the same time, insulin resistance increases hepatic glucose production, which ultimately impairs insulin action and promotes hyperinsulinemia [54]. A high level of blood insulin induces myocyte growth *via* increased FFA levels as well as activating Phosphatidylinositol-3-Kinase Ak strain transforming-1 (PI3K/Akt-1) pathway, resulting in cardiac hypertrophy and contractile dysfunction [55].

Role of Glycemic Control in Diabetes and CVD

It has been observed that early diagnosis and treatment of hyperglycemic patients when they have a short period with diabetes, low cardiovascular risk profile, and glycated hemoglobin levels below 7%, then a long-term significant cardiovascular benefit may result in. However, in older patients, having hyperglycemia for a longer period and a higher cardiovascular risk profile, tighter glycemic control could not bring many benefits. Scientists named this phenomenon "metabolic memory," which explains the capacity of remembering the influence of a previous glycemic exposure environment to the target tissues [56], causing long-term detrimental or protecting outcomes. This fact is explained by the epigenetic and metabolic alterations responsible for oxidative stress, low-grade inflammation, and endothelial dysfunction [56].

Role of Dyslipidemia in Diabetes and CVD

Dyslipidemia is a condition when the blood contains an inappropriate amount of lipid, especially triglycerides (TG), low-density lipoprotein cholesterol (VLDL), and high-density lipoprotein (HDL) cholesterol. During T2DM, dyslipidemia may happen with a high VLDL, TG, and small and dense LDL levels; on the other hand, diminished HDL level. These altered lipid molecules aggravate cardiovascular risk due to their increased tendency for oxidation and glycosylation, causing a significant reduction of vascular compliance, prompting early and aggressive atherosclerosis [57]. Although in T1DM, patients are usually young and occasionally have lipid abnormalities, they encounter similar difficulties. However, in T1DM, the atherogenic complications are not exclusively caused by abnormal lipid levels, but hyperglycemia also plays pivotal role in that process [58]. Other studies also support that both hyperlipidemia and hyperglycemia contribute to distinct atherogenesis phases in DM [59]. Similarly, in a diabetic-mouse model, intensive glycemic control with insulin can prevent dyslipidemia mediated start of the atherosclerotic injury [59]. Several clinical trials also unveil the importance of lipid control in DM patients, including the Collaborative Atorvastatin Diabetes Study (CARDS), which first studied T2DM patients without any past CVD incidences. Interestingly, this study showed that treatment with 10 mg atorvastatin could cause a 37% drop in cardiovascular cases and a 48% drop in stroke compared to control [60].

Role of Hypertension in Diabetes and CVD

Hypertension is highly prevalent worldwide and most common among DM patients. It is a condition when blood pressure (BP) in the arteries is persistently elevated. Reports showed that around 10-30% of T1DM and approximately 60% of T2DM patients have hypertension [61].

Unfortunately, patients who have both DM and hypertension, having a higher possibility of developing macrovascular (myocardial infarction, stroke) and/or microvascular complications (nephropathy and retinopathy) [62]. However, initiation of hypertension is quite diverse in different forms of diabetes. For example, in T1DM patients, hypertension starts years later to DM detection, typically during the progress of diabetic nephropathy [61]. It was found that BP tends to get higher three years after the onset of microalbuminuria [63]. In contrast, T2DM patients may already have hypertension existing at diagnosis or starts even earlier the rise of blood glucose levels [64]. Therefore, the management of hypertension in diabetic patients primarily focuses on preventing CVD, diminishing the advancement of renal disease and diabetic retinopathy. The United Kingdom Prospective Diabetes Study (UKPDS) stated that persons with T2DM might take advantage of proper BP management by nonpharmacological actions than with firm regulation of blood glucose concentration [65]. However, diabetics patients with persistent BP higher than 130/80 mmHg and now experiencing a modification in lifestyle executed for three months or the maximum BP levels are already greater than 140/90 mmHg at diagnosis-should pharmacological therapy [66].

BIOCHEMICAL ASPECTS BETWEEN DIABETES AND CVDS

Most of the DM patients died due to cerebrocardiovascular diseases, like atherosclerosis, that have been initiated due to diabetes-related metabolic abnormalities like insulin resistance and hyperglycemia [67 - 69]. This is called diabetic macroangiopathy, defined as a condition when atherosclerosis is diagnosed secondary to DM. Endothelial and vascular smooth muscle cell dysfunction instigated this situation, and as a result, vascular homeostasis gets altered. Although insulin resistance and hyperglycemia can initiate low-grade confined inflammations in the vascular wall, chronic enhancement of oxidative stress due to DM can ultimately initiate endothelial dysfunction and promoting atherogenesis [70]. Interestingly, insulin resistance can alone produce ROS and potentiate the reaction further [71]. This situation also increases adhesion molecules' expression; the release of different humoral components like cytokines (IL-1β, IL-6, TNF-α), chemokines, and CRP from vascular endothelial cells strengthen the progressive nature of the vascular injury, leading to atherosclerosis [68, 72, 73]. Moreover, blood monocytes migrate to the injured site *via* chemotaxis and attach to the endothelium through interaction with adhesion molecules [69]. These monocytes differentiated and matured into macrophages upon their penetration to the subendothelial space and again release cytokines. ROS oxidizes and modifies high LDL-cholesterol and remnant lipoproteins, further exacerbating the atherogenic condition [74]. In the case of high LDL, LDL cholesterol infiltrates in the subendothelial area, stayed in the intima, and can be oxidized or otherwise altered [71]. Unluckily, macrophages acquire as well as accrue oxidized LDL cholesterol and convert themselves to foam cell [75]. Foam cells in the presence of oxidized lipids trigger the further secretion of various growth factors by the endothelium, which transforms vascular smooth muscle cells of the media and causes its migration to the intima, where they multiply and dynamically create an extracellular matrix. These malformed vascular smooth muscle cells also acquire oxidized LDL cholesterol and change to foam cells that accelerate the atherogenesis [76]. Simultaneously, the growth of vascular smooth muscle cells and an expansion of the extracellular matrix may cause intimal thickening and sclerosis.

Interestingly, DM patients have high levels of small dense LDL (sd-LDL) cholesterol, which has a small particle size and low antioxidant content. Moreover, it has a lower affinity to LDL receptors, a greater tendency to be transported into the subendothelial space, and more propensity to be oxidized or otherwise degraded. All these properties make them very atherogenic [77]. Interestingly, lifestyle modifications, such as physical activity and weight loss, can reduce the sd-LDL level, thus CVD risk factors in prediabetic individuals [78].

AGEs can also initiate foam cell formation *via* accelerating monocytes' migration to the subendothelial space and the expression of adhesion molecules on the endothelial cells. Tissue macrophages then use their scavenger receptors to uptake either the circulating oxidized LDL cholesterols or oxidized AGE-modified LDL cholesterols to become foam cells and release cytokines [79]. Moreover, AGEs inhibit reverse cholesterol transport by reducing the expression of ATP-binding membrane cassette transporter-A1 (ABCA1) and ABCG1 on monocytes. AGEs also induce vasoconstriction by increasing endothelin-1 levels, reducing vasodilation by decreasing nitric oxide levels and enhancing extracellular matrix modifications to accelerate atherosclerosis progression. Furthermore, AGEs induce pathological neovascularization *via* autocrine production of vascular endothelial growth factor (VEGF). Unfortunately, inappropriate neovascularization is involved in the bleeding and instability of plaques which may lead to stroke and myocardial infarction. Moreover, AGEs can accelerate the synthesis of tissue factors and suppress fibrinolysis by stimulating the production of PAI-1 to induce clot formation. Interestingly, scientists reported that experimentally induced atherosclerosis progression is relatively slow in the RAGE knockout mouse model. Moreover, myocardial infarction after experimental coronary artery ligation is small in this RAGE knockout mouse model [80]. Another animal study showed that administration of soluble RAGE molecules, as a ligand decoy, can inhibit the AGE-mediated Extracellular Signal-Regulated Kinase (ERK) phosphorylation and the expression of VEGF [81], which reduce the size of atherosclerotic injuries in the aorta of Apolipoprotein E (Apo E) knockout diabetes mice [82] and diminished the growth of neoendothelium after femoral artery injury in mice [83].

MOLECULAR ASPECTS BETWEEN DIABETES AND CVDS

Although a mutation in a single gene can trigger diseases, both DM and CVDs are multi-gene associated diseases [84]. Heterozygous alterations in any of these genes can be the source of familial forms of the disease Table **1** [85]. However, mutations in some of these genes may have a beneficial role in diseases. For example, impaired intracellular cholesterol transport due to mutation in the LDL receptor or Apo B gene has described a protective role against T2DM; this suggests a mechanistic role of cholesterol metabolism in T2DM [86].

Table 1. Gene variants commonly associated with T2DM and CVD (modified from Brunetti *et al.* [9].

Gene	Cellular Involvement	Role	Refs.
Adiponectin	exerts anti-inflammatory and antiatherogenic function	↑ Risk	[83]
ADIPOR1 (Adiponectin receptor)	involved in fatty acids and glucose metabolism	↑ Risk	[91, 92]
ApoE (Apolipoprotein E)	involved in lipoprotein transport	↑ Risk	[96, 97]
CDKN2A/2B (Cyclin-dependent kinase inhibitor 2B)	regulate cell cycle *via* Cadherin EGF LAG seven-pass G-type receptor 2	↑ Risk	[93]
CELSR2-PSRC1-SORT1 (CELSR2: cadherin, EGF LAG seven-pass G-type receptor 2, PSRC1: proline/serine rich coiled coil 1, and SORT1: sortilin 1)	CELSR2 is part of the cadherin superfamily, involved in contact-mediated communication. Proline- and serine-rich coiled-coil 1 plays an important role in mitosis. Sortilin 1 is involved in transferring distinct proteins to either cell surface or subcellular compartments.	↓ Risk	[93]
GLUL (Glutamine synthetase)	enzyme implicated in ammonia and glutamate detoxification, acid-base homeostasis, cell signaling, and cell proliferation High-mobility	↑ Risk	[98, 99]
HMGA1 (High-mobility group A1)	involved in architectural transcription factor with a role in cell growth, differentiation, and glucose metabolism	↑ Risk	[80, 100]
HNF1A (Hepatic nuclear factor 1A)	involved in the development and metabolic homeostasis	↑ Risk	[93]
HP (Haptoglobin)	hemoglobin-binding capacity. Implicated in angiogenesis and in cholesterol-crystallizatio--promoting activity	↑ Risk	[101, 102]
Paraoxonase	an enzyme that protects against lipid oxidation Proprotein	↑ Risk	[103]
PCSK9 (Proprotein convertase subtilisin/Kexin type 9)	plasma cholesterol metabolism	↓ Risk	[93])
PHACTR1 (Phosphatase and actin regulator 1)	binds actin and plays a role in the reorganization of the actin cytoskeleton	↑ Risk	[93]
SOD2 (Superoxide dismutase 2)	transforms toxic superoxide into hydrogen peroxide and diatomic oxygen	↑ Risk	[89]
TCF7L2 (Transcription factor 7-like 2)	member of the Wnt signaling pathway	↑ Risk	[104]

Genetic Loci Linked with T2DM and CVD

It has been observed that when diseases are linked phenotypically, they might have some genetic linkage. As T2DM and CVD are phenotypically linked in many aspects, therefore, distinctive groups used diverse approaches— for example, comprising candidate gene studies, linkage analyses, and Genome-Wide Association Study (GWAS)— to identify different genes influencing the diseases Table 1 [87]. It has been found that at least 83 loci are linked with T2DM [81], and more than 30 loci with CVD [82].

Among the candidate genes, the paraoxonase gene encodes an enzyme that binds to HDL particles and protects LDL from oxidation and proatherogenic modifications. Several polymorphic variants of this protein have been reported, which may be responsible for the circulating enzyme's reduced level of activity. When considering the paraoxonase variants, Gln192Arg or Met54Leu is independently associated with T2DM and CVD [88]. Similar to this, diabetic women having the Ala16Val (rs4880) variant of the antioxidant enzyme superoxide dismutase (SOD) may experience a higher risk of developing CVD [89]. The risk for T2DM and CVD is also high in patients with a low level of obesity-associated protein adiponectin (an adipokine, which has anti-inflammatory and antiatherogenic effects). In contrast, an increased level of this protein can diminish the risk of CVD in diabetes [90]. Moreover, the report showed a G>T mutation in the adiponectin gene at position 276 has also been associated with CAD in patients with T2DM [83]. In addition to adiponectin, its receptor, the adiponectin receptor 1 (ADIPOR1) gene, is also intensively studied as a candidate gene for CVD in diabetic subjects. Specifically, the presence of a haplotype in T2DM, defined with rs7539542, rs10920531, and rs4950894 SNPs, caused a reduction in ADIPOR1 gene expression and were found significantly associated with CAD [91]. The same is true for its promoter variant (rs266729) in T2DM subjects, which has also been linked with oxidative stress and cardiovascular risk [92].

Five other gene variants of CDKN2A/2B (Cyclin-dependent kinase inhibitor, rs4977574), CELSR2-PSRC1-SORT1 (cadherin, EGF LAG seven-pass G-type receptor- proline/serine rich coiled coil- sortilin, rs646776), PHACTR1 (Phosphatase and actin regulator, rs12526453), HNF1A (Hepatic nuclear factor, rs2259816), and PCSK9 (Proprotein convertase subtilisin/Kexin, rs11206510), in T2DM patients also showed significant associations with the risk for CAD [93]. Interestingly, GWAS identified another novel T2DM susceptibility gene, Transcription factor 7-like 2 (TCF7L2) [94]. Some of its variants are associated with CVD [92], but not all [95]. Scientists subsequently analyzed these genes in more detail among 1,650 patients who experienced coronary angiography and revealed that these variants were more strongly linked with diabetic patients having CVD compared to non-diabetics [104].

Polymorphism in the TNF-α gene is another example of genetic variation that may confer CAD risk in persons with T2DM than in non-diabetic subjects. Among the variants, a TNF-α promoter region (−308) variation has a stronger association with CAD in diabetic women [105]. ApoE polymorphisms can also modulate the risk for CVD in T2DM. Among the isotypes, reports showed that the ApoE4 allele can significantly increase the susceptibility for CVD in the presence of T2DM [97]. This is also true for the haptoglobin (HP) gene, which is a serum protein that interacts with free hemoglobin and prevents hemoglobin-induced oxidation. This gene has two alleles, HP1 and HP2, generated by duplications of exons 3 and 4. Researchers found that HP2 has a reduced ability to prevent oxidative stress-driven changes to hemoglobin compared to HP1 and, therefore, is strongly related to CVD in T2DM patients [101, 106]. In another study of T2DM patients of American-European origin, the HP2-2 phenotype was strongly linked with triglyceride levels, subclinical atherosclerosis in the form of increased carotid-media thickness, but not of calcified arterial plaques, and CVD mortality [102].

DNA or Histone Modifications in T2DM and CVDs

In vitro exposition of aortic endothelial cells to a high amount of glucose showed reduced H3K9/K14 acetylation of histone and an altered DNA methylation pattern [107]. In another study, the activity and expression of histone deacetylases (HDACs) of T2DM patients were evaluated with glycemia, inflammation, and insulin resistance. Results showed that HDAC3 expression and activity were induced by insulin resistance and chronic low-grade inflammation. Moreover, different circulating pro-inflammatory markers, such as TNF-α, and IL-6 were positive, whereas Sirt1 expression was negatively correlated with HDAC3 expression and activity [108]. Studies also figured out the other associations between epigenetic modifications and CVD risks with cardio-metabolic phenotypes, such as obesity, dyslipidemia, insulin resistance, inflammation, and hypertension [109]. It has been reported that the alpha-ketoglutarate-dependent dioxygenase encoding gene can be hypermethylated at rs8050136 or rs9939609 and, therefore, increased the risk for obesity and CVD [110, 111]. In a different study, insulin-like growth factor 2 (IGF2) hypermethylation was found to be linked with increased triglyceride/HDL-cholesterol ratio among obese children, demonstrating an epigenetic marker of metabolic threat [112]. When whole-cell transcriptomes of insulin-resistant patients were compared with control, many distinctly-methylated CpG islands were detected in adipose tissue samples, which includes IL18, a cluster of differentiation 44 (CD44), CD48, CD38, CD37,

CX3CL1 (CXC-type chemokine receptor), CXCR1, CXCR2, CXCL1, IGF1R, and APOB48R genes [113]. Furthermore, experiments with obese mice showed that methylation at the Peroxisome proliferator-activated receptor delta (PPARγ) gene promoter could cause the preference of adipose tissue macrophages from an anti-inflammatory (M2) to a pro-inflammatory phenotype (M1), and thus, increasing the risk of CVD. The influence of these epigenetic changes can be further realized from the observation that some of these changes that occurred in the prenatal stage can increase the probability of future MI [114].

Association of HMGA1 with T2DM and CVD Risk

One of the non-histone small nuclear proteins, called high-mobility group A1 (HMGA1), can bind at the minor groove of DNA and ultimately alter the chromatin conformation. Upon binding, it can facilitate the assembly and stability of stereospecific DNA–protein complexes called "enhanceosomes," thus potentiating regulation of different genes involved in glucose metabolism, *via* modulating the insulin-like growth factor-binding protein 1 (IGFBP1), insulin receptor (INSR), RBP4, and insulin (INS) genes [9, 115, 116], as well as *via* insulin action [117]. One of the HMGA1 variants, rs139876191, can diminish INSR expression and increase trans-ethnic vulnerabilities to either T2DM [118] or other metabolic disorders [119]. Likewise, another variant, rs139876191, is associated with BMI and diminished HDL levels in patients with metabolic syndrome and T2DM [119]. Besides, HMGA1 can also promote the growth, expansion, and relocation of VSMCs to the neointima and induces the synthesis of different inflammatory cytokines, adhesion molecules, including CD44 and chemokines. Therefore, accelerating the development and progression of the atherosclerotic plaque [120]. In contrast, the absence or reduced activity of HMGA1 is involved in the impairment of vascular repair and neoangiogenesis because of the lack of activation of the matrix metalloproteinase 9 (MMP-9), and VEGF [121].

Association of MicroRNAs (miRNA) with T2DM and CVD Risk

miRNAs are small single-strand RNA molecules regulating many biological processes *via* altering target genes at the post-transcriptional level. Researchers found that several of these miRNAs have also been related to T2DM and CVD [122], where they control beta-cell function, insulin response, glucose homeostasis, as well as vascular pathogenesis [123]. Several studies demonstrated that high blood glucose could increase oxidative stress *via* inducing miR-185 expression that suppresses the glutathione peroxidase-1 (GPx-1) gene expression. This enzyme involves hydrogen peroxide detoxification, and thus, inhibition of this enzyme induces oxidative stress to the cell [124]. Besides, hyperglycemia can impair SIRT-1 expression and function *via* upregulating miR-34a and miR-204, thus contributing to the endothelial cell senescence [125]. Another report showed, endothelial progenitor cells (EPCs) can increase miR-134 and miR-130a expression under the hyperglycemic situation to affect cell motility and apoptosis, respectively [126]. During hyperglycemia, miR-145 impairs myocardial gene expression *via* kruppel-like factor 4 (KLF4) and accelerates VSMC proliferation *via* downgrading its level [127]. Moreover, high blood glucose can also reduce the level of miR-504 and miR-24. Therefore VSMC proliferation and migration have been severely impaired in diabetes [128]. Impaired vascular contractility and augmented proliferative and migratory properties of VSMC may, therefore, accelerating the probability of CVD-related diseases [129]. In contrast, miR-126 can exert proangiogenic and anti-inflammatory activities in the endothelium. miR-126 can also inhibit TNF-α, ROS, and Nicotinamide adenine dinucleotide phosphate (NADPH) oxidase *via* HMGB1 to suppresses inflammation [130]. It also maintains vascular integrity and angiogenesis *via* enhancing VEGF and fibroblast growth factor activities [131], recruiting progenitor cells through the chemokine CXCL12 [132]. Interestingly, both the T2DM patients [133] and patients with CAD [134] showed a reduced level of miR-126 equally in myocardial tissue and plasma, suggesting that its role as a potential new diagnostic marker for DM and CVD.

Probable molecular links between lipid metabolism and miRNAs were also studied in diabetic CVD patients. Animal studies revealed impairment of numerous important lipid metabolism-associated genes, like FoxA2 (Forkhead box), Ppargc1a (Peroxisome proliferator-activated receptor gamma coactivator 1-alpha), and Hmgcs2 (hydroxy-Methylglutaryl-Coa Synthase) by miR-29 in Zucker diabetic fatty rats [135]. In contrast, miR-122 upregulates the level of HNF-4 alpha in both diabetic mice and insulin-resistant HepG2 cells. Upregulation of miR-122 and HNF-4 alpha can increase the expression of SREBP-1 (Sterol Regulatory Element-binding Proteins) and fatty acid synthesis genes, therefore, increases the risk of CVD *via* facilitating fatty acid and triglyceride synthesis, in addition to altered cholesterol homeostasis [136]. In contrast, obese mice showed a reduced level of miR-26a that upregulated fatty acid synthesis and therefore initiated several CVDs and other obesity-related pathophysiology [137].

Reports found a reduced level of miR- 223, 126, or 146a in diabetic and hyperglycemic patients is associated with increased platelet reactivity and aggregation [138, 139]. Moreover, inhibition of miR-223 in the animal model also showed a similar hyper-reactive and -adhesive platelet phenotype due to beta1 integrin, kindlin-3, and factor XIII mediated increase calpain activation [140]. Interestingly, diabetic patients showed diminished plasma miR-223 and miR-126 levels [139]. Lower levels of these miRNA in plasma are responsible for platelet dysfunction in diabetic patients due to the P-selectin and P2Y12 receptors' upregulation. They, therefore, cause an even more activation of platelets in T2DM [141, 142]. Circulating miR-223 levels is thus considered as an independent predictor of increased on-treatment platelet reactivity [143]. Moreover, platelets release different kinds of RNA molecules in the blood, including intronic transcripts and non-coding RNAs *via* microvesicles, which play an important role in thrombosis [142]. These secreting RNAs can facilitate the horizontal transfer of localized molecular signals to specific sites and increase the chance of thrombosis [144]. Furthermore, prediabetes or overt diabetic patients have increased platelet-derived miR-103b, responsible for the downregulation of pancreatic islets derived Frizzled-Related Protein-4 (SFRP4) [145], which support the role of miR-103b as an innovative marker of prediabetes/diabetes and prospective therapeutic option in T2DM.

The role of macrophages in the development of atherosclerotic plaques in diabetic patients is well documented, where a shift to M1 phenotype and accumulation to the vessel wall was observed. Reports showed this is due to the excess production of pro-inflammatory molecules from adipose tissue [146]. Interestingly, *in vitro* and *in vivo* experiments found a diminished miR-181b expression by endothelial cells under both hyperglycemic and insulin-resistant states. Moreover, increased production of miR-181b, due to decreased AKT Ser 473 phosphorylation, was observed, responsible for an anti-inflammatory M2 response [147]. Therefore, indicating a protective role of miR-181b in atherosclerosis.

There are a few miRNAs include miR-1, and miR-206, and miR133a, associated with both CVD and hyperglycemia. It has been reported that some of these miRNAs negatively regulate the heat shock protein 60 to suppress cardiomyocytes' apoptosis [148]. More recently, scientists described the involvement of miR-208, miR- 499, miR-1, and miR-133 in the differentiation of stem cells to cardiomyocytes [149]. Furthermore, the involvement of miR-133a in cardiac contractility was recently revealed in streptozotocin-induced diabetic rats [150], where upregulation of miR-133a increases the expression of tyrosine aminotransferase (a regulator of norepinephrine production and β-adrenergic receptors) to improve cardiac contractility [150]. Unfortunately, not sufficient data is available to show the involvement of miR-208 in diabetic heart disease. However, scientists proposed a mechanism where miR-208 may involve regulating myosin heavy chain gene expression to provide cardiac protection [151]. Another study showed that miR-499 could suppress the calcineurin-mediated dephosphorylation of dynamin-related protein-1 to keep cardiomyocytes safe from ischemic damage and apoptosis [152].

In contrast, few miRNAs, including miR-1 and miR-133a, have critical roles in cardiomyocytes and disease prevention. It is believed that alteration of different proteins, like the suppression of serum response factor (plays a role in myoblast proliferation), RhoA (Ras homolog family member A, protein involved in GDP-GTP cycling), Cdc42 (Cell division control, kinase implicated in hypertrophy), and Nelf-A (Negative elongation factor A) nuclear factor [153], may involve with this protective response. Evidence showed that these miRNAs' level gets reduced in diabetic cardiomyopathy, ischemic myocardial tissue, and left ventricular hypertrophy, which further supports this hypothesis [154].

Association of Long Non-Coding RNA (lncRNAs) with T2DM and CVD Risk

Long non-coding RNAs (lncRNAs) are more than 200 nucleotides long, non-protein-coding transcripts [155]. They are involved in several biological functions, including signal amplification as well as regulation of gene expression [156]. *In vitro* studies revealed its involvement in smooth muscle cell (SMC) proliferation, endothelial function, inflammation, lipid metabolism, and obesity, as well as insulin resistance [157]. In contrast, *in vivo* studies found similar involvements where T2DM [158] or the CVD outcome [159] can be easily predicted using the circulating lncRNAs. For example, Metastasis-associated lung adenocarcinoma transcript 1 (MALAT1) lncRNA is predominantly expressed in the nucleus of endothelial cells to regulate its function by targeting serum amyloid antigen 3 (a pro-inflammatory ligand) to stimulate the expression of IL-6, TNF-α, and ROS synthesis [160]. Moreover, at high blood glucose concentration, the expression of this lncRNA also got altered, leading to micro- and macrovascular damages [161]. Another interesting lncRNA is lncRNA H19 that can regulate cell proliferation and limit body weight gain. Under the hyperglycemic condition, this lncRNA level was reduced and induced cardiomyocyte apoptosis *via* miR-675 that targets VDAC1 (Voltage-dependent anion-selective channel 1), a porin involved in mitochondrial ATP transport, in a mouse model of diabetic cardiomyopathy [162]. Moreover, lncRNAs can also modulate macrophages to induce inflammation to initiate diabetic vascular complications. When bone marrow-derived macrophages of db/db and diet-induced insulin-resistant type 2 diabetic mice were used for transcriptome profiling, it was found that increased lncRNA E330013P06 can induce the expression of inflammatory genes (*e.g* ., Nos2, IL6, and Prostaglandin-Endoperoxide Synthase 2 (ptgs2)) to promote the foam cell formation and endothelial dysfunction [163]. In contrast, another lncRNA Lethe can prevent the NF-kB transcription factor's translocation to the nucleus and, therefore, show an anti-inflammatory effect. Interestingly, at hyperglycemic condition, the level of lncRNA Lethe was reduced, which causes an increase in NOX2 (NADPH oxidases) gene expression and ultimately induce oxidative stress [164].

PRIMARY PREVENTION OF CARDIOVASCULAR DISEASE IN DIABETES MELLITUS

Although enormous efforts were given to improve DM-associated mortality, the incidence of obesity, metabolic syndrome, and CVD continue to rise. It is projected that by 2050, around 1 in 3 people will have T2DM in certain parts of the world [165]. Therefore, it is very much urgent to prevent CVD probabilities in DM patients, especially in T2DM, *via* lifestyle and risk factors management (Table **2**). Under the lifestyle management schemes, daily exercise, balanced diet, weight management (by focusing on dietary habits, especially *via* caloric restriction and increased energy expenditure), and behavior modifications related to lifestyle (*ss* ., smoking cessation) are the key points. For example, many reports documented that cigarette smoking is strongly associated with CVD and other poor health outcomes [166]. Thus, a routine and comprehensive assessment of tobacco use with cessation advocating and pharmacotherapy for CVD prevention among patients with and without T2DM are very much urgent to perform. On the other hand, CVD risk factor management considers the impact of aspirin and similar drugs, controlling blood glucose, BP, cholesterol levels, directions for risk stratification, and prevention of CVD in patients with T2DM.

CVD complications among the patients with DM are getting difficult because the most accepted and reasonable target for DM control, Hb A1C, does not go hand in hand with CVD morbidity and mortality reduction [169]. It has been found that few hypoglycemic drugs can reduce the Hb A1C level but are unable to show any CVD benefits, while others can do so. That's why it has been requested by the US Food and Drug Administration (FDA) that each and every new glucose-lowering agent must prove CV safety [170]. Interestingly, scientists have already reported newer DM medications, although with modest HbA1c reduction, could show significant CVD benefits in the clinical trials (CVD outcome trials, CVOTs) [171].

Among the pharmacological agents, CVDs are associated with generalized insulin intake. Insulin intake alters several systemic and neurohumoral signaling that alters metabolic pathways in the heart and leads to MI as well as heart failure. The changes range from activation of proximal insulin signaling pathways that may contribute to adverse left ventricular remodeling and mitochondrial dysfunction to repress distal elements of insulin signaling pathways such as forkhead transcriptional signaling or glucose transport which may also impair cardiac metabolism, structure, and function. In contrast, aspirin provides a significant advantage for the secondary prevention of CVD among patients with and without T2DM [172], although its primary prevention is still questionable. Moreover, It has been found that 70-80% of T2DM patients have comorbid hypertension that increases the risk of MI, stroke, nephropathy, different microvascular outcomes, and all-cause mortality [173]. Diabetic patients controlling BP, specifically the systolic blood pressure (SBP), can get superior benefits against the CVD risks. Epidemiological studies found that T2DM patients having SBP from approximately 115 mm Hg or above are at a progressively higher risk of developing micro- and macrovascular complications [174].

Table 2. Management for CVD Prevention for Patients with Diabetes Mellitus Risk (modified from Newman *et al.* [165].

Key Factor	Recommendation	Refs.
Physical activity	150 min/week moderate intensity (50%70% MPHR) over 3 days/week with 2 consecutive days without exercise	[166]
Nutrition	consumption of Mediterranean style diet, especially fruits, vegetables, legumes, whole grains, and dairy in place of other carbohydrate sources	[166]
Weight management	lifestyle changes by a sustained 3%–5% rate of weight loss that confers a clinically meaningful health benefit	[167]
Cigarette Smoking	not to use cigarettes, other tobacco products, or e-cigarettes	[166]
Glycemic control	consider HbA1c <6.5% for patients with diabetes of short duration, long life expectancy, and no significant CVD if it can be achieved safely	[166]
Blood pressure	a target of <140/90 mm Hg is appropriate for most diabetic patients assuming the target can be safely achieved using either an ACE inhibitor or an ARB or both	[166, 168]
Cholesterol	Diabetic patients 40–75 yrs of age with CV risk factors can receive high-intensity statin	[166, 168]
Antiplatelet therapy	Aspirin 75–162 mg is reasonable for diabetic patients with at one or more CV risk factors without increased GI bleeding risk	[166]

ACE= Angiotensin-converting-enzyme; ARB= Angiotensin II receptor blockers; CV=cardiovascular; CVD=cardiovascular disease; GI=gastrointestinal; HbA1c=glycosylated hemoglobin; LDL=low density lipoprotein; MPHR=maximum predicted heart rate.

Statin: Statin is a 3-hydroxy methylglutaryl Coenzyme A (HMG-CoA) reductase inhibitor used to lower blood lipid concentration in the treatment of diabetic patients having a tendency of dyslipidemia as well as cardiovascular diseases. Thus, preventing the primary and secondary occurrence of CVD and associated death [175 - 177]. Research showed statin could activate ATP-dependent K^+ channels in the endothelium as well as in the myocardium that improves vascular and cardiac function. A large meta-analysis considering 14 randomized trials of statin therapy having more than 18,000 patients with diabetes (>95% T2DM) monitored for around 4.3 years exhibited almost a 9% proportional decrease in all-cause death and a 13% decrease in vascular death per 1 mmol/l (39 mg/dl) reduction in LDL-C [178]. However, pleiotropic activation of these channels by statin in the beta cells of the pancreas leads to inhibition of insulin release and, ultimately, aggravated diabetes [179].

Metformin: Metformin is a biguanide derivative (dimethyl biguanide) used to treat T2DM. It acts on the liver to reduce hepatic glucose release and, to a lower extent, on peripheral tissues to promote glucose uptake. Thus, it exerts a hypoglycemic effect on the patient [180]. It activates AMP-activated kinase (AMPK) directly and indirectly to show the molecular level results. In the direct pathway, metformin directly binds to AMPK, causes a conformation change that is much more preferable by the upstream kinases. Thus, it increases phosphorylated AMPK without altering the total AMPK level in both acute and chronic metformin treatment [181]. In the indirect pathway, metformin alters AMP/ADP-to-ATP ratio either by blocking AMP-deaminase [182] or by inhibiting complex 1 of the mitochondrial respiratory chain [183]. Upon inhibition, mitochondria cannot produce ATP from AMP/ADP, therefore, activates AMPK.

In addition to these, metformin can improve endothelial function, protect from oxidative stress, inflammation, and the harmful effects of angiotensin II at the tissue level. Some of these activities are mediated by reducing ROS production, deterring protein kinase C-NAD(P)H oxidase signaling, promoting anti-inflammatory macrophage differentiation, inducing antioxidant gene expressions as well as eNOS activity. On the cardiac tissue, metformin attenuates ischemia-reperfusion mediated cardiac tissue damage as well as detrimental cardiac remodeling induced by humoral and hemodynamic factors. All these ideas support the hypothesis that metformin may reduce the risk of cardiovascular events, at least with respect to sulphonylureas [181].

Sulfonylureas: Sulfonylureas is considered as one of the most used anti-diabetic agents because of its low cost, mono-dosing, and the possibility of mixing with metformin in the same tablet. However, due to their tendency to create hypoglycemia and induce cardiovascular risks, first-generation sulfonylureas are now replaced with newer prolonged-release forms of sulfonylureas. Because of their slow-release, these preparations are much safer and preferable to maintain blood glucose levels [184].

When pancreatic β-cells are present, sulfonylureas can raise the plasma insulin concentrations *via* direct and indirect mechanisms. It stimulates pancreatic β-cells for insulin secretion and simultaneously causes a decrease in insulin metabolism and clearance by the liver cells [185]. When it binds to specific receptors on β-pancreatic cells, sulfonylurea blocks the ATP-dependent potassium (K^+) channel and depolarizes the cell. This opens the Ca^{2+} channel and causes a flow of calcium to enter into β-cells. Intracellular Ca^{2+} then initiates contraction of the actomyosin filaments for the exocytosis of insulin-containing vesicles to secrete insulin in large amounts. Although to a lesser extent, the main side effect of sulfonylurea is weight gain. Luckily, metformin can balance the tendency of weight gain initiated by sulfonylurea [185] when taken together.

Moreover, sulfonylureas affect cardiac function *via* their receptor on cardiomyocytes and vascular smooth muscle. This is maybe the reason why patients using sulfonylurea show poorer outcomes after myocardial infarction [186]. During MI, sulfonylureas may inhibit ATP-dependent K+ channels present on cardiomyocytes and coronary vessels, thus impairing adequate coronary vasodilatation, resulting in massive cardiac damage [187]. It can also damage cardiac tissue by interfering with ischemic preconditioning, arrhythmogenesis, and reverse cholesterol transport [188].

Dipeptidyl Peptidase-4 (DPP-4) Inhibitors: Dipeptidyl peptidase-4 is an enzyme expressed in most cells and tissues and can degrade two gut-derived incretin hormones GLP-1 (Glucagon-like peptide-1), and GIP (glucose-dependent insulinotropic polypeptide) [189]. Upon binding to pancreatic β-cell receptors, these two hormones stimulate insulin release, increase glucose sensitivity, and promote β-cell health. At the same time, these hormones inhibit glucagon secretion and gastric emptying [190]. DPP- 4 is widely expressed in most cells and tissues. It exhibits enzymatic activity against dozens of peptide hormones and chemokines with roles in vascular pathophysiology, inflammation, stem cell homing, and cell survival [191 - 193]. Chemical compounds that can inhibit DPP-4 are known as DPP-4 inhibitors. Upon inhibiting the enzyme, these inhibitors lower blood glucose levels by lengthening the above mentioned hormones' activities. Although they have shown modest HbA1C reductions, because of their other effects, such as less weight gain, easy intake (usually one tablet a day, without titration), and safety profiles, DPP-4 inhibitors gradually occupy the place in the management of T2DM by replacing sulfonylureas [194 - 196]. Reports showed that these inhibitors ameliorate different CV risk factors in addition to hypoglycemia and weight gains, such as improve blood pressure (without an increase in heart rate), post-prandial lipemia, and endothelial function, at the same time reduce inflammation and oxidative stress in T2DM patients [191, 193, 197, 198]. Moreover, they are not associated with fluid retention or lipid disturbances responsible for HF. Molecular studies found that DPP-4 can inhibit the degradation of SDF-1α (stromal cell-derived factor-1α). Thus, enhance homing of endothelial progenitor cells and thereby exert vascular protection [199]. Luckily, few of the recent variants of DPP- 4 even do not require dose adjustments because of their biliary excretion rather than renal excretion. This makes it even useable in patients with moderate to severe chronic kidney disease (CKD) [200]. Unfortunately, none of the DPP-4 inhibitors showed any sorts of adverse or beneficial CVD events or all-cause mortality in large CVD outcome trials [201 - 203]. In contrast, few of its group member drugs even showed increased hospitalizations for HF patients [204].

Sodium-glucose-linked Transporter 2 (SGLT-2) Inhibitors: SGLT-2 inhibitors can lower the blood glucose level by enhancing glucosuria without taking help from insulin [205]. This ultimately inhibits the development of hypoglycemia and helps to lose body weight. β-cells, therefore, get relief from the excess amount of glucose, which helps to improve their function and insulin sensitivity [205, 206]. All these properties make SGLT-2 inhibitors useful in all stages of T2DM patients having any sort of kidney disease [207, 208]. SGLT-2 inhibitors can also favorably influence CV prognosis [205, 207]. In addition to weight reduction, they are responsible for dropping arterial blood pressure by natriuresis and a diuretic effect [209, 210]. At the same time, it enhances urinary excretion of uric acid to reduce serum uric acid levels [211]. Furthermore, SGLT-2 increases erythropoiesis which may also exert positive CV effects [212]. However, it has minimal impact on serum lipid profile and electrolyte levels, especially on magnesium, potassium, and phosphate levels with unknown CV protection roles [213, 214]. In addition to these, reports showed that SGLT-2 could reduce inflammation and oxidative stress, decrease albuminuria in diabetic nephropathy, and diminish fatty liver disease [215]. It is now believed that positive CV roles of SGLT-2 are mostly implemented by the improvement in renal outcomes and functions by direct and indirect effects of SGLT-2 on the renal system [216]. When compared, it was found that SGLT-2 inhibitors have superiority compared to DPP-4 inhibitors *versus* placebo. Therefore, SGLT-2 inhibitors are preferred by the cardiologist, at least, to the T2DM patients with high CV risk [217].

Glucagon-like Peptide 1 (GLP-1) Analogs: Like GLP-1, several of its chemical analogs can bind and activate the endogenous GLP-1 receptor to exert their hypoglycemic effect. GLP-1 analogs can promote glucose-dependent insulin release, inhibit glucagon secretion, and delay gastric emptying to maintain proper blood glucose levels. Moreover, they show a low hypoglycemic risk, even when basal insulin is present [218]. GLP-1 analogs modulate pancreatic β-cells in such a way so that a sustained reduction in HbA1C level can be achieved. Interestingly, GLP-1 mediated delayed gastric emptying can suppress appetite. Thus, these analogs can cause weight loss compared to basal insulin rather than weight gain [219]. Additionally, this class of drugs can control BP [220], improve systolic function, exercise capacity, and healthy living standards in diabetic and non-diabetic patients [221].

LESSONS LEARNED AND FUTURE DIRECTIONS

As the global drug market is rapidly evolving, it is urgent to continue the CVD safety trials to identify and keep potentially harmful hypoglycemic agents away from the market. This will not only provide a new set to the clinicians about the potential anti-diabetic drugs with CVD benefit but also helps to prevent secondary CVD development. Considering the individual differences, recent guidelines accentuate on personalization of glycemic goals. Therefore, both higher (>6.5%) or lower (<8%) level of HbA1c is acceptable considering the patient features and medical record [166]. However, clinicians have suggested an HbA1c of <7% for most patients with T2DM to diminish the probability of microvascular disease incidents [222]. Moreover, depending on better primary prevention of macrovascular disease of T2DM patients, metformin is accepted as the initial treatment for glycemic control [223]. The latest trials have also suggested other pharmacological approaches to diminish the vascular risk for diabetes patients.

Few drugs show superior performance in patients with either diabetes and pre-existing CVD or multiple CVD risk factors by improving both CVD-associated mortality and all-cause mortality, for example, SGLT2 inhibitor (empagliflozin) or GLP-1 analog (liraglutide) [224, 225]. Moreover, recent findings show that SGLT2 inhibitors reduce HF hospitalizations. However, a detailed assessment aiming at an extensive comparison of DM medications rather than merely establishing efficacy against placebo is a must to identify potential new medications with proven CVD benefits to validate whether these agents are superior or additive to the CVD risk reduction described with the use of metformin.

CONCLUSION

This review presents an overview of the critical genetic and epigenetic factors linking DM and CVD, with particular importance on the pathophysiological mechanisms involved. We focused on accepted genetic variants shared by both situations and the most significant epigenetic mechanisms involved in their interplay. A greater understanding of gene networks, intracellular pathways, and cell-to-cell communication mechanisms will permit the identification of unique biomarkers and innovative therapeutic targets to practice in the management of CVD in patients with DM.

CONSENT FOR PUBLICATION

Not applicable.

CONFLICT OF INTEREST

The author declares no conflict of interest, financial or otherwise.

ACKNOWLEDGEMENTS

The authors are grateful to the Department of Biochemistry and Molecular Biology, the University of Dhaka, to support the review.

REFERENCES

[1]   Stumvoll M, Goldstein BJ, van Haeften TW. Type 2 diabetes: principles of pathogenesis and therapy. Lancet 2005; 365(9467): 1333-46.
        [http://dx.doi.org/10.1016/S0140-6736(05)61032-X] [PMID: 15823385]

[2]   Hossain P, Kawar B, El Nahas M. Obesity and diabetes in the developing world--a growing challenge. N Engl J Med 2007; 356(3): 213-5.
        [http://dx.doi.org/10.1056/NEJMp068177] [PMID: 17229948]

[3]   Twomey PJ, Viljoen A, Reynolds TM, Wierzbicki AS. http://care.diabetesjournals.org/content/27/10/2569.12004. abstract

[4]   Guariguata L, Whiting DR, Hambleton I, Beagley J, Linnenkamp U, Shaw JE. Global estimates of diabetes prevalence for 2013 and projections for 2035. Diabetes Res Clin Pract 2014; 103(2): 137-49.
        [http://dx.doi.org/10.1016/j.diabres.2013.11.002] [PMID: 24630390]

[5]   Krolewski AS, Warram JH, Freire MBS. Epidemiology of late diabetic complications. A basis for the development and evaluation of preventive programs. Endocrinol Metab Clin North Am 1996; 25(2): 217-42.http://www.sciencedirect.com/science/article/pii/S0889852905703224
        [http://dx.doi.org/10.1016/S0889-8529(05)70322-4] [PMID: 8799698]

[6]   Benjamin EJ, Muntner P, Alonso A, *et al.* Heart Disease and Stroke Statistics-2019 Update: A Report From the American Heart Association. Circulation 2019; 139(10): e56-e528.
        [http://dx.doi.org/10.1161/CIR.0000000000000659] [PMID: 30700139]

[7]   Kim JA, Koh KK, Quon MJ. The union of vascular and metabolic actions of insulin in sickness and in health. Arterioscler Thromb Vasc Biol 2005; 25(5): 889-91.
        [http://dx.doi.org/10.1161/01.ATV.0000164044.42910.6b] [PMID: 15863720]

[8]   Grundy SM, Benjamin IJ, Burke GL, *et al.* Diabetes and cardiovascular disease: a statement for healthcare professionals from the American Heart Association. Circulation 1999; 100(10): 1134-46.
        [http://dx.doi.org/10.1161/01.CIR.100.10.1134] [PMID: 10477542]

[9]   Brunetti A, Indolfi C. Type 2 Diabetes Mellitus and Cardiovascular Disease : Genetic and epigenetic. Links 2018; 9(January): 1-13.

[10]   Mozaffarian D, Benjamin EJ, Go AS, *et al.* Heart disease and stroke statistics--2015 update: a report from the American Heart Association. Circulation 2015; 131(4): e29-e322.
        [http://dx.doi.org/10.1161/CIR.0000000000000152] [PMID: 25520374]

[11]   Prevalence of self-reported cardiovascular disease among persons aged > or =35 years with diabetes--United States, 1997-2005. MMWR Morb Mortal Wkly Rep 2007; 56(43): 1129-32.
        [PMID: 17975525]

[12]   Huxley RR, Filion KB, Konety S, Alonso A. Meta-analysis of cohort and case-control studies of type 2 diabetes mellitus and risk of atrial fibrillation. Am J Cardiol 2011; 108(1): 56-62.
        [http://dx.doi.org/10.1016/j.amjcard.2011.03.004] [PMID: 21529739]

[13]   Rao Kondapally Seshasai S, Kaptoge S, Thompson A, *et al.* Diabetes mellitus, fasting glucose, and risk of cause-specific death. N Engl J Med 2011; 364(9): 829-41.

[http://dx.doi.org/10.1056/NEJMoa1008862] [PMID: 21366474]

[14] Regensteiner JG, Golden S, Huebschmann AG, *et al.* Sex differences in the cardiovascular consequences of diabetes mellitus: a scientific statement from the american heart association. Circulation 2015; 132(25): 2424-47.
[http://dx.doi.org/10.1161/CIR.0000000000000343] [PMID: 26644329]

[15] Peters SAE, Huxley RR, Woodward M. Diabetes as risk factor for incident coronary heart disease in women compared with men: a systematic review and meta-analysis of 64 cohorts including 858,507 individuals and 28,203 coronary events. Diabetologia 2014; 57(8): 1542-51.
[http://dx.doi.org/10.1007/s00125-014-3260-6] [PMID: 24859435]

[16] Peters SAE, Huxley RR, Woodward M. Diabetes as a risk factor for stroke in women compared with men: a systematic review and meta-analysis of 64 cohorts, including 775,385 individuals and 12,539 strokes. Lancet 2014; 383(9933): 1973-80.
[http://dx.doi.org/10.1016/S0140-6736(14)60040-4] [PMID: 24613026]

[17] Bai J, Ding X, Du X, Zhao X, Wang Z, Ma Z. Diabetes is associated with increased risk of venous thromboembolism: a systematic review and meta-analysis. Thromb Res 2015; 135(1): 90-5.
[http://dx.doi.org/10.1016/j.thromres.2014.11.003] [PMID: 25434631]

[18] Zaccardi F, Khan H, Laukkanen JA. Diabetes mellitus and risk of sudden cardiac death: a systematic review and meta-analysis. Int J Cardiol 2014; 177(2): 535-7.
[http://dx.doi.org/10.1016/j.ijcard.2014.08.105] [PMID: 25189500]

[19] Levelt E, Pavlides M, Banerjee R, *et al.* Ectopic and Visceral Fat Deposition in Lean and Obese Patients With Type 2 Diabetes. J Am Coll Cardiol 2016; 68(1): 53-63.
[http://dx.doi.org/10.1016/j.jacc.2016.03.597] [PMID: 27364051]

[20] Levelt E, Mahmod M, Piechnik SK, Ariga R, Francis JM, Rodgers CT, *et al.* Ectopic and visceral fat deposition in lean and obese patients with type 2 diabetes. J Am Coll Cardiol 2016.

[21] Falcão-Pires I, Hamdani N, Borbély A, *et al.* Diabetes mellitus worsens diastolic left ventricular dysfunction in aortic stenosis through altered myocardial structure and cardiomyocyte stiffness. Circulation 2011; 124(10): 1151-9.
[http://dx.doi.org/10.1161/CIRCULATIONAHA.111.025270] [PMID: 21844073]

[22] Wong TC, Piehler KM, Kang IA, *et al.* Myocardial extracellular volume fraction quantified by cardiovascular magnetic resonance is increased in diabetes and associated with mortality and incident heart failure admission. Eur Heart J 2014; 35(10): 657-64.
[http://dx.doi.org/10.1093/eurheartj/eht193] [PMID: 23756336]

[23] Shimizu I, Minamino T, Toko H, *et al.* Excessive cardiac insulin signaling exacerbates systolic dysfunction induced by pressure overload in rodents. J Clin Invest 2010; 120(5): 1506-14.
[http://dx.doi.org/10.1172/JCI40096] [PMID: 20407209]

[24] Levelt E, Rodgers CT, Clarke WT, *et al.* Cardiac energetics, oxygenation, and perfusion during increased workload in patients with type 2 diabetes mellitus. Eur Heart J 2016; 37(46): 3461-9.
[http://dx.doi.org/10.1093/eurheartj/ehv442] [PMID: 26392437]

[25] Basta G, Schmidt AM, De Caterina R. Advanced glycation end products and vascular inflammation: implications for accelerated atherosclerosis in diabetes. Cardiovasc Res 2004; 63(4): 582-92.
[http://dx.doi.org/10.1016/j.cardiores.2004.05.001] [PMID: 15306213]

[26] Sowers JR, Epstein M, Frohlich ED. Diabetes, hypertension, and cardiovascular disease: an update. Hypertens (Dallas, Tex 1979) [Internet] 2001; 37(4): 1053-9.
[http://dx.doi.org/10.1161/01.HYP.37.4.1053]

[27] Ramasamy R, Schmidt AM. Receptor for advanced glycation end products (RAGE) and implications for the pathophysiology of heart failure. Curr Heart Fail Rep 2012; 9(2): 107-16.
[http://dx.doi.org/10.1007/s11897-012-0089-5] [PMID: 22457230]

[28] Bonapace S, Valbusa F, Bertolini L, *et al.* Early impairment in left ventricular longitudinal systolic

function is associated with an increased risk of incident atrial fibrillation in patients with type 2 diabetes. J Diabetes Complications 2017; 31(2): 413-8.
[http://dx.doi.org/10.1016/j.jdiacomp.2016.10.032] [PMID: 27884663]

[29] Rijzewijk LJ, Jonker JT, van der Meer RW, *et al*. Effects of hepatic triglyceride content on myocardial metabolism in type 2 diabetes. J Am Coll Cardiol 2010; 56(3): 225-33.
[http://dx.doi.org/10.1016/j.jacc.2010.02.049] [PMID: 20620743]

[30] Ertunc ME, Hotamisligil GS. Lipid signaling and lipotoxicity in metaflammation: indications for metabolic disease pathogenesis and treatment. J Lipid Res 2016; 57(12): 2099-114.
[http://dx.doi.org/10.1194/jlr.R066514] [PMID: 27330055]

[31] Lowell BB, Shulman GI. Mitochondrial Dysfunction and Type 2 Diabetes. Science (80-) 2005; 307(5708): 384-7.

[32] Glass CK, Olefsky JM. Inflammation and lipid signaling in the etiology of insulin resistance. Cell Metab 2012; 15(5): 635-45.
[http://dx.doi.org/10.1016/j.cmet.2012.04.001] [PMID: 22560216]

[33] Fink BD, Bai F, Yu L, Sivitz WI. Impaired utilization of membrane potential by complex II-energized mitochondria of obese, diabetic mice assessed using ADP recycling methodology. Am J Physiol Regul Integr Comp Physiol 2016; 311(4): R756-63.
[http://dx.doi.org/10.1152/ajpregu.00232.2016] [PMID: 27558314]

[34] Lehrke M, Marx N. Diabetes Mellitus and Heart Failure. Am J Med 2017; 130(6S): S40-50.
[http://dx.doi.org/10.1016/j.amjmed.2017.04.010] [PMID: 28526183]

[35] El-Osta A, Brasacchio D, Yao D, *et al*. Transient high glucose causes persistent epigenetic changes and altered gene expression during subsequent normoglycemia. J Exp Med 2008; 205(10): 2409-17.http://www.ncbi.nlm.nih.gov/pubmed/18809715
[http://dx.doi.org/10.1084/jem.20081188] [PMID: 18809715]

[36] Giacco F, Brownlee M, Marie SA. Oxidative stress and diabetic complications. Circ Res 2010; 107(9): 1058-70.
[http://dx.doi.org/10.1161/CIRCRESAHA.110.223545] [PMID: 21030723]

[37] Sverdlov AL, Elezaby A, Qin F, *et al*. Mitochondrial Reactive Oxygen Species Mediate Cardiac Structural, Functional, and Mitochondrial Consequences of Diet-Induced Metabolic Heart Disease. J Am Heart Assoc 2016; 5(1): e002555.
[http://dx.doi.org/10.1161/JAHA.115.002555] [PMID: 26755553]

[38] Neubauer S. The failing heart--an engine out of fuel. N Engl J Med 2007; 356(11): 1140-51.
[http://dx.doi.org/10.1056/NEJMra063052] [PMID: 17360992]

[39] Chokshi A, Drosatos K, Cheema FH, *et al*. Ventricular assist device implantation corrects myocardial lipotoxicity, reverses insulin resistance, and normalizes cardiac metabolism in patients with advanced heart failure. Circulation 2012; 125(23): 2844-53.
[http://dx.doi.org/10.1161/CIRCULATIONAHA.111.060889] [PMID: 22586279]

[40] Doehner W, Frenneaux M, Anker SD. Metabolic impairment in heart failure: the myocardial and systemic perspective. J Am Coll Cardiol 2014; 64(13): 1388-400.
[http://dx.doi.org/10.1016/j.jacc.2014.04.083] [PMID: 25257642]

[41] Doehner W, Rauchhaus M, Ponikowski P, *et al*. Impaired insulin sensitivity as an independent risk factor for mortality in patients with stable chronic heart failure. J Am Coll Cardiol 2005; 46(6): 1019-26.
[http://dx.doi.org/10.1016/j.jacc.2005.02.093] [PMID: 16168285]

[42] Bedi KC Jr, Snyder NW, Brandimarto J, *et al*. Evidence for Intramyocardial Disruption of Lipid Metabolism and Increased Myocardial Ketone Utilization in Advanced Human Heart Failure. Circulation 2016; 133(8): 706-16.
[http://dx.doi.org/10.1161/CIRCULATIONAHA.115.017545] [PMID: 26819374]

[43] Aubert G, Martin OJ, Horton JL, *et al.* The Failing Heart Relies on Ketone Bodies as a Fuel. Circulation 2016; 133(8): 698-705.
[http://dx.doi.org/10.1161/CIRCULATIONAHA.115.017355] [PMID: 26819376]

[44] Müller MJ, Lagerpusch M, Enderle J, Schautz B, Heller M, Bosy-Westphal A. Beyond the body mass index: tracking body composition in the pathogenesis of obesity and the metabolic syndrome. Obes Rev 2012; 13 (Suppl. 2): 6-13.
[http://dx.doi.org/10.1111/j.1467-789X.2012.01033.x] [PMID: 23107255]

[45] Dagenais GR, Auger P, Bogaty P, *et al.* Increased occurrence of diabetes in people with ischemic cardiovascular disease and general and abdominal obesity. Can J Cardiol 2003; 19(12): 1387-91.
[PMID: 14631473]

[46] Menke A, Casagrande S, Geiss L, Cowie CC. Prevalence of and Trends in Diabetes Among Adults in the United States, 1988-2012. JAMA 2015; 314(10): 1021-9. http://www.ncbi.nlm.nih.gov/pubmed/26348752
[http://dx.doi.org/10.1001/jama.2015.10029] [PMID: 26348752]

[47] Prevalence of overweight and obesity among adults with diagnosed diabetes--United States, 1988-1994 and 1999-2002. MMWR Morb Mortal Wkly Rep 2004; 53(45): 1066-8. http://www.ncbi.nlm.nih.gov/pubmed/15549021
[PMID: 15549021]

[48] Tuomilehto J, Lindström J, Eriksson JG, *et al.* Prevention of type 2 diabetes mellitus by changes in lifestyle among subjects with impaired glucose tolerance. N Engl J Med 2001; 344(18): 1343-50.
[http://dx.doi.org/10.1056/NEJM200105033441801] [PMID: 11333990]

[49] Diabetes Prevention Program Research Group; Knowler WC, Fowler SE, Hamman RF, Christophi CA, Hoffman HJ, *et al.* 10-year follow-up of diabetes incidence and weight loss in the Diabetes Prevention Program Outcomes Study. Lancet 2009; 374(9702): 1677-86. http://www.ncbi.nlm.nih.gov/pubmed/19878986

[50] Duncan BB, Schmidt MI, Pankow JS, *et al.* Atherosclerosis Risk in Communities Study. Low-grade systemic inflammation and the development of type 2 diabetes: the atherosclerosis risk in communities study. Diabetes 2003; 52(7): 1799-805.
[http://dx.doi.org/10.2337/diabetes.52.7.1799] [PMID: 12829649]

[51] Shoelson SE, Lee J, Goldfine AB. Inflammation and insulin resistance. J Clin Invest 2006; 116(7): 1793-801.
[http://dx.doi.org/10.1172/JCI29069] [PMID: 16823477]

[52] Vicenová B, Vopálenský V, Buryšek L, Pospíšek M. Emerging role of interleukin-1 in cardiovascular diseases. Physiol Res 2009; 58(4): 481-98.
[http://dx.doi.org/10.33549/physiolres.931673] [PMID: 19093736]

[53] Wellen KE, Hotamisligil GS. Inflammation, stress, and diabetes. J Clin Invest 2005; 115(5): 1111-9.
[http://dx.doi.org/10.1172/JCI25102] [PMID: 15864338]

[54] DeFronzo RA. Pathogenesis of type 2 diabetes mellitus. Med Clin North Am 2004; 88(4): 787-835, ix.
[http://dx.doi.org/10.1016/j.mcna.2004.04.013] [PMID: 15308380]

[55] Poornima IG, Parikh P, Shannon RP. Diabetic cardiomyopathy: the search for a unifying hypothesis. Circ Res 2006; 98(5): 596-605.
[http://dx.doi.org/10.1161/01.RES.0000207406.94146.c2] [PMID: 16543510]

[56] Ceriello A, Ihnat MA, Thorpe JE. Clinical review 2: The "metabolic memory": is more than just tight glucose control necessary to prevent diabetic complications? J Clin Endocrinol Metab 2009; 94(2): 410-5.
[http://dx.doi.org/10.1210/jc.2008-1824] [PMID: 19066300]

[57] Watts GF, Playford DA. Dyslipoproteinaemia and hyperoxidative stress in the pathogenesis of endothelial dysfunction in non-insulin dependent diabetes mellitus: an hypothesis. Atherosclerosis

1998; 141(1): 17-30.
[http://dx.doi.org/10.1016/S0021-9150(98)00170-1] [PMID: 9863535]

[58]   Matheus AS de M, Cobas RA, Gomes MB RA, Gomes MB. Dislipidemias no diabetes melito tipo 1: abordagem atual. Arquivos Brasileiros de Endocrinologia & Metabologia scielo 2008; 52: 334-9.

[59]   Renard CB, Kramer F, Johansson F, *et al.* Diabetes and diabetes-associated lipid abnormalities have distinct effects on initiation and progression of atherosclerotic lesions. J Clin Invest 2004; 114(5): 659-68.
[http://dx.doi.org/10.1172/JCI200417867] [PMID: 15343384]

[60]   Colhoun HM, Betteridge DJ, Durrington PN, *et al.* Primary prevention of cardiovascular disease with atorvastatin in type 2 diabetes in the Collaborative Atorvastatin Diabetes Study (CARDS): multicentre randomised placebo-controlled trial. Lancet 2004; 364(9435): 685-96.
[http://dx.doi.org/10.1016/S0140-6736(04)16895-5] [PMID: 15325833]

[61]   Saldanha A, Matheus DM, Righeti L, Tannus M, Cobas RA, Palma CCS, *et al.* Effect of diuretic-based antihypertensive treatment on cardiovascular disease risk in older diabetic patients with isolated systolic hypertension. Systolic Hypertension in the Elderly Program Cooperative Research Group 1996; 276(23): 1886-92.
[PMID: 8968014]

[62]   Curb JD, Pressel SL, Cutler JA, *et al.* Effect of diuretic-based antihypertensive treatment on cardiovascular disease risk in older diabetic patients with isolated systolic hypertension. JAMA 1996; 276(23): 1886-92.
[http://dx.doi.org/10.1001/jama.1996.03540230036032] [PMID: 8968014]

[63]   Mogensen CE, Hansen KW, Pedersen MM, Christensen CK. Renal factors influencing blood pressure threshold and choice of treatment for hypertension in IDDM. Diabetes Care 1991; 14 (Suppl. 4): 13-26.
[http://dx.doi.org/10.2337/diacare.14.4.13] [PMID: 1748053]

[64]   Hypertension in Diabetes Study (HDS). Hypertension in Diabetes Study (HDS): I. Prevalence of hypertension in newly presenting type 2 diabetic patients and the association with risk factors for cardiovascular and diabetic complications. J Hypertens 1993; 11(3): 309-17.
[http://dx.doi.org/10.1097/00004872-199303000-00012] [PMID: 8387089]

[65]   UK Prospective Diabetes Study Group. Tight blood pressure control and risk of macrovascular and microvascular complications in type 2 diabetes: UKPDS 38. BMJ 1998; 317(7160): 703-13.
[http://dx.doi.org/10.1136/bmj.317.7160.703] [PMID: 9732337]

[66]   The sixth report of the Joint National Committee on prevention, detection, evaluation, and treatment of high blood pressure. Arch Intern Med 1997; 157(21): 2413-46.
[http://dx.doi.org/10.1001/archinte.1997.00440420033005] [PMID: 9385294]

[67]   Stamler J, Vaccaro O, Neaton JD, Wentworth D. Diabetes, Other Risk Factors, and 12-Yr Cardiovascular Mortality for Men Screened in the Multiple Risk Factor Intervention Trial. Diabetes Care 1993; 16(2): 434.

[68]   Haffner SM, Lehto S, Rönnemaa T, Pyörälä K, Laakso M. Mortality from coronary heart disease in subjects with type 2 diabetes and in nondiabetic subjects with and without prior myocardial infarction. N Engl J Med 1998; 339(4): 229-34.
[http://dx.doi.org/10.1056/NEJM199807233390404] [PMID: 9673301]

[69]   Emerging Risk Factors Collaboration; Sarwar N, Gao P, Seshasai SRK, Gobin R, Kaptoge S, *et al.* Diabetes mellitus, fasting blood glucose concentration, and risk of vascular disease: a collaborative meta-analysis of 102 prospective studies. Lancet (London, England). 2010; 375(9733): 2215–22.
[PMID: 20609967]

[70]   Hsueh WA, Law R. The central role of fat and effect of peroxisome proliferator-activated receptor-gamma on progression of insulin resistance and cardiovascular disease. Am J Cardiol 2003; 92(4A): 3J-9J.

[http://dx.doi.org/10.1016/S0002-9149(03)00610-6] [PMID: 12957321]

[71]   Bornfeldt KE, Tabas I. Insulin resistance, hyperglycemia, and atherosclerosis. Cell Metab 2011; 14(5): 575-85.
[http://dx.doi.org/10.1016/j.cmet.2011.07.015] [PMID: 22055501]

[72]   Carr ME. Diabetes mellitus: a hypercoagulable state. J Diabetes Complications 2001; 15(1): 44-54.
[http://dx.doi.org/10.1016/S1056-8727(00)00132-X] [PMID: 11259926]

[73]   Grundy SM. Pre-diabetes, metabolic syndrome, and cardiovascular risk. J Am Coll Cardiol 2012; 59(7): 635-43.
[http://dx.doi.org/10.1016/j.jacc.2011.08.080] [PMID: 22322078]

[74]   Libby P, Ridker PM, Hansson GK. Progress and challenges in translating the biology of atherosclerosis. Nature 2011; 473(7347): 317-25.
[http://dx.doi.org/10.1038/nature10146] [PMID: 21593864]

[75]   Jeong-a K, Monica M, Kon KK, Reciprocal Relationships Between Insulin Resistance J QM. Circulation 2006; 113(15): 1888-904.
[http://dx.doi.org/10.1161/CIRCULATIONAHA.105.563213] [PMID: 16618833]

[76]   Cubbon RM, Rajwani A, Wheatcroft SB. The impact of insulin resistance on endothelial function, progenitor cells and repair. Diab Vasc Dis Res 2007; 4(2): 103-11.
[http://dx.doi.org/10.3132/dvdr.2007.027] [PMID: 17654443]

[77]   Berneis KK, Krauss RM. Metabolic origins and clinical significance of LDL heterogeneity. J Lipid Res 2002; 43(9): 1363-79.
[http://dx.doi.org/10.1194/jlr.R200004-JLR200] [PMID: 12235168]

[78]   Greco M, Chiefari E, Montalcini T, Accattato F, Costanzo FS, Pujia A, *et al.* 2014.
[http://dx.doi.org/10.1155/2014/750860]

[79]   Stern MP. Diabetes and cardiovascular disease. The "common soil" hypothesis. Diabetes 1995; 44(4): 369-74.
[http://dx.doi.org/10.2337/diab.44.4.369] [PMID: 7698502]

[80]   Chiefari E, Tanyolaç S, Paonessa F, *et al.* Functional variants of the HMGA1 gene and type 2 diabetes mellitus. JAMA 2011; 305(9): 903-12.
[http://dx.doi.org/10.1001/jama.2011.207] [PMID: 21364139]

[81]   Wang X, Strizich G, Hu Y, Wang T, Kaplan RC, Qi Q. Genetic markers of type 2 diabetes: Progress in genome-wide association studies and clinical application for risk prediction. J Diabetes 2016; 8(1): 24-35.
[http://dx.doi.org/10.1111/1753-0407.12323] [PMID: 26119161]

[82]   Ashar FN, Arking DE. Genomics of complex cardiovascular disease. Genomic Med Princ Pract 2014; p. 316.

[83]   Bacci S, Menzaghi C, Ercolino T, *et al.* The +276 G/T single nucleotide polymorphism of the adiponectin gene is associated with coronary artery disease in type 2 diabetic patients. Diabetes Care 2004; 27(8): 2015-20.
[http://dx.doi.org/10.2337/diacare.27.8.2015] [PMID: 15277433]

[84]   Classification and Diagnosis of Diabetes: *Standards of Medical Care in Diabetes-2020.* Diabetes Care 2020; 43 (Suppl. 1): S14-31.
[http://dx.doi.org/10.2337/dc20-S002] [PMID: 31862745]

[85]   O'Donnell CJ, Nabel EG. Genomics of cardiovascular disease. N Engl J Med 2011; 365(22): 2098-109.
[http://dx.doi.org/10.1056/NEJMra1105239] [PMID: 22129254]

[86]   Besseling J, Kastelein JJP, Defesche JC, Hutten BA, Hovingh GK. Association between familial hypercholesterolemia and prevalence of type 2 diabetes mellitus. JAMA 2015; 313(10): 1029-36.

[http://dx.doi.org/10.1001/jama.2015.1206] [PMID: 25756439]

[87]   Kathiresan S, Srivastava D. Genetics of human cardiovascular disease. Cell 2012; 148(6): 1242-57.
       [http://dx.doi.org/10.1016/j.cell.2012.03.001] [PMID: 22424232]

[88]   Pfohl M, Koch M, Enderle MD, *et al.* Paraoxonase 192 Gln/Arg gene polymorphism, coronary artery
       disease, and myocardial infarction in type 2 diabetes. Diabetes 1999; 48(3): 623-7.
       [http://dx.doi.org/10.2337/diabetes.48.3.623] [PMID: 10078566]

[89]   Jones DA, Prior SL, Tang TS, *et al.* Association between the rs4880 superoxide dismutase 2 (C>T)
       gene variant and coronary heart disease in diabetes mellitus. Diabetes Res Clin Pract 2010; 90(2): 196-
       201.
       [http://dx.doi.org/10.1016/j.diabres.2010.07.009] [PMID: 20728955]

[90]   Schulze MB, Shai I, Rimm EB, Li T, Rifai N, Hu FB. Adiponectin and future coronary heart disease
       events among men with type 2 diabetes. Diabetes 2005; 54(2): 534-9.
       [http://dx.doi.org/10.2337/diabetes.54.2.534] [PMID: 15677512]

[91]   Soccio T, Zhang Y-Y, Bacci S, *et al.* Common haplotypes at the adiponectin receptor 1 (ADIPOR1)
       locus are associated with increased risk of coronary artery disease in type 2 diabetes. Diabetes 2006;
       55(10): 2763-70.
       [http://dx.doi.org/10.2337/db06-0613] [PMID: 17003341]

[92]   Sousa AG, Selvatici L, Krieger JE, Pereira AC. Association between genetics of diabetes, coronary
       artery disease, and macrovascular complications: exploring a common ground hypothesis. Rev Diabet
       Stud 2011; 8(2): 230-44.
       [http://dx.doi.org/10.1900/RDS.2011.8.230] [PMID: 22189546]

[93]   Qi L, Parast L, Cai T, *et al.* Genetic susceptibility to coronary heart disease in type 2 diabetes: 3
       independent studies. J Am Coll Cardiol 2011; 58(25): 2675-82.
       [http://dx.doi.org/10.1016/j.jacc.2011.08.054] [PMID: 22152955]

[94]   Grant SFA, Thorleifsson G, Reynisdottir I, *et al.* Variant of transcription factor 7-like 2 (TCF7L2)
       gene confers risk of type 2 diabetes. Nat Genet 2006; 38(3): 320-3.
       [http://dx.doi.org/10.1038/ng1732] [PMID: 16415884]

[95]   Bielinski SJ, Pankow JS, Folsom AR, North KE, Boerwinkle E. TCF7L2 single nucleotide
       polymorphisms, cardiovascular disease and all-cause mortality: the Atherosclerosis Risk in
       Communities (ARIC) study. Diabetologia 2008; 51(6): 968-70.
       [http://dx.doi.org/10.1007/s00125-008-1004-1] [PMID: 18437354]

[96]   Ukkola O, Kervinen K, Salmela PI, von Dickhoff K, Laakso M, Kesäniemi YA. Apolipoprotein E
       phenotype is related to macro- and microangiopathy in patients with non-insulin-dependent diabetes
       mellitus. Atherosclerosis 1993; 101(1): 9-15.
       [http://dx.doi.org/10.1016/0021-9150(93)90096-D] [PMID: 8216506]

[97]   El-Lebedy D, Raslan HM, Mohammed AM. Apolipoprotein E gene polymorphism and risk of type 2
       diabetes and cardiovascular disease. Cardiovasc Diabetol 2016; 15(1): 12.
       [http://dx.doi.org/10.1186/s12933-016-0329-1] [PMID: 26800892]

[98]   Qi L, Qi Q, Prudente S, *et al.* Association between a genetic variant related to glutamic acid
       metabolism and coronary heart disease in individuals with type 2 diabetes. JAMA 2013; 310(8): 821-
       8.
       [http://dx.doi.org/10.1001/jama.2013.276305] [PMID: 23982368]

[99]   Beaney KE, Cooper JA, McLachlan S, *et al.* Variant rs10911021 that associates with coronary heart
       disease in type 2 diabetes, is associated with lower concentrations of circulating HDL cholesterol and
       large HDL particles but not with amino acids. Cardiovasc Diabetol 2016; 15(1): 115.
       [http://dx.doi.org/10.1186/s12933-016-0435-0] [PMID: 27549350]

[100] De Rosa S, Chiefari E, Salerno N, *et al.* HMGA1 is a novel candidate gene for myocardial infarction
       susceptibility. Int J Cardiol 2017; 227: 331-4.

[http://dx.doi.org/10.1016/j.ijcard.2016.11.088] [PMID: 27839822]

[101] Levy AP. Haptoglobin: a major susceptibility gene for diabetic cardiovascular disease. Isr Med Assoc J 2004; 6(5): 308-10.
[PMID: 15151377]

[102] Adams JN, Cox AJ, Freedman BI, Langefeld CD, Carr JJ, Bowden DW. Genetic analysis of haptoglobin polymorphisms with cardiovascular disease and type 2 diabetes in the Diabetes Heart Study. Cardiovasc Diabetol 2013; 12(1): 31.
[http://dx.doi.org/10.1186/1475-2840-12-31] [PMID: 23399657]

[103] Ruiz J, Blanché H, James RW, *et al.* Gln-Arg192 polymorphism of paraoxonase and coronary heart disease in type 2 diabetes. Lancet 1995; 346(8979): 869-72.
[http://dx.doi.org/10.1016/S0140-6736(95)92709-3] [PMID: 7564671]

[104] Muendlein A, Saely CH, Geller-Rhomberg S, *et al.* Single nucleotide polymorphisms of TCF7L2 are linked to diabetic coronary atherosclerosis. PLoS One 2011; 6(3): e17978.
[http://dx.doi.org/10.1371/journal.pone.0017978] [PMID: 21423583]

[105] Vendrell J, Fernandez-Real J-M, Gutierrez C, *et al.* A polymorphism in the promoter of the tumor necrosis factor-α gene (-308) is associated with coronary heart disease in type 2 diabetic patients. Atherosclerosis 2003; 167(2): 257-64.
[http://dx.doi.org/10.1016/S0021-9150(02)00429-X] [PMID: 12818408]

[106] Asleh R, Marsh S, Shilkrut M, *et al.* Genetically determined heterogeneity in hemoglobin scavenging and susceptibility to diabetic cardiovascular disease. Circ Res 2003; 92(11): 1193-200.
[http://dx.doi.org/10.1161/01.RES.0000076889.23082.F1] [PMID: 12750308]

[107] Pirola L, Balcerczyk A, Tothill RW, *et al.* Genome-wide analysis distinguishes hyperglycemia regulated epigenetic signatures of primary vascular cells. Genome Res 2011; 21(10): 1601-15.
[http://dx.doi.org/10.1101/gr.116095.110] [PMID: 21890681]

[108] Sathishkumar C, Prabu P, Balakumar M, *et al.* Augmentation of histone deacetylase 3 (*HDAC3*) epigenetic signature at the interface of proinflammation and insulin resistance in patients with type 2 diabetes. Clin Epigenetics 2016; 8(1): 125.
[http://dx.doi.org/10.1186/s13148-016-0293-3] [PMID: 27904654]

[109] Aslibekyan S, Claas SA, Arnett DK. Clinical applications of epigenetics in cardiovascular disease: the long road ahead. Transl Res 2015; 165(1): 143-53.
[http://dx.doi.org/10.1016/j.trsl.2014.04.004] [PMID: 24768945]

[110] Bell CG, Finer S, Lindgren CM, *et al.* Integrated genetic and epigenetic analysis identifies haplotype-specific methylation in the FTO type 2 diabetes and obesity susceptibility locus. PLoS One 2010; 5(11): e14040.
[http://dx.doi.org/10.1371/journal.pone.0014040] [PMID: 21124985]

[111] Liu C, Mou S, Pan C. The FTO gene rs9939609 polymorphism predicts risk of cardiovascular disease: a systematic review and meta-analysis. PLoS One 2013; 8(8): e71901.
[http://dx.doi.org/10.1371/journal.pone.0071901] [PMID: 23977173]

[112] Deodati A, Inzaghi E, Liguori A, *et al.* IGF2 methylation is associated with lipid profile in obese children. Horm Res Paediatr 2013; 79(6): 361-7.
[http://dx.doi.org/10.1159/000351707] [PMID: 23774180]

[113] Benton MC, Johnstone A, Eccles D, *et al.* An analysis of DNA methylation in human adipose tissue reveals differential modification of obesity genes before and after gastric bypass and weight loss. Genome Biol 2015; 16(1): 8.
[http://dx.doi.org/10.1186/s13059-014-0569-x] [PMID: 25651499]

[114] Talens RP, Jukema JW, Trompet S, *et al.* Hypermethylation at loci sensitive to the prenatal environment is associated with increased incidence of myocardial infarction. Int J Epidemiol 2012; 41(1): 106-15.

[http://dx.doi.org/10.1093/ije/dyr153] [PMID: 22101166]

[115] Paonessa F, Foti D, Costa V, Chiefari E, Brunetti G, Leone F, *et al.* Activator Protein-2 Overexpression Accounts for Increased Insulin Receptor Expression in Human Breast Cancer 2006. [http://dx.doi.org/10.1158/0008-5472.CAN-05-3678]

[116] Arcidiacono B, Iiritano S, Chiefari E, Brunetti FS, Gu G, Foti DP, *et al.* Cooperation between HMGA1, PDX-1, and MafA is Essential for Glucose-Induced Insulin Transcription in Pancreatic Beta Cells. Front Endocrinol 2015; 5: 237.

[117] Chiefari E, Nevolo MT, Arcidiacono B, *et al.* HMGA1 is a novel downstream nuclear target of the insulin receptor signaling pathway. Sci Rep 2012; 2(1): 251. [http://dx.doi.org/10.1038/srep00251] [PMID: 22355763]

[118] Bianco A, Chiefari E, Nobile CGA, Foti D, Pavia M, Brunetti A. The Association between HMGA1 rs146052672 Variant and Type 2 Diabetes: A Transethnic Meta-Analysis. PLoS One 2015; 10(8): e0136077. [http://dx.doi.org/10.1371/journal.pone.0136077] [PMID: 26296198]

[119] Chiefari E, Tanyolaç S, Iiritano S, *et al.* A polymorphism of HMGA1 is associated with increased risk of metabolic syndrome and related components. Sci Rep 2013; 3(1): 1491. [http://dx.doi.org/10.1038/srep01491] [PMID: 23512162]

[120] Schlueter C, Hauke S, Loeschke S, Wenk HH, Bullerdiek J. HMGA1 proteins in human atherosclerotic plaques. Pathol Res Pract 2005; 201(2): 101-7. [http://dx.doi.org/10.1016/j.prp.2004.11.010] [PMID: 15901130]

[121] Chiefari E, Ventura V, Capula C, *et al.* A polymorphism of HMGA1 protects against proliferative diabetic retinopathy by impairing HMGA1-induced VEGFA expression. Sci Rep 2016; 6(1): 39429. [http://dx.doi.org/10.1038/srep39429] [PMID: 27991577]

[122] Hashimoto N, Tanaka T. Role of miRNAs in the pathogenesis and susceptibility of diabetes mellitus. J Hum Genet 2017; 62(2): 141-50. [http://dx.doi.org/10.1038/jhg.2016.150] [PMID: 27928162]

[123] Ding Y, Sun X, Shan PF. MicroRNAs and Cardiovascular Disease in Diabetes Mellitus. Biomed Res Int 2017.

[124] La Sala L, Cattaneo M, De Nigris V, *et al.* Oscillating glucose induces microRNA-185 and impairs an efficient antioxidant response in human endothelial cells. Cardiovasc Diabetol 2016; 15(1): 71. [http://dx.doi.org/10.1186/s12933-016-0390-9] [PMID: 27137793]

[125] Arunachalam G, Lakshmanan AP, Samuel SM, Triggle CR, Ding H. Molecular Interplay between microRNA-34a and Sirtuin1 in Hyperglycemia-Mediated Impaired Angiogenesis in Endothelial Cells: Effects of Metformin. J Pharmacol Exp Ther 2016; 356(2): 314-23.

[126] Wang H-W, Su S-H, Wang Y-L, *et al.* MicroRNA-134 Contributes to Glucose-Induced Endothelial Cell Dysfunction and This Effect Can Be Reversed by Far-Infrared Irradiation. PLoS One 2016; 11(1): e0147067. [http://dx.doi.org/10.1371/journal.pone.0147067] [PMID: 26799933]

[127] Cordes KR, Sheehy NT, White MP, *et al.* miR-145 and miR-143 regulate smooth muscle cell fate and plasticity. Nature 2009; 460(7256): 705-10. [http://dx.doi.org/10.1038/nature08195] [PMID: 19578358]

[128] Reddy MA, Das S, Zhuo C, *et al.* Regulation of Vascular Smooth Muscle Cell Dysfunction Under Diabetic Conditions by miR-504. Arterioscler Thromb Vasc Biol 2016; 36(5): 864-73. [http://dx.doi.org/10.1161/ATVBAHA.115.306770] [PMID: 26941017]

[129] Lars M. J. RK, J. LN. MicroRNA Regulation of Vascular Smooth Muscle Function and Phenotype. Arterioscler Thromb Vasc Biol 2015; 35(1): 2-6. [http://dx.doi.org/10.1161/ATVBAHA.114.304877] [PMID: 25520518]

[130] Tang ST, Wang F, Shao M, Wang Y, Zhu HQ. MicroRNA-126 suppresses inflammation in endothelial cells under hyperglycemic condition by targeting HMGB1. Vascul Pharmacol 2017; 88: 48-55.
[http://dx.doi.org/10.1016/j.vph.2016.12.002] [PMID: 27993686]

[131] Wang S, Aurora AB, Johnson BA, *et al.* The endothelial-specific microRNA miR-126 governs vascular integrity and angiogenesis. Dev Cell 2008; 15(2): 261-71.
[http://dx.doi.org/10.1016/j.devcel.2008.07.002] [PMID: 18694565]

[132] Zernecke A, Bidzhekov K, Noels H, Shagdarsuren E, Gan L, Denecke B, *et al.* Delivery of MicroRNA-126 by Apoptotic Bodies Induces CXCL12-Dependent Vascular Protection. Sci Signal 2009; 2(100): ra81.

[133] Rawal S, Munasinghe PE, Shindikar A, *et al.* Down-regulation of proangiogenic microRNA-126 and microRNA-132 are early modulators of diabetic cardiac microangiopathy. Cardiovasc Res 2017; 113(1): 90-101.
[http://dx.doi.org/10.1093/cvr/cvw235] [PMID: 28065883]

[134] Fichtlscherer S, De Rosa S, Fox H, *et al.* Circulating microRNAs in patients with coronary artery disease. Circ Res 2010; 107(5): 677-84.
[http://dx.doi.org/10.1161/CIRCRESAHA.109.215566] [PMID: 20595655]

[135] Kurtz CL, Peck BCE, Fannin EE, Beysen C, Miao J, Landstreet SR, *et al.* MicroRNA-29 Fine-tunes the Expression of Key FOXA2-Activated Lipid Metabolism Genes and Is Dysregulated in Animal Models of Insulin Resistance and Diabetes. Diabetes 2014; 63(9): 3141-8.

[136] Wei S, Zhang M, Yu Y, *et al.* HNF-4α regulated miR-122 contributes to development of gluconeogenesis and lipid metabolism disorders in Type 2 diabetic mice and in palmitate-treated HepG2 cells. Eur J Pharmacol 2016; 791: 254-63.
[http://dx.doi.org/10.1016/j.ejphar.2016.08.038] [PMID: 27592052]

[137] Fu X, Dong B, Tian Y, *et al.* MicroRNA-26a regulates insulin sensitivity and metabolism of glucose and lipids. J Clin Invest 2015; 125(6): 2497-509.
[http://dx.doi.org/10.1172/JCI75438] [PMID: 25961460]

[138] Carino A, De Rosa S, Sorrentino S, Polimeni A, Sabatino J, Caiazzo G, *et al.* Modulation of circulating microRNAs levels during the switch from clopidogrel to ticagrelor. Biomed Res Int 2016.
[http://dx.doi.org/10.1155/2016/3968206]

[139] Zampetaki A, Kiechl S, Drozdov I, *et al.* Plasma microRNA profiling reveals loss of endothelial miR-126 and other microRNAs in type 2 diabetes. Circ Res 2010; 107(6): 810-7.
[http://dx.doi.org/10.1161/CIRCRESAHA.110.226357] [PMID: 20651284]

[140] Elgheznawy A, Shi L, Hu J, *et al.* Dicer cleavage by calpain determines platelet microRNA levels and function in diabetes. Circ Res 2015; 117(2): 157-65.
[http://dx.doi.org/10.1161/CIRCRESAHA.117.305784] [PMID: 25944670]

[141] Fejes Z, Póliska S, Czimmerer Z, *et al.* Hyperglycaemia suppresses microRNA expression in platelets to increase P2RY12 and SELP levels in type 2 diabetes mellitus. Thromb Haemost 2017; 117(3): 529-42.
[http://dx.doi.org/10.1160/TH16-04-0322] [PMID: 27975100]

[142] Landry P, Plante I, Ouellet DL, Perron MP, Rousseau G, Provost P. Existence of a microRNA pathway in anucleate platelets. Nat Struct Mol Biol 2009; 16(9): 961-6.
[http://dx.doi.org/10.1038/nsmb.1651] [PMID: 19668211]

[143] Zhang Y-Y, Zhou X, Ji W-J, *et al.* Decreased circulating microRNA-223 level predicts high on-treatment platelet reactivity in patients with troponin-negative non-ST elevation acute coronary syndrome. J Thromb Thrombolysis 2014; 38(1): 65-72.
[http://dx.doi.org/10.1007/s11239-013-1022-9] [PMID: 24202700]

[144] Iaconetti C, Sorrentino S, De Rosa S, Indolfi C. Exosomal miRNAs in heart disease. Physiology (Bethesda) 2016; 31(1): 16-24.

[http://dx.doi.org/10.1152/physiol.00029.2015] [PMID: 26661525]

[145] Luo M, Li R, Deng X, *et al.* Platelet-derived miR-103b as a novel biomarker for the early diagnosis of type 2 diabetes. Acta Diabetol 2015; 52(5): 943-9.
[http://dx.doi.org/10.1007/s00592-015-0733-0] [PMID: 25820527]

[146] Mills CD. M1 and M2 macrophages: oracles of health and disease. Crit Rev Immunol 2012; 32(6): 463-88.
[http://dx.doi.org/10.1615/CritRevImmunol.v32.i6.10] [PMID: 23428224]

[147] Sun X, Lin J, Zhang Y, *et al.* MicroRNA-181b improves glucose homeostasis and insulin sensitivity by regulating endothelial function in white adipose tissue. Circ Res 2016; 118(5): 810-21.
[http://dx.doi.org/10.1161/CIRCRESAHA.115.308166] [PMID: 26830849]

[148] Shan Y-X, Liu T-J, Su H-F, Samsamshariat A, Mestril R, Wang PH. Hsp10 and Hsp60 modulate Bcl-2 family and mitochondria apoptosis signaling induced by doxorubicin in cardiac muscle cells. J Mol Cell Cardiol 2003; 35(9): 1135-43.
[http://dx.doi.org/10.1016/S0022-2828(03)00229-3] [PMID: 12967636]

[149] Rawal S, Manning P, Katare R. Cardiovascular microRNAs: as modulators and diagnostic biomarkers of diabetic heart disease. Cardiovasc Diabetol 2014; 13(1): 44.
[http://dx.doi.org/10.1186/1475-2840-13-44] [PMID: 24528626]

[150] Nandi SS, Zheng H, Sharma NM, Shahshahan HR, Patel KP, Mishra PK. Lack of miR-133a decreases contractility of diabetic hearts: a role for novel cross talk between tyrosine aminotransferase and tyrosine hydroxylase. Diabetes 2016; 65(10): 3075-90.
[http://dx.doi.org/10.2337/db16-0023] [PMID: 27411382]

[151] Babiarz JE, Ravon M, Sridhar S, *et al.* Determination of the human cardiomyocyte mRNA and miRNA differentiation network by fine-scale profiling. Stem Cells Dev 2012; 21(11): 1956-65.
[http://dx.doi.org/10.1089/scd.2011.0357] [PMID: 22050602]

[152] Wang J-X, Jiao J-Q, Li Q, *et al.* miR-499 regulates mitochondrial dynamics by targeting calcineurin and dynamin-related protein-1. Nat Med 2011; 17(1): 71-8.
[http://dx.doi.org/10.1038/nm.2282] [PMID: 21186368]

[153] Carè A, Catalucci D, Felicetti F, *et al.* MicroRNA-133 controls cardiac hypertrophy. Nat Med 2007; 13(5): 613-8.
[http://dx.doi.org/10.1038/nm1582] [PMID: 17468766]

[154] Kuwabara Y, Ono K, Horie T, *et al.* Increased microRNA-1 and microRNA-133a levels in serum of patients with cardiovascular disease indicate myocardial damage. Circ Cardiovasc Genet 2011; 4(4): 446-54.
[http://dx.doi.org/10.1161/CIRCGENETICS.110.958975] [PMID: 21642241]

[155] Fatica A, Bozzoni I. Long non-coding RNAs: new players in cell differentiation and development. Nat Rev Genet 2014; 15(1): 7-21.
[http://dx.doi.org/10.1038/nrg3606] [PMID: 24296535]

[156] Wang KC, Chang HY. Molecular mechanisms of long noncoding RNAs. Mol Cell 2011; 43(6): 904-14.
[http://dx.doi.org/10.1016/j.molcel.2011.08.018] [PMID: 21925379]

[157] Li H, Zhu H, Ge J. Long noncoding RNA: recent updates in atherosclerosis. Int J Biol Sci 2016; 12(7): 898-910.
[http://dx.doi.org/10.7150/ijbs.14430] [PMID: 27314829]

[158] Carter G, Miladinovic B, Patel AA, Deland L, Mastorides S, Patel NA. Circulating long noncoding RNA GAS5 levels are correlated to prevalence of type 2 diabetes mellitus. BBA Clin 2015; 4: 102-7.
[http://dx.doi.org/10.1016/j.bbacli.2015.09.001] [PMID: 26675493]

[159] Kumarswamy R, Bauters C, Volkmann I, *et al.* Circulating long noncoding RNA, LIPCAR, predicts survival in patients with heart failure. Circ Res 2014; 114(10): 1569-75.

[http://dx.doi.org/10.1161/CIRCRESAHA.114.303915] [PMID: 24663402]

[160] Puthanveetil P, Chen S, Feng B, Gautam A, Chakrabarti S. Long non-coding RNA MALAT1 regulates hyperglycaemia induced inflammatory process in the endothelial cells. J Cell Mol Med 2015; 19(6): 1418-25.
[http://dx.doi.org/10.1111/jcmm.12576] [PMID: 25787249]

[161] Michalik KM, You X, Manavski Y, *et al.* Long noncoding RNA MALAT1 regulates endothelial cell function and vessel growth. Circ Res 2014; 114(9): 1389-97.
[http://dx.doi.org/10.1161/CIRCRESAHA.114.303265] [PMID: 24602777]

[162] Li X, Wang H, Yao B, Xu W, Chen J, Zhou X. lncRNA H19/miR-675 axis regulates cardiomyocyte apoptosis by targeting VDAC1 in diabetic cardiomyopathy. Sci Rep 2016; 6(1): 36340.
[http://dx.doi.org/10.1038/srep36340] [PMID: 27796346]

[163] Reddy MA, Chen Z, Park JT, Wang M, Lanting L, Zhang Q, *et al.* Regulation of Inflammatory Phenotype in Macrophages by a Diabetes-Induced Long Noncoding RNA. Diabetes 2014; 63(12): 4249-61.
[http://dx.doi.org/10.2337/db14-0298]

[164] Zgheib C, Hodges MM, Hu J, Liechty KW, Xu J. Long non-coding RNA Lethe regulates hyperglycemia-induced reactive oxygen species production in macrophages. PLoS One 2017; 12(5): e0177453.
[http://dx.doi.org/10.1371/journal.pone.0177453] [PMID: 28494015]

[165] Newman JD, Schwartzbard AZ, Weintraub HS, Goldberg IJ, Berger JS. Primary Prevention of Cardiovascular Disease in Diabetes Mellitus. J Am Coll Cardiol 2017; 70(7): 883-93.
[http://dx.doi.org/10.1016/j.jacc.2017.07.001] [PMID: 28797359]

[166] Introduction. Diabetes Care. 2016; 39(Supplement 1): S1 LP-S2..

[167] Jensen MD, Ryan DH, Apovian CM, *et al.* 2013 AHA/ACC/TOS guideline for the management of overweight and obesity in adults: a report of the American College of Cardiology/American Heart Association Task Force on Practice Guidelines and The Obesity Society. J Am Coll Cardiol 2014; 63 (25 Pt B): 2985-3023.
[http://dx.doi.org/10.1016/j.jacc.2013.11.004] [PMID: 24239920]

[168] Stone NJ, Robinson JG, Lichtenstein AH, *et al.* 2013 ACC/AHA guideline on the treatment of blood cholesterol to reduce atherosclerotic cardiovascular risk in adults: a report of the American College of Cardiology/American Heart Association Task Force on Practice Guidelines. J Am Coll Cardiol 2014; 63 (25 Pt B): 2889-934.
[http://dx.doi.org/10.1016/j.jacc.2013.11.002] [PMID: 24239923]

[169] Benjamin EJ, Blaha MJ, Chiuve SE, *et al.* Heart Disease and Stroke Statistics-2017 Update: A Report From the American Heart Association. Circulation 2017; 135(10): e146-603.
[http://dx.doi.org/10.1161/CIR.0000000000000485] [PMID: 28122885]

[170] Goldfine AB. Assessing the cardiovascular safety of diabetes therapies. N Engl J Med 2008; 359(11): 1092-5.
[http://dx.doi.org/10.1056/NEJMp0805758] [PMID: 18784098]

[171] Acharya T, Deedwania P. Cardiovascular outcome trials of the newer anti-diabetic medications. Prog Cardiovasc Dis 62(4): 342-8.
[http://dx.doi.org/10.1016/j.pcad.2019.08.003]

[172] Antithrombotic Trialists' (ATT) Collaboration. Aspirin in the primary and secondary prevention of vascular disease: collaborative meta-analysis of individual participant data from randomised trials. Lancet (London, England) 2009; 373(9678): 1849-60.
[PMID: 9482214]

[173] Fox CS, Golden SH, Anderson C, *et al.* Update on Prevention of Cardiovascular Disease in Adults With Type 2 Diabetes Mellitus in Light of Recent Evidence: A Scientific Statement From the

American Heart Association and the American Diabetes Association. Circulation 2015; 132(8): 691-718.
[http://dx.doi.org/10.1161/CIR.0000000000000230] [PMID: 26246173]

[174] Adler AI, Stratton IM, Neil HA, *et al.* Association of systolic blood pressure with macrovascular and microvascular complications of type 2 diabetes (UKPDS 36): prospective observational study. BMJ 2000; 321(7258): 412-9.
[http://dx.doi.org/10.1136/bmj.321.7258.412] [PMID: 10938049]

[175] Soran H, Durrington PN. Susceptibility of LDL and its subfractions to glycation. Curr Opin Lipidol 2011; 22(4): 254-61.
[http://dx.doi.org/10.1097/MOL.0b013e328348a43f] [PMID: 21734572]

[176] Collins R, Reith C, Emberson J, *et al.* Interpretation of the evidence for the efficacy and safety of statin therapy. Lancet 2016; 388(10059): 2532-61.
[http://dx.doi.org/10.1016/S0140-6736(16)31357-5] [PMID: 27616593]

[177] Shepherd J, Barter P, Carmena R, *et al.* Effect of lowering LDL cholesterol substantially below currently recommended levels in patients with coronary heart disease and diabetes: the Treating to New Targets (TNT) study. Diabetes Care 2006; 29(6): 1220-6.
[http://dx.doi.org/10.2337/dc05-2465] [PMID: 16731999]

[178] Cholesterol Treatment Trialists' (CTT) Collaborators. 2008.
[PMID: 18191683]

[179] Sehra D, Sehra S, Sehra ST. Cardiovascular pleiotropic effects of statins and new onset diabetes: is there a common link: do we need to evaluate the role of KATP channels? Expert Opin Drug Saf 2017; 16(7): 823-31.
[http://dx.doi.org/10.1080/14740338.2017.1338269] [PMID: 28571494]

[180] Natali A, Ferrannini E. Effects of metformin and thiazolidinediones on suppression of hepatic glucose production and stimulation of glucose uptake in type 2 diabetes: a systematic review. Diabetologia 2006; 49(3): 434-41.
[http://dx.doi.org/10.1007/s00125-006-0141-7] [PMID: 16477438]

[181] Nesti L, Natali A. Metformin effects on the heart and the cardiovascular system: A review of experimental and clinical data. Nutr Metab Cardiovasc Dis 2017; 27(8): 657-69.
[http://dx.doi.org/10.1016/j.numecd.2017.04.009] [PMID: 28709719]

[182] Ouyang J, Parakhia RA, Ochs RS. Metformin activates AMP kinase through inhibition of AMP deaminase. J Biol Chem 2011; 286(1): 1-11.
[http://dx.doi.org/10.1074/jbc.M110.121806] [PMID: 21059655]

[183] Owen MR, Doran E, Halestrap AP. Evidence that metformin exerts its anti-diabetic effects through inhibition of complex 1 of the mitochondrial respiratory chain. Biochem J 2000; 348(Pt 3): 607-14.
[http://dx.doi.org/10.1042/bj3480607] [PMID: 10839993]

[184] Sola D, Rossi L, Schianca GPC, *et al.* Sulfonylureas and their use in clinical practice. Arch Med Sci 2015; 11(4): 840-8.
[http://dx.doi.org/10.5114/aoms.2015.53304] [PMID: 26322096]

[185] Derosa G, Limas CP, Macías PC, Estrella A, Maffioli P. Dietary and nutraceutical approach to type 2 diabetes. Arch Med Sci 2014; 10(2): 336-44.
[http://dx.doi.org/10.5114/aoms.2014.42587] [PMID: 24904670]

[186] Rao AD, Kuhadiya N, Reynolds K, Fonseca VA. Is the combination of sulfonylureas and metformin associated with an increased risk of cardiovascular disease or all-cause mortality?: a meta-analysis of observational studies. Diabetes Care 2008; 31(8): 1672-8.
[http://dx.doi.org/10.2337/dc08-0167] [PMID: 18458139]

[187] Garratt KN, Brady PA, Hassinger NL, Grill DE, Terzic A, Holmes DR Jr. Sulfonylurea drugs increase early mortality in patients with diabetes mellitus after direct angioplasty for acute myocardial

infarction. J Am Coll Cardiol 1999; 33(1): 119-24.
[http://dx.doi.org/10.1016/S0735-1097(98)00557-9] [PMID: 9935017]

[188] Terao Y, Ayaori M, Ogura M, *et al.* Effect of sulfonylurea agents on reverse cholesterol transport *in vitro* and *in vivo.* J Atheroscler Thromb 2011; 18(6): 513-30.
[http://dx.doi.org/10.5551/jat.7641] [PMID: 21636950]

[189] Drucker DJ, Nauck MA. The incretin system: glucagon-like peptide-1 receptor agonists and dipeptidyl peptidase-4 inhibitors in type 2 diabetes. Lancet 2006; 368(9548): 1696-705.
[http://dx.doi.org/10.1016/S0140-6736(06)69705-5] [PMID: 17098089]

[190] Gupta A, Jelinek HF, Al-Aubaidy H. Glucagon like peptide-1 and its receptor agonists: Their roles in management of Type 2 diabetes mellitus. Diabetes Metab Syndr 2017; 11(3): 225-30.
[http://dx.doi.org/10.1016/j.dsx.2016.09.003] [PMID: 27884496]

[191] Mulvihill EE, Drucker DJ. Pharmacology, physiology, and mechanisms of action of dipeptidyl peptidase-4 inhibitors. Endocr Rev 2014; 35(6): 992-1019.
[http://dx.doi.org/10.1210/er.2014-1035] [PMID: 25216328]

[192] Ussher JR, Drucker DJ. Cardiovascular biology of the incretin system. Endocr Rev 2012; 33(2): 187-215.
[http://dx.doi.org/10.1210/er.2011-1052] [PMID: 22323472]

[193] Ussher JR, Drucker DJ. Cardiovascular actions of incretin-based therapies. Circ Res 2014; 114(11): 1788-803.
[http://dx.doi.org/10.1161/CIRCRESAHA.114.301958] [PMID: 24855202]

[194] Garber AJ, Abrahamson MJ, Barzilay JI, *et al.* Consensus statement by the american association of clinical endocrinologists and american college of endocrinology on the comprehensive type 2 diabetes management algorithm - 2018 executive summary. Endocr Pract 2018; 24(1): 91-120.
[http://dx.doi.org/10.4158/CS-2017-0153] [PMID: 29368965]

[195] Scheen AJ. A review of gliptins for 2014. Expert Opin Pharmacother 2015; 16(1): 43-62.
[http://dx.doi.org/10.1517/14656566.2015.978289] [PMID: 25381751]

[196] Scheen AJ. Safety of dipeptidyl peptidase-4 inhibitors for treating type 2 diabetes. Expert Opin Drug Saf 2015; 14(4): 505-24.
[http://dx.doi.org/10.1517/14740338.2015.1006625] [PMID: 25630605]

[197] Scheen AJ. Cardiovascular effects of gliptins. Nat Rev Cardiol 2013; 10(2): 73-84.
[http://dx.doi.org/10.1038/nrcardio.2012.183] [PMID: 23296071]

[198] Nauck MA, Meier JJ, Cavender MA, Abd El Aziz M, Drucker DJ. Cardiovascular Actions and Clinical Outcomes With Glucagon-Like Peptide-1 Receptor Agonists and Dipeptidyl Peptidase-4 Inhibitors. Circulation 2017; 136(9): 849-70.
[http://dx.doi.org/10.1161/CIRCULATIONAHA.117.028136] [PMID: 28847797]

[199] Anderluh M, Kocic G, Tomovic K, Kocic R, Deljanin-Ilic M, Smelcerovic A. Cross-talk between the dipeptidyl peptidase-4 and stromal cell-derived factor-1 in stem cell homing and myocardial repair: Potential impact of dipeptidyl peptidase-4 inhibitors. Pharmacol Ther 2016; 167: 100-7.
[http://dx.doi.org/10.1016/j.pharmthera.2016.07.009] [PMID: 27484974]

[200] Scheen AJ. Pharmacokinetics and clinical use of incretin-based therapies in patients with chronic kidney disease and type 2 diabetes. Clin Pharmacokinet 2015; 54(1): 1-21.
[http://dx.doi.org/10.1007/s40262-014-0198-2] [PMID: 25331711]

[201] Scirica BM, Bhatt DL, Braunwald E, *et al.* Saxagliptin and cardiovascular outcomes in patients with type 2 diabetes mellitus. N Engl J Med 2013; 369(14): 1317-26.
[http://dx.doi.org/10.1056/NEJMoa1307684] [PMID: 23992601]

[202] White WB, Cannon CP, Heller SR, *et al.* Alogliptin after acute coronary syndrome in patients with type 2 diabetes. N Engl J Med 2013; 369(14): 1327-35.
[http://dx.doi.org/10.1056/NEJMoa1305889] [PMID: 23992602]

[203] Green JB, Bethel MA, Armstrong PW, *et al.* Effect of Sitagliptin on Cardiovascular Outcomes in Type 2 Diabetes. N Engl J Med 2015; 373(3): 232-42.
[http://dx.doi.org/10.1056/NEJMoa1501352] [PMID: 26052984]

[204] Zannad F, Cannon CP, Cushman WC, *et al.* Heart failure and mortality outcomes in patients with type 2 diabetes taking alogliptin *versus* placebo in EXAMINE: a multicentre, randomised, double-blind trial. Lancet 2015; 385(9982): 2067-76.
[http://dx.doi.org/10.1016/S0140-6736(14)62225-X] [PMID: 25765696]

[205] Abdul-Ghani MA, Norton L, Defronzo RA. Role of sodium-glucose cotransporter 2 (SGLT 2) inhibitors in the treatment of type 2 diabetes. Endocr Rev 2011; 32(4): 515-31.
[http://dx.doi.org/10.1210/er.2010-0029] [PMID: 21606218]

[206] Scheen AJ, Paquot N. Metabolic effects of SGLT-2 inhibitors beyond increased glucosuria: A review of the clinical evidence. Diabetes Metab 2014; 40(6) (Suppl. 1): S4-S11.
[http://dx.doi.org/10.1016/S1262-3636(14)72689-8] [PMID: 25554070]

[207] Scheen AJ. Pharmacodynamics, efficacy and safety of sodium-glucose co-transporter type 2 (SGLT2) inhibitors for the treatment of type 2 diabetes mellitus. Drugs 2015; 75(1): 33-59.
[http://dx.doi.org/10.1007/s40265-014-0337-y] [PMID: 25488697]

[208] Scheen AJ. Pharmacokinetics, Pharmacodynamics and Clinical Use of SGLT2 Inhibitors in Patients with Type 2 Diabetes Mellitus and Chronic Kidney Disease. Clin Pharmacokinet 2015; 54(7): 691-708.
[http://dx.doi.org/10.1007/s40262-015-0264-4] [PMID: 25805666]

[209] Mazidi M, Rezaie P, Gao HK, Kengne AP. Effect of Sodium-Glucose Cotransport-2 Inhibitors on Blood Pressure in People With Type 2 Diabetes Mellitus: A Systematic Review and Meta-Analysis of 43 Randomized Control Trials With 22 528 Patients. J Am Heart Assoc 2017; 6(6): e004007.
[http://dx.doi.org/10.1161/JAHA.116.004007] [PMID: 28546454]

[210] Baker WL, Buckley LF, Kelly MS, *et al.* Effects of Sodium-Glucose Cotransporter 2 Inhibitors on 24-Hour Ambulatory Blood Pressure: A Systematic Review and Meta-Analysis. J Am Heart Assoc 2017; 6(5): e005686.
[http://dx.doi.org/10.1161/JAHA.117.005686] [PMID: 28522675]

[211] Zhao Y, Xu L, Tian D, *et al.* Effects of sodium-glucose co-transporter 2 (SGLT2) inhibitors on serum uric acid level: A meta-analysis of randomized controlled trials. Diabetes Obes Metab 2018; 20(2): 458-62.
[http://dx.doi.org/10.1111/dom.13101] [PMID: 28846182]

[212] Sano M, Takei M, Shiraishi Y, Suzuki Y. Increased Hematocrit During Sodium-Glucose Cotransporter 2 Inhibitor Therapy Indicates Recovery of Tubulointerstitial Function in Diabetic Kidneys. J Clin Med Res 2016; 8(12): 844-7.
[http://dx.doi.org/10.14740/jocmr2760w] [PMID: 27829948]

[213] Bays HE, Sartipy P, Xu J, Sjöström CD, Underberg JA. Dapagliflozin in patients with type II diabetes mellitus, with and without elevated triglyceride and reduced high-density lipoprotein cholesterol levels. J Clin Lipidol 2017; 11(2): 450-8.
[http://dx.doi.org/10.1016/j.jacl.2017.01.018] [PMID: 28502502]

[214] Filippatos TD, Tsimihodimos V, Liamis G, Elisaf MS. SGLT2 inhibitors-induced electrolyte abnormalities: An analysis of the associated mechanisms. Diabetes Metab Syndr 2018; 12(1): 59-63.
[http://dx.doi.org/10.1016/j.dsx.2017.08.003] [PMID: 28826578]

[215] Imprialos K, Faselis C, Boutari C, *et al.* SGLT-2 Inhibitors and Cardiovascular Risk in Diabetes Mellitus: A Comprehensive and Critical Review of the Literature. Curr Pharm Des 2017; 23(10): 1510-21.
[http://dx.doi.org/10.2174/1381612823666170124123927] [PMID: 28120716]

[216] Heerspink HJL, Perkins BA, Fitchett DH, Husain M, Cherney DZI. Sodium Glucose Cotransporter 2

Inhibitors in the Treatment of Diabetes Mellitus: Cardiovascular and Kidney Effects, Potential Mechanisms, and Clinical Applications. Circulation 2016; 134(10): 752-72.
[http://dx.doi.org/10.1161/CIRCULATIONAHA.116.021887] [PMID: 27470878]

[217] American Diabetes Association. 8. Pharmacologic Approaches to Glycemic Treatment: *Standards of Medical Care in Diabetes-2018.* Diabetes Care 2018; 41 (Suppl. 1): S73-85.
[http://dx.doi.org/10.2337/dc18-S008] [PMID: 29222379]

[218] Cimmaruta D, Maiorino M, Scavone C, Sportiello L, Rossi F, Giugliano D, *et al.* Efficacy and safety of insulin-GLP-1 receptor agonists combination in type 2 diabetes mellitus: a systematic review 2016.
[http://dx.doi.org/10.1080/14740338.2016.1221402]

[219] Bunck MC, Cornér A, Eliasson B, *et al.* Effects of exenatide on measures of β-cell function after 3 years in metformin-treated patients with type 2 diabetes. Diabetes Care 2011; 34(9): 2041-7.
[http://dx.doi.org/10.2337/dc11-0291] [PMID: 21868779]

[220] von Scholten BJ, Lajer M, Goetze JP, Persson F, Rossing P. Time course and mechanisms of the anti-hypertensive and renal effects of liraglutide treatment. Diabet Med 2015; 32(3): 343-52.
[http://dx.doi.org/10.1111/dme.12594] [PMID: 25251901]

[221] Sokos GG, Nikolaidis LA, Mankad S, Elahi D, Shannon RP. Glucagon-like peptide-1 infusion improves left ventricular ejection fraction and functional status in patients with chronic heart failure. J Card Fail 2006; 12(9): 694-9.
[http://dx.doi.org/10.1016/j.cardfail.2006.08.211] [PMID: 17174230]

[222] Skyler JS, Bergenstal R, Bonow RO, *et al.* Intensive glycemic control and the prevention of cardiovascular events: implications of the ACCORD, ADVANCE, and VA diabetes trials: a position statement of the American Diabetes Association and a scientific statement of the American College of Cardiology Foundation and the American Heart Association. Circulation 2009; 119(2): 351-7.
[http://dx.doi.org/10.1161/CIRCULATIONAHA.108.191305] [PMID: 19095622]

[223] UK Prospective Diabetes Study (UKPDS) Group. Effect of intensive blood-glucose control with metformin on complications in overweight patients with type 2 diabetes (UKPDS 34). Lancet 1998; 352(9131): 854-65.
[http://dx.doi.org/10.1016/S0140-6736(98)07037-8] [PMID: 9742977]

[224] Marso SP, Daniels GH, Brown-Frandsen K, *et al.* LEADER Steering Committee; LEADER Trial Investigators. Liraglutide and Cardiovascular Outcomes in Type 2 Diabetes. N Engl J Med 2016; 375(4): 311-22.
[http://dx.doi.org/10.1056/NEJMoa1603827] [PMID: 27295427]

[225] Marso SP, Bain SC, Consoli A, *et al.* Semaglutide and Cardiovascular Outcomes in Patients with Type 2 Diabetes. N Engl J Med 2016; 375(19): 1834-44.
[http://dx.doi.org/10.1056/NEJMoa1607141] [PMID: 27633186]

SUBJECT INDEX

A

Abnormal heart pumping 29
ACE inhibitors 103, 107, 108, 127, 209
Acid(s)
  amino 55
  arachidonic (AA) 59, 142
  base homeostasis 201
  fatty 31, 194, 196, 201, 205
  free fatty (FFA) 194, 197
  hypochlorous 77
  nucleic 69
  salvianolic 82
  uric 212
Actin 73, 75, 201
  cytoskeleton 201
  nucleation 67
  regulator, cytoskeleton 67
Action
  cardiac cell 2, 3
  myocardial 30
Activation 54, 55, 56, 72, 73, 74, 76, 77, 81,
    83, 141, 142, 143, 144, 148
  calpain 205
  hepatic 146
  metabolic 146
  pleiotropic 210
Active metabolite formation 172
Activity 57, 61, 66, 68, 75, 76, 82, 202, 203,
    210, 211
  anti-inflammatory 205
  catalytic 59
  effective anti-tumor cytotoxic 25
  enzymatic 211
  fibroblast growth factor 205
  plasma antioxidant enzymes 64
Acute
  coronary syndrome (ACS) 14, 21, 22, 23,
    141, 149, 153, 154, 155, 158, 160, 162,
    164, 167, 168, 176
  leukemia 64
  lymphoblastic 25

Adenosine diphosphate (ADP) 141, 142, 143,
    145, 149
Adenosquamous carcinoma 72
Adiponectin
  gene 202
  obesity-associated protein 202
Adriamycin 25, 64, 65
  ameliorated 65
  anthracycline antibiotic 64
  induced heart injury 55, 64
Agents 110, 111, 120, 124, 125, 146, 152,
    161, 213
  antiarrhythmic 26, 120
  anti-diabetic 210
  antineoplastic 110
  anti-platelet 119
  antithrombotic 111, 132
  hypoglycemic 2, 213
  inhibitory 147
  therapeutic 69
Aggregation 71, 142, 143, 145, 149, 205
  integrin 143
  macrophage 63
Airway 71, 72, 73
  chronic 71
  infiltration 71
  inflammation 71
Albuminuria 78, 212
Alcohol consumption 196
Aldosterone, inhibiting 60
AMP-activated kinase 210
AMPK 210
  phosphorylated 210
Amyloid antigen 207
Analysis, economic 123
Anemia 7, 78
Angina 1, 4, 13, 14, 15, 16, 19, 20, 22, 26, 27,
    30, 33, 38, 39
  symptoms 13, 14, 15
Angioedema 7, 107
Angiogenesis 201, 205
Angiotensin 103, 197

www.ingramcontent.com/pod-product-compliance
Lightning Source LLC
Chambersburg PA
CBHW050823220326

41598CB00006B/303